NURSING HISTORY REVIEW

OFFICIAL JOURNAL OF THE AMERICAN ASSOCIATION FOR THE HISTORY OF NURSING

1993 • Volume 1

CONTENTS

upp University of Pennsylvania Press, Philadelphia
ISSN 1062-8061

BOOK REVIEWS

Volume 1 1993

Nursing History Review

Nursing History Review is published annually for the American Association for the History of Nursing, Inc., by the University of Pennsylvania Press.

International Standard Serial Number ISSN 1062-8061
International Standard Book Number ISBN 0-8122-1450-1 (Volume 1)
Printed in the United States of America

All inquiries concerning subscriptions or advertising should be sent to:

Marketing Department
University of Pennsylvania Press
418 Service Drive
Philadelphia, Pa. 19104-6097
Attention: Subscription Manager

Yearly subscription rates are: $35.00, individuals; $50.00, institutions and libraries.

Members of the American Association for the History of Nursing, Inc. (AAHN) receive *Nursing History Review* on payment of $60.00 annual membership dues. Applications and other correspondence relating to AAHN membership should be directed to:

Dr. Rosemary McCarthy, Executive Director
American Association for the History of Nursing, Inc.
P.O. Box 90803
Washington, D.C. 20090-0803

Please direct all submissions and editorial correspondence to:

Joan E. Lynaugh, Editor
Nursing History Review
University of Pennsylvania
420 Guardian Drive, Room 307
Philadelphia, Pa. 19104-6096

NURSING HISTORY REVIEW

JOAN E. LYNAUGH, Editor
BARBARA BRODIE, Book Review Editor
CARLA CASTILLO, Assistant Editor

EDITORIAL

This first volume of *Nursing History Review* marks a significant next step toward assuring vigorous and useful scholarship in nursing history. In 1980 a small band of committed people gathered together to form what was at first called the International History of Nursing Society. Ten years ago the society's members renamed themselves the American Association for the History of Nursing; now they are ready to sponsor this annual journal. This first volume thus celebrates more than a decade of achievement in the field; at the same time it inaugurates a new era of historical research and writing. Scholars from inside and outside nursing trace various roads to historical understanding of the complex and vitally important phenomenon we call nursing. *Nursing History Review* is the critical vehicle bringing their work to health professionals, historians, other scholars, and to the public we serve.

The *Review* publishes historical studies, commentary, historiographic essays, and book reviews. This first volume reflects our intent: to help all those interested in health care history to keep in touch with new and ongoing work, gain ready access to related historiography, and analyze the historical perspective on contemporary health care concerns. We believe our readers will read all of the *Review* because the history of nursing deals with the most central aspects of life—birth and death, health and illness. We hope to hear from you.

JOAN E. LYNAUGH
Center for the Study of the History of Nursing
University of Pennsylvania

Restraining the Troublesome Patient

A Historical Perspective on a Contemporary Debate

NEVILLE E. STRUMPF
School of Nursing
University of Pennsylvania

NANCY TOMES
History Department
State University of New York at Stony Brook

Introduction

In recent years the American public and the nursing profession have confronted what might aptly be termed a restraint crisis. A steady stream of articles in newspapers and magazines has provided readers with horror stories of elderly, mentally ill, and retarded patients physically confined for long periods of time in hospitals and nursing homes. For example, a *Wall Street Journal* article chronicling a week in a Florida nursing home described a seventy-six-year-old former schoolteacher "struggling to free herself from a belt tying her to what looks like an adult highchair mounted on small wheels."[1]

Based on statistical evidence for restraint use among the elderly, such incidents of individual abuse are probably repeated many times. In 1977 a national survey of nursing homes indicated that 25 percent of 1,303,000 residents were regularly restrained. By 1988 the figure had risen to 41.3 percent of skilled nursing home residents and 31.7 percent of intermediate care facility residents restrained at some point in a twenty-four hour period. Reports also showed that up to 22 percent of patients above age seventy were restrained during a stay in an acute care hospital. Thus, in a widely cited paper published in 1989, two nurse researchers at the University of

Nursing History Review 1 (1993): 3–24.

Pennsylvania estimated that 500,000 older persons were daily tied to their beds or chairs in American hospitals and nursing homes.[2]

Contemporary observers often assume that this modern restraint crisis is a peculiar product of the late twentieth century, with its large population of aged and chronically ill, fiscal crises, institutional overcrowding, and staff turnover. While these factors are undeniably important, explanations that focus only on current conditions neglect more subtle forces at work and fail to account for the fact that staff in other countries where circumstances are similar to those in the United States offer care to patients with little physical restraint.

In fact, for over a century, health care professionals in the United States have differed from their British counterparts over the use of restraint. Many of the contemporary dilemmas involving physical restraint can be traced back to an earlier "restraint crisis" that occurred during the middle of the nineteenth century. Then, as now, Americans and Britons debated the advisability of restraint use; then, as now, American practices differed significantly from the commitment to a "nonrestraint" philosophy that came to characterize English and Scottish mental hospitals. Understanding the reasons for this difference requires more than knowledge of structural constraints on patient care; it necessitates reflection on the historical and cultural influences on restraint use as well.

As we will demonstrate in this article, nurses in the United States are heir to a persistent but largely unexamined set of attitudes about the use of physical restraint for management of troublesome patients. These attitudes were already evident when the first generation of American psychiatrists presided over the expansion of private and public mental hospitals in the decades from 1830 to 1880. Through incorporation into nursing practice in the late nineteenth century, a philosophy of restraint still influences care not only of the mentally ill, but of other groups as well, including the aged. By bringing this historical legacy to light, we hope that American nurses will shape a more independent and humane policy regarding the use of restraints.

An examination of nineteenth-century beliefs about violence and the mentally ill—particularly cultural differences between Americans and Britons concerning the need for mechanical restraint to control behavior—presents many parallels to the present debate over restraint. As with earlier attempts to promote philosophy and practice aimed at nonrestraint, the movement of the last decade to eliminate use of physical restraints with elderly persons in nursing homes in the United States is also, increasingly, "a watchword, a battle-cry, a symbol . . . publicly proclaimed as a new system."[3]

This article represents a joint collaboration between a historian who has studied the nineteenth-century controversy over restraint of mental patients and a nurse researcher who has studied the current use of restraint with frail, elderly adults. Our purposes are to examine the origins of restraint use in nineteenth-century psychiatry, to trace the growing prominence of its use with frail, elderly adults as standard nursing practice in this country, and to analyze the implications of a complex historical legacy. First we examine the earlier restraint crisis, which occurred in the mid- to late nineteenth century, and the reasons American psychiatrists rejected the ideal of nonrestraint; next, the resolution of that crisis and its impact on nursing texts and practice from the late 1800s to the 1960s; and last, the forces contributing to concerns today about restraint, especially among the frail elderly.

The Nineteenth-Century Nonrestraint Movement

The nonrestraint movement was an offshoot of a broader crusade to reform care of the mentally ill through "moral treatment." Moral treatment reflected a general trend of the Enlightenment that favored gentler, more humane attitudes toward the poor and deviant classes of society. From its inception, reduction in the amount of restraint for control of the mentally ill was a central tenet of moral treatment. Among the most powerful images of that reform was Philippe Pinel removing chains and fetters in 1794 from his charges at the Bicetre Hospital in Paris. Concurrently, the Society of Friends began to introduce similar measures in England. A major impetus for reform was the publication in 1813 of an account by the Quaker Samuel Tuke of the Retreat at York. The specific methods of Tuke's humane approach toward the mentally ill, characterized in his words by "calmness and kindness," were widely disseminated in England and the United States.[4]

While insisting that humane treatment was incompatible with extensive use of physical restraints, early advocates of moral treatment never envisioned the entire abolition of devices such as straitjackets or leather cuffs. In fact, during the 1820s, restraint was used sparingly, but regularly, at the famed York Retreat and at another exemplar of moral treatment, the Friends Asylum in Philadelphia.[5] The contradiction between the goals of moral treatment and the use of restraint devices soon came to trouble some

British physicians. First E. P. Charlesworth and Robert Gardiner Hill at the small Lincoln Asylum, followed by John Conolly at the much larger Hanwell Asylum, began to experiment with general abandonment of restraint devices. In Conolly's words, they came to believe that "restraints and neglect may be considered as synonymous, for restraints are merely a general substitute for the thousand attentions required by troublesome patients."[6]

Conolly, called the "father of nonrestraint," and his followers evolved a philosophy of patient management whereby mechanical restraints such as straitjackets and cuffs were replaced by less coercive measures, chiefly seclusion. As the change in management proved successful, many restrictive aspects of the asylum were dismantled, including locked wards and barred windows. More generous patient furloughs were available as well. The underlying premise was simple: If patients were not physically coerced, they would become less violent. Once openness and trust were an established part of the asylum regimen, the need for security would lessen.

With support from a national regulatory board known as the Lunacy Commission, which began to operate in the mid-1840s, the ideal of nonrestraint became a powerful force in British psychiatry, especially in the public asylums. While physical restraint continued in so-called exceptional cases, usage became much circumscribed by bureaucratic scrutiny. Rates of restraint were dramatically reduced; at the same time, seclusion and sedation also declined, suggesting that these methods were not substitute forms of control. In other words, with introduction of the nonrestraint system, the overall level of violence and physical coercion in the asylum also declined. The system of nonrestraint by no means ended all violence against patients; incidents of rib-breaking and physical abuse of patients by attendants still plagued English mental institutions. On the whole, however, institutions gained a reputation for unusual order and tranquility during this period.[7]

In sharp contrast to their British counterparts, American asylum physicians opposed the system of nonrestraint from its inception in the early 1840s. Although in agreement with those tenets of moral treatment requiring minimal restraint and patient well-being, American physicians nevertheless felt that English reformers went too far in proscribing its therapeutic value. At the very first meeting in 1844 of the American Psychiatric Association (then known as the Association of Medical Superintendents of American Institutions for the Insane), members expressed opposition to the English system of nonrestraint, and for the next four decades the leadership campaigned actively against it.[8]

American hostility to nonrestraint was grounded in markedly different assumptions about the need for institutional control of the mentally ill. In general, American physicians believed that security and restraint were essential for the proper care of asylum patients. Their arguments, initially brought forward in 1844 by Dr. Isaac Ray, at the time superintendent of the Maine Insane Asylum, and later by others, have been summarized by Alfred Deutsch:

> The ideal of non-restraint could never be completely realized. . . . Some forms of forcible restraint would always be necessary. . . . The abolition of mechanical restraint meant merely the substitution of another form of coercion. . . . To supplant mechanical restraint by attendants would necessitate large staffs and consequently greater expense. Suicidal, destructive and unmanageable patients required some form of personal restraints. . . . Mechanical restraints were also required for patients who were prone to exhaust their energy and to lower their vitality. . . . The patients of European institutions . . . might willingly submit to "moral" restraint, but not your liberty-loving American who . . . could be restrained only by mechanical means. In certain institutions where the abolition of mechanical restraint had been tried, it had resulted in dismal failure, and the old restraints had been resumed.[9]

In 1863 Ray, now head of the prestigious Butler Hospital in Providence, Rhode Island, continued as an ardent spokesman for the necessity of restraint. "In some shape or other, restriction is an essential element in all hospital management of insanity," he wrote. Not surprisingly, given the views held by leaders such as Ray, American hospitals of the period had more barred windows and locked wards, and granted fewer patient liberties, than did their British counterparts.[10]

American physicians justified their greater reliance on restraint by arguing that patients in the United States were simply more aggressive than their British counterparts. The circumstances of American life, so they claimed, increased the incidence of mental disorders characterized by violent excitement. As citizens of a democratic nation, American patients did not respond to authority as quickly and quietly as did the more subservient British. In the words of Isaac Ray, "The patient is accustomed to obeying the voice of his superior, and the voice of a superior is a different thing in England from what it is here." His colleague John Butler of the Hartford Retreat in Connecticut put the matter even more bluntly: "The great secret of non-restraint [is] the stupidity of their patients." Thus, at the heart of American resistance to the ideal of nonrestraint was a conception of the American patient as inherently boisterous, freedom-loving, and aggressive in defense of personal liberty.[11]

In addition, debate over nonrestraint revealed a very different conception of patient *risk* on the part of British and American physicians. English physicians admitted that the system of nonrestraint required subordination of patient safety to the greater moral good of elimination of mechanical restraint. As an anonymous editorialist put it in the British *Journal of Mental Science* in 1858, "It is better to submit to defeat from the unmanageable exceptions than to break the rule of kindness." Likewise, an English alienist wrote to an American reformer, Charles Folsom, "It seems to me that the only way we are ahead of you is this: We run risks, you endeavor not to do so."[12]

Greater willingness by the English superintendents to accept apparently riskier styles of patient management may have been related to differences in class status of their clientele. In general, British mental hospitals of the period were more sharply divided along private/public lines than were their American counterparts. The nonrestraint system originated in public hospitals where the vast majority of inmates were pauper wards of the state. It could be argued that physicians associated with the public asylums had less to answer for if their pauper charges suffered bruises or other mishaps under a nonrestraint system. Significantly, private asylums in England, which had a higher ranking clientele, consistently used more restraint than the public institutions.[13]

In comparison to English hospitals, both public and private hospital boards in the United States were more concerned about patronage and public relations. While many public hospitals had a large pauper contingent supported by the state, they had as well a more "mixed" class of clients than the English. To retain the patronage of middle class families, state hospital and private asylum superintendents alike did not want the adverse publicity of a patient suicide or injury. The fear of lawsuits seemed to haunt American physicians far more than it did the British.

For whatever reason, the American psychiatric profession believed that a more repressive asylum order, including the use of mechanical restraint, would assure anxious families that the mentally ill were better off in a hospital than at home. To their way of thinking, the benefits of nonrestraint simply did not balance the potential for adverse publicity from patient accidents. When criticized for insistence on security first, American physicians invariably replied that the risk of patient harm far outweighed any gains from open wards or personal furloughs. As Thomas Story Kirkbride of the Pennsylvania Hospital for the Insane put it, "No slight advantage can compensate the loss of a single life, for the destruction of property or the hundred kinds of mischief that may be perpetuated by insane thus given their freedom." Although a firm believer in moral treatment, Kirkbride could nevertheless endorse what he considered the mildest form of mechanical restraint—wristlets, mittens, and the bedstrap, for use in exceptional cases.[14]

Thus, in the United States, reduction of physical restraint never became a compelling professional ideal. Out of individual conviction, some asylum physicians did indeed work to limit use only to the most serious cases. For these reformers, prominent among them Kirkbride who was often called the "American Conolly," practice was consistent with the increasingly mainstream idea of English nonrestraint.[15] In general, however, American mental hospitals continued to accept a wider range of reasons for restraint than their British colleagues.

Even more important, the issue of restraint in America never became a matter of collective professional soul-searching, as it did in Britain. In America, views of restraint practice at the end of the nineteenth century could be summed up as follows: Moderate use was therapeutically and morally sound; it was required by the peculiar violence of American insanity; and it prevented tragic accidents and injuries. As a result, restraint practices in the United States remained both more extensive and more diverse into the twentieth century.

In the meantime, the "great restraint controversy" gradually diminished in the late 1880s and 1890s, and by turn of the century British and American opinion concerning restraint use converged. For complex reasons, the system of nonrestraint gained some favor among the younger physicians who took over American asylums during this period. These advocates of a new "scientific psychiatry" endorsed the general principles of nonrestraint as consistent with a more modern point of view concerning mental disease. At the same time, British physicians felt less compelled to condemn the occasional use of restraint as a grave moral threat. As the more somatic approaches of late nineteenth century psychiatry eclipsed the reform spirit of moral treatment, restraint became much less central to the profession's agenda for uplifting the specialty. Instead, the philosophy and practice of restraint use was ceded to the profession of nursing, which came into existence only as the restraint controversy was nearing its end.[16]

Nursing Care for the Troublesome Patient

While controversy over restraint usage raged in the medical and psychiatric communities, nursing began establishing itself as a new profession for care of the sick. In short order, a literature detailing the techniques of nursing intervention emerged, with telling descriptions of appropriate means for handling the problematic behaviors of patients. A review of representative texts beginning in 1885 and nursing journals starting in 1900 confirms the influence of attitudes, largely unexamined by the nursing profession, of American psychiatrists in the decades from 1830 to 1880.

At the outset, it is important to note that professional nurses had no role in developing this American philosophy of restraint use. Nineteenth-century mental hospitals operated under the sole professional direction of the asylum physician. Untrained attendants, often young immigrants looking for a steady job, carried out the physician's treatment philosophy with little input of their own.[17] By the time professional nursing became a presence in the hospital (toward the end of the nineteenth century), the matter of restraint practice was generally established. If nursing can be faulted for acceptance of this heritage, the profession nevertheless bears no responsibility for its creation.

The management of behavior, and the justification of restraint in specific circumstances, is well illustrated by examples from nursing's earliest literature to that of the present day. Although it will be evident from examination of this literature that restraint was reserved for unusual circumstances, its early incorporation into nursing practice has remained a potent influence on care.

In the first general text for nurses, Clara Weeks's *Textbook of Nursing* (1885), the point is made that restraint "only aggravates the trouble" in delirium. Weeks suggested that patients be allowed "as much freedom as is compatible with safety" and urged diversion rather than opposition, along with gentleness, forbearance, firmness, and vigilance.[18]

From 1900 onward, texts and procedure manuals of nursing emphasized avoidance of restraints yet increasingly described available devices and methods for applying them. A 1909 text briefly listed restraint sheets and jackets but stated as well that the "nurse should . . . by using her brains and general resources . . . get beyond the necessity of . . . restraining appliances." Minnie Goodnow's *Textbook for Pupils During Their First Year of Hospital Work* made no mention of *mechanical* restraints in the 1921 edition (other than showing two pictures of a nurse *manually* restraining a struggling patient), and in the 1926 edition noted only that "forcible restraint exhausts the patient and is very harmful." By the mid-1920s, however, information concerning restraint of patients was considerably more detailed.[19]

A Manual of Nursing Procedures, published in 1923, indicated that the purpose of restraint was "to prevent irresponsible patients from doing themselves injury." Among restraining methods outlined were the bed-board, considered especially well suited to old people who may continually try to get out of bed, and various forms of sheets or jackets. Likewise, Maxwell and Pope's *Practical Nursing* (1923), in a section concerning "procedures incidental to the comfort and care of patients," gave as requisites to restraining the delirious a camisole, a pair of handcuffs and anklets, four pieces of gauze, two draw sheets or one sheet and one canvas thigh restrainer, four soft pads to fit under the handcuffs, and sideboards.[20]

Guidelines governing restraint use appeared in Kelley's 1926 *Text-book of Nursing Techniques*. These guidelines included prohibiting restraint without a physician's order; making restraint as inconspicuous as possible and no more than necessary; never leaving a patient unattended; checking circulation, chest, and comfort of arms and legs and watching general condition; using padding appliances; and fastening restraints so that patients cannot undo them. The 1927 procedure manual for Philadelphia General Hospital (PGH) noted that restraints are to be removed three times in twenty-four hours, twice during the day and once at night. To the usual list of appliances the PGH manual added leather restraints, for use only with "*special* order of the doctor." Of further interest in the PGH manual is another early reference to "extreme old age." In this case, "a thin, smooth flannel pad" was to be placed about the limb or body part before application of the restraint.[21]

Still insisting that the nurse avoid restraint if possible, Pope and Young's 1934 edition of *The Art and Principles of Nursing* described "padded leather cuffs fashioned for locking around the wrists and ankles and provided with an attachment through which a strap is passed"; the clove hitch, a commonly used substitute with women or children; the camisole, featuring a slit to allow exposure of the chest, in order that the physician might listen to breath sounds; and ropes for tying around bars at the head and foot of the bed to prevent wrinkling of the sheets. In a typed set of notes based on a Maxwell and Pope textbook, a student nurse at the Mount Sinai Hospital in Philadelphia, circa 1934, was advised not to go off duty carrying the key to locked restraining buckles.[22]

The 1941 edition of Harmer and Henderson's well-known *Textbook of the Principles and Practice of Nursing* noted the psychological distress caused by limitations in movement from restraints and urged efforts to reduce restraints, except in cases necessary for protection from injury. Still, pictures of devices, including canvas and metal sides on beds (possibly one of the first pictures of siderails), and various types of jackets are shown. Harmer and Henderson reported that "the word *restraint* is seldom heard because of its distasteful connotation"; shortly thereafter Young, in a discussion of patient safety, noted a trend toward using the word "protector" instead of restraint. Using peculiar logic, Young went on to say in the next sentence: "Restraining devices often arouse great resentment in the patient, but since protectors are sometimes necessary, a nurse should know the indications for the use of all types of protectors." Purposes of protectors included, among other things, prevention of injury to aged patients. Types of devices described were a folded sheet placed under the patient's shoulders and fastened to the top of the bed, a clove hitch gauze protector, and a leather cuff and strap with lock. By 1943 the manual of nursing procedures for Philadelphia General Hospital described the need to chart details concerning restraint: Type, time of application and removal, nursing care given, and condition of the patient. Unlike the earlier edition of the PGH manual, wrist and ankle restraints were now always to be used together.[23]

Although restraints were not even mentioned in the first textbook devoted exclusively to geriatric nursing, published in 1950, a review of fundamentals texts from this point onward provides explicit evidence for the use of physical restraints as part of standard practice for managing certain kinds of behavior. In contrast to this prevailing standard, however, authors of specialized texts in gerontological nursing, most of which have emerged in the last decade, rarely mention restraints or describe the devices as unacceptable and a treatment of last resort. In a chapter on physical restraint of the elderly appearing in *Clinical Gerontological Nursing*, the creation of restraint-free facilities in the United States is called "one of the great challenges for those who nurse and care deeply about older people in our society."[24]

Nursing journals covering the same span of years as the aforementioned texts also reflect the existence of restraints, ambivalence toward them, and over time, their growing usage with the elderly. Prior to 1940, mention of physical restraint pertained mainly to the mentally ill. However, the 1940s appeared to mark a period of growing concern for the aged as potential victims of broken bones resulting from a fall from bed. Interventions included a cloth harness to insure security; the "geri-chair" with locked tray table, specifically designed "to overcome the hazards of getting aged and paralyzed patients out of bed" and "to promote better digestion, improve morale, self-help, and an earlier convalescence"; and a "protective vest" to prevent older confused patients from falling out of bed and wheel chairs. It was increasingly apparent that the confused or forgetful elderly patient was considered a special problem among medical and surgical patients and that sheet restraints, cribsides, or a cloth wrist restraint might be warranted. Against this growing tide of opinion, Edith Marsh's success, in 1944, of eliminating restraints in a county nursing home—by using psychology in handling the old who were mentally off-balance, administering no barbiturates, permitting no coercion or mechanical restraints, giving patients a sense of stability with bedrails, and keeping the wards at twenty-five beds—was remarkable indeed.[25]

The regular appearance of advertisements for restraints, especially after 1950, suggests a growing preoccupation with patient safety. The J. T. Posey Company, still in business, began manufacturing "patient self-help and protection devices" in 1937; numerous examples for such items as the safety belt, patient support, McDonald restraint, wrist or ankle restraint, "V" restraint, and "tidy gown" are amply illustrated in pages of *Nursing Outlook*. Concern for liability in the case of injury also grew more apparent during the 1950s and 1960s, with stronger recommendations for bedrails and restraints. One description of accident prevention in a geriatric setting (in 1963) began with: "Sing a song of safety / Seek it everywhere / Daily pray for safety / Of patients in your care."[26]

Little information exists on the actual prevalence of restraint use for the decades 1900–1970 in the United States, but the preceding description of the literature confirms entrenched views on the necessity of restraint in certain circumstances, a deliberate pattern of educating nurses about the types and uses of such devices, and limited debate concerning the efficacy of physical restraint. As the population of frail elders in hospitals and nursing homes increased, concern for safety and protection intensified. Few alternatives to physical restraint were proposed. Thus were laid the foundations for widespread use of the devices beginning in 1970—and the resurgence of a new movement, not unlike its nineteenth century predecessor, to minimize or eliminate physical restraints. This time, however, the call for action came from consumer advocates and the nursing profession.[27]

The Rediscovery of Nonrestraint

Over the last five years, a new generation of institutional reformers has focused attention on the misuse of restraints in hospitals and nursing homes. Patient advocates have aligned with investigative journalists to draw public attention to restraint use as a regular, albeit disturbing, method of patient management. In an account from the *New York Times*, jail inmates with AIDS at Bellevue Hospital Center's psychiatric unit were reported "shackled to their beds without regard to physical condition." Editorials in the *Times* also deplored conditions permitting the "sick to lie in chains" and urged that "oldsters be set free" in compliance with new regulations established by the federal government.[28]

Several stories in the *Philadelphia Inquirer* have documented conditions at Byberry, a state hospital in Pennsylvania often compared with England's notorious Bedlam. Typical is the story of Billy Kirsch, a twenty-seven-year-old mildly retarded resident who was finally freed by order of a federal judge in 1988. According to the press, his wrists and ankles had been bound twenty-four hours a day for fourteen months. Along very different lines, the *Inquirer* also reported the difficult moral and ethical dilemmas faced by physicians and nurses in critical care units at the Hospital of the University of Pennsylvania. A large picture on the front page in January of 1989 was captioned "A MICU team restrains a patient. Frightened patients can become agitated, pulling loose IV lines and monitor wires."[29]

The *Washington Post* in 1989 described the fatal burning of a twenty-seven-year-old female AIDS patient at Southern Maryland Hospital Center. When found, the patient was strapped to her bed with leather restraints that could be opened only with a key, a package of cigarettes lying beneath her burned body. In another story covering New York's beleaguered hospital system, the *Post* described the scene in an emergency room at Bronx Municipal Hospital where a "demented woman had been lashed to a chair for more than five days" because there was nowhere else for her to go.[30]

A report on committed youth appearing in *Newsweek* in July of 1989 gave details concerning the treatment of teens in mental hospitals, including restraint for those deemed as uncooperative or as having a poor attitude. In an extraordinary piece of investigative journalism, the *Minneapolis Star Tribune* ran a four-part series in December 1990 concerning death from vest restraints, estimating that as many as two hundred such deaths were occurring annually. Since then, several court cases concerning death by asphyxiation from a vest restraint have resulted in multimillion dollar awards for the plaintiffs.[31]

Clearly, these illustrations reinforce our analysis of the historical evidence—namely, that reduction of mechanical restraint never became a compelling professional ideal in the United States and, further, that a therapeutic philosophy of control characterizes most health care institutions. Physical restraint and locked seclusion remain a reality in the management of many troublesome patients, despite renewed acceptance over the past thirty years of a "therapeutic milieu" supporting greater freedom. Although it may sound barbaric and out-of-date to tie people up, the circumstances for justifiable restraint versus the dangers and abuses of these devices are still debated in the psychiatric literature. In a recent study of psychiatric wards at one metropolitan public hospital, E. F. Morrison confirmed a "tradition of toughness" as a unit norm, with emphasis on "control" of behavior and recognition of the need for physical restraint of difficult patients, especially by nonprofessional staff.[32]

Analysis of Current Practice and Impetus for Change

While entrenched American habits for managing problematic behaviors no doubt contribute to the widespread use of physical restraints, other converging forces might explain the especially high prevalence of their use with the elderly. In the last two decades, the aging population has expanded dramatically, and faster than any adjustment in values by society toward this large group. Since 1965 the number of nursing home beds has also risen, and residents frequently are those with mental impairment. Staff believe in the efficacy of restraints for all the cultural reasons enumerated earlier, and have little knowledge and skill about alternatives. As is constantly noted in the nursing literature, a medical rather than a psychosocial model of care is widely accepted. At the heart of much practice in health care remain concerns about litigation when perceived needs for safety are unmet. That restraints neither prevent falls nor injuries, and probably exacerbate them, is generally ignored. The approach advised by "risk managers" is always safety first.[33]

In 1987, two nurse researchers, having heard that physical restraints were rarely used in the United Kingdom, conducted a descriptive study of care practices in nine geriatric facilities in Scotland, including four general hospitals with large geriatric services, four psychiatric hospitals with psychogeriatric services, and one small, freestanding geriatric hospital. Consistently, the investigators were told by geriatricians and nursing staff, "we never restrain," or "restraints are rarely used." A tour of thirty-one wards and observation of 826 patients revealed no vest, wrist, or ankle restraints; no hand mitts; one cotside (bedrail) for a patient in an intensive care unit; two seat belts; ten geriatric chairs, and nineteen Buxton (tilting) chairs, for an overall prevalence, by counting the belts and chairs as restraints, of only 3.8 percent.[34]

This markedly lower prevalence of restraint, compared to the United States for the same period of time, immediately reminds us of contrasting views held by British and Americans concerning the subject of physical restraint during the nineteenth century. Clearly there remain to this day some differences in therapeutic belief and style, despite the fact that Scottish patients receiving long-term care are remarkably similar in disability and illness to their counterparts in the United States, and furthermore, that relative numbers of staff are no greater in Scotland than in this country. The assumptions made by our British colleagues about managing and controlling behavior, however, are different: Their focus is on rehabilitation, not restriction in mobility, and fears concerning liability are minimal. A general attitude prevails that restraints are "bad" and "against the law" (in actuality, there is no such law). Technology, especially the imposition of various tubes in the body, is kept to a minimum, eliminating the need for restraint because of interference with treatment. Professional staff with some knowledge of geriatrics are in greater evidence and few restraining devices are available. Architecturally, many open spaces permit easy visibility of patients and the environment features low beds and special chairs, thus reducing the need for physical restraint.

Scottish nurses employed a wide range of alternatives to physical restraint, including companionship and supervision, change in treatment to promote greater comfort, physical and diversionary activity, psychosocial interventions, and environmental modification. These efforts were clearly augmented by administrative support and staff training. No evidence was given for excessive injury from falls or increased episodes of violence and disruptiveness. Appalled by the investigators' accounts of restraint practices in the United States, one Scottish nurse asked incredulously, "But who *forces* you to do it?" Another was prompted to write: "The routine use of physical restraint . . . is morally repugnant. It could only be tolerated by those societies, institutions, and individuals who neither care for, nor about, their frail elderly."

Since 1987 attitudes have shifted considerably in the United States regarding the use of physical restraints with older persons in nursing homes, and there appears to be a collective professional soul-searching such as that which occurred in Britain a century ago. This soul-searching has been sparked by nurses associated with the Quaker-operated Kendal Corporation in Kennett Square, Pennsylvania; consumer advocacy groups, especially the National Citizens' Coalition for Nursing Home Reform in

Washington, D.C.; and a growing number of researchers from nursing and other disciplines. These collective efforts no doubt contributed to greater media attention and to a U.S. Senate hearing in December of 1989.[35]

Without question, however, the strongest impetus for change came with the passage of the Nursing Home Reform Act, part of the Omnibus Budget Reconciliation Act (OBRA) of 1987.[36] As a result of this legislation, which was fully implemented in October of 1990, physical restraints cannot be applied unless required for treatment of a medical condition, and then only with consent of the patient or surrogate. Failure to comply could mean citation by state regulatory agencies and, without correction of the problem, ineligibility for funds from Medicare or Medicaid, the sources for much of the reimbursement to nursing homes. Although a comparison of the efforts of the Health Care Financing Administration (HCFA), the agency that oversees the procedures and guidelines for nursing home surveys, with those of the Lunacy Commission of the 1840s may be overdrawn, it is clear that enforced compliance can produce change.

Even with its numerous proponents, a change toward nonrestraint is unlikely to occur easily. In the current debate, many continue to argue that restraints can never be entirely abolished, that staffing will need to be increased drastically, and that mechanical means assure safety, reduce risk, and prevent troublesome behaviors. The manufacturers of restraints are marketing new products that are allegedly less restrictive in nature; for example, belts with velcro ties at the front. Many are suggesting that such products should not be considered restraints, but "postural supports" or "enablers." The U.S. Food & Drug Administration has warned that physical restraints must be used safely to avoid harm but refuses to conduct tests it says are the responsibility of the manufacturers. The nursing home industry continues to lobby forcefully for a change in HCFA's requirements concerning residents in nursing homes—specifically, altering the circumstances that allow the imposition of physical restraints for physical, emotional, and behavioral problems. Many states, with California leading the way, believe that provisions of the Nursing Home Reform Act cannot be implemented, including the use of fewer restraints, without more money to hire additional staff.[37]

Conclusion

The final outcome of this renewed debate about physical restraint and the legislation limiting physical restraints in nursing homes remains to be seen.

Viewed historically, the nineteenth-century restraint controversy highlights several important elements in the current debate. First, the matter of controlling behavior remains, now as it was then, a central issue in clinical practice. Second, the need to manage behavior, both physically and psychologically, emphasizes safety as a chief characteristic of the institution. And third, the predominant management style in the United States continues to emphasize minimal risk-taking. The American practice of restraint, while almost always justified as being "for the patient's own good," nevertheless serves institutional desires to minimize perceived risks of accidents and injuries that could deter paying clients or lead to expensive litigation.

Thus, if the current movement toward nonrestraint, or at least less restraint, is not to become a casualty of limited institutional horizons as it did in the late nineteenth century, American beliefs will need to change. Fundamental assumptions about control are involved. This means nothing less than a shift from the longstanding paradigm emphasizing "management of behavior" to a model more attuned to individual needs.

The practice of physically restraining the elderly, as was true in the past with the mentally ill, remains very much a function of cultural, social, and economic forces. It presents to nursing and society the task of reconciling conflicting claims on the ways in which patients will be treated. If earlier reformers offered no "magic bullet" but rather alternatives aimed chiefly at improving the environment—enhancing restorative activities and promoting greater efforts toward structured kindliness—today's experts also champion similar interventions for the "difficult," "uncooperative," or "confused" person. Despite a legislative mandate, legal and ethical debates favoring greater autonomy and resident rights, and research documenting the harms of restraint, change away from past practice will require new responses to behaviors traditionally seen as troublesome. For a different "therapeutic philosophy" to take hold, perceptions and habits developed and reinforced over decades will have to be replaced.

In examining the forces currently at work, however, we can take heart that this may be a new moment for change. Renewed debate concerning the "great restraint controversy" may at last mean realization of Annie Goodrich's dream of reform and humanity, as stated in her address to the Congress of the International Council of Nurses held in Montreal, Canada, in 1929:

> Today may be found in truly beautiful surroundings many who in another time might, probably would, have lain manacled and unattended in loathsome cells. Here we see frenzy reduced to serenity, hope restored to the despairing,

> inconsequence effectively motivated; and this is but the beginning of things that are to be.[38]

If history repeats itself, we may not get total abolition of restraints with the elderly. But, in successfully limiting their use, we will have advanced considerably toward a new vision of professional practice.

NEVILLE E. STRUMPF, PhD, RN, C, FAAN
Doris Schwartz Term Professor
School of Nursing
University of Pennsylvania
Nursing Education Building
420 Guardian Drive
Philadelphia, Pa. 19104-6096
Phone: (215) 898-8802

NANCY TOMES, PhD
Associate Professor
History Department
State University of New York at Stony Brook
Stony Brook, N.Y. 11794-4340
Phone: (516) 632-7500

Acknowledgments

Grateful acknowledgment is made to Catherine M. Stevenson for assistance in collecting materials for this article, and to Lois K. Evans for her significant contribution to current research aimed at limiting the use of physical restraints.

Notes

1. "A Week in a Florida Nursing Home Shows a Week of Sorrow and Strain," *Wall Street Journal*, 29 January 1988.

2. Data are drawn from Department of Health, Education, and Welfare, *National Nursing Home Survey: 1977* (Hyattsville, Md.: National Center for Health Statistics, 1979), PHS 79–1794; Health Care Financing Administration, *Medicare/Medicaid Nursing Home Information: 1987–1988* (Washington, D.C.: U.S. Government Printing Office, 1988); L. Mion, J. D. Frengley, and M. Adams, "Nursing Patients 75 Years and Older," *Nursing Management* 17 (September 1986): 24–28; and L. K. Evans and N. E. Strumpf, "Tying Down the Elderly: A Review of the Literature on Physical Restraint," *Journal of the American Geriatrics Society* 37 (January 1989): 65–74.

3. Alexander Walk, "Lincoln and Non-Restraint," *British Journal of Psychiatry* 117 (1970): 481.

4. For a description of these reforms, see Albert Deutsch, *The Mentally Ill in America*, 2nd ed. (New York: Columbia University Press, 1960), 213–28; Anne Digby, "Moral Treatment at the Retreat, 1796–1846," in *The Anatomy of Madness: Essays in the History of Psychiatry*, ed. W. F. Bynum, Roy Porter, and Michael Shepherd (London and New York: Tavistock, 1985), 2:52–72; and Paul H. Soloff, "Historical Notes on Seclusion and Restraint," in *The Psychiatric Uses of Seclusion and Restraint*, ed. K. Tardiff (Washington, D.C.: APA Press, 1984), 5–9.

5. The discussion of the nonrestraint movement in England and the United States presented in the following pages is drawn from Nancy Tomes, "The Great Restraint Controversy: A Comparative Perspective on Anglo-American Psychiatry in the Nineteenth Century," in *The Anatomy of Madness: Essays in the History of Psychiatry*, ed. W. F. Bynum, Roy Porter, and Michael Shepherd (London and New York: Routledge, 1988), 3:190–225. On restraint use at the York Retreat, see Anne Digby, *Madness, Morality, and Medicine: A Study of the York Retreat, 1796–1914* (New York: Cambridge University Press, 1985), especially pages 78–84. On restraint use at the Friends Asylum, see Patricia O'Brien D'Antonio, "Staff Needs and Patient Care: Seclusion and Restraint in a Nineteenth Century Insane Asylum," *Transactions and Studies of the College of Physicians of Philadelphia*, ser. V, 13:4 (December 1991): 411–23.

6. The quote comes from Andrew Scull, "Insanity in the Eighteenth and Nineteenth Centuries—John Conolly: A Reconsideration," *Journal of the Royal Society of Medicine* 81 (February 1988): 67. For additional background on the English nonrestraint movement, see Andrew Scull, "A Victorian Alienist: John Conolly, FRCP, DCL," in *The Anatomy of Madness: Essays in the History of Psychiatry*, 1:103–50 (see note 4, above).

7. Tomes, "The Great Restraint Controversy," 196–99.

8. Ibid., 202.

9. Deutsch, *The Mentally Ill in America*, 216–17.

10. Isaac Ray is quoted in "Reports of American Asylums," *American Journal of Insanity* 20 (1863–64): 488 (hereafter cited as *AJI*). On the more repressive style of American mental hospitals, see Tomes, "The Great Restraint Controversy," 202–5; and Tomes, *A Generous Confidence* (New York: Cambridge University Press, 1984).

11. Isaac Ray, "Association of Medical Superintendents of American Institutions for the Insane Proceedings," *AJI* 19 (1862–63): 59 (hereafter cited as AMSAII); and, John Butler, "AMSAII Proceedings," *AJI* 12 (1855–56): 90.

12. "Annual Reports of Lunatic Asylums," *Journal of Mental Science* (1858–59): 191; and Charles Folsom, "Treatment of Insanity," *Boston Medical and Surgical Journal* 94 (1876): 228.

13. Tomes, "The Great Restraint Controversy," 215–16.

14. Kirkbride is quoted in the "AMSAII Proceedings," *AJI* 32 (1875–76): 338–39.

15. Tomes, *A Generous Confidence*, especially pages 197–98, 378, note 20.

16. Tomes, "The Great Restraint Controversy," 217.

17. On nursing in the early asylum, see Ellen Dwyer, *Homes for the Mad: Life*

Inside Two Nineteenth Century Asylums (New Brunswick, N.J.: Rutgers University Press, 1987), 163–85; and Tomes, *A Generous Confidence*, especially pages 179–87.

18. Clara S. Weeks, *A Textbook of Nursing* (New York: Appleton, 1885), 302.

19. See Charlotte A. Aikens, *Clinical Studies for Nurses* (Philadelphia: W. B. Saunders and Co., 1909), 435; Minnie Goodnow, *A Textbook for Pupils During Their First Year of Hospital Work* (Philadelphia: W. B. Saunders and Co., 1921), 314–15, 249.

20. See E. Priscilla Reid, Mabel E. Hoffman, Hazel L. Jennings, and Lillian A. Read, *A Manual of Nursing Procedures* (Philadelphia: W. B. Saunders and Co., 1923), 165–66; and Anne C. Maxwell and Amy E. Pope, *Practical Nursing—A Textbook for Nurses*, 4th ed. (New York: G. P. Putnam's Sons, 1923), 156–57.

21. See Irene V. Kelley, *Text-Book of Nursing Techniques* (Philadelphia: W. B. Saunders and Co., 1926), 329; and *Nursing Procedures*, 2nd ed. (1927), Philadelphia General Hospital School of Nursing Records, Center for the Study of the History of Nursing, School of Nursing, University of Pennsylvania, pp. 59–60.

22. Amy E. Pope and Verna M. Young, *The Art and Principles of Nursing* (New York: G. P. Putnam's Sons, 1934), 105–6; and Lecture Notes from The Mount Sinai Hospital School of Nursing, Philadelphia, 1934–37, Edna La Porte Strumpf Papers, Center for the Study of the History of Nursing, School of Nursing, University of Pennsylvania.

23. Bertha Harmer and Virginia Henderson, *Textbook of the Principles and Practice of Nursing*, 4th ed. (New York: Macmillan Co., 1941), 364–67; Helen Young, *Essentials of Nursing* (New York: G. P. Putnam's Sons, 1942), 70–72; and *Nursing Procedures*, 8th ed. (1943), Philadelphia General Hospital School of Nursing Records, Center for the Study of the History of Nursing, School of Nursing, University of Pennsylvania, p. 96.

24. Kathleen Newton's *Geriatric Nursing* (St. Louis: Mosby, 1950) was the first such text explicitly devoted to nursing care of the elderly. Only in the last decade have specialty texts in gerontological nursing become more common. The following were examined for any mention of restraint use: Irene Burnside, *Psychosocial Nursing and the Aged*, 2nd ed. (New York: McGraw-Hill, 1980), 307–8; May Futrell, Stephen Brovender, Elizabeth McKinnon-Mullet, and H. Terri Brower, *Primary Health Care of the Older Adult* (North Scituate, Mass.: Duxbury Press, 1980); Ann Gera Yurick, Susanne S. Robb, Barbara Elliott Spier, and Nancy J. Ebert, *The Aged Person and the Nursing Process* (New York: Appleton-Century-Crofts, 1980); Elizabeth Jane Forbes and Virginia Macken Fitzsimmons, *The Older Adult* (St. Louis: C. V. Mosby, 1981); Doris L. Carnevali and Maxine Patrick, *Nursing Management for the Elderly*, 2nd ed. (Philadelphia: J. B. Lippincott, 1986); Irene Burnside, *Nursing and the Aged*, 3rd ed. (New York: McGraw-Hill, 1988), 412–13; Mary Anne Matteson and Eleanor S. McConnell, *Gerontological Nursing* (Philadelphia: W. B. Saunders and Co., 1988), 705, 742–43; Virginia Burggraf and Mickey Stanley, *Nursing the Elderly* (Philadelphia: J. B. Lippincott, 1989). The quote comes from Neville E. Strumpf, Lois K. Evans, and Doris Schwartz, "Physical Restraint of the Elderly," in *Clinical Gerontological Nursing*, ed. C. Chenitz, J. Stone, and S. Salisbury (Philadelphia: W. B. Saunders and Co., 1991), 342.

A long list of fundamental texts from 1950 onward suggests by their descriptions of restraint use that it is standard practice: Mildred L. Montag and Margaret

Filson, *Nursing Arts*, 2nd ed. (Philadelphia: W. B. Saunders and Co., 1953), 310–14; Alice L. Price, *The Art, Science and Spirit of Nursing* (Philadelphia: W. B. Saunders and Co., 1954), 231–33; Elinor V. Fuerst, LuVerne Wolff, and Marlene Weitzel, *Fundamentals of Nursing*, 5th and 6th eds. (Philadelphia: J. B. Lippincott, 1974 and 1979), chapters 17 and 18, respectively; Eunice M. King, Lynn Wieck, and Marilyn Dyer, *Illustrated Manual of Nursing Techniques*, 1st and 3rd eds. (Philadelphia: J. B. Lippincott, 1977 and 1986), chapter 58 and pages 627–32, respectively; Norma Dison, *Clinical Nursing Techniques*, 4th ed. (St. Louis: Mosby, 1979), 134–43; Pamela Holsclaw Mitchell and Anne Loustau, *Concepts Basic to Nursing*, 3rd ed. (New York: McGraw-Hill, 1981), 292–93; Jane Hirsch and Leslie Hancock, *Mosby's Manual of Clinical Nursing Procedures* (St. Louis: C. V. Mosby, 1981), 171–73; Sandra F. Smith and Donna Duell, *Nursing Skills and Evaluation* (Los Altos, Calif.: National Nursing Review, 1982), 344–47; Katherine Carey, ed., *Nursing Photobook* (Springhouse, Pa.: Intermed Communications, Inc., 1982), 95–97; Beverly J. Rambo and Lucille A. Wood, *Nursing Skills for Clinical Practice*, 3rd ed. (Philadelphia: W. B. Saunders and Co., 1982), 627–37; Lynda J. Carpenito, *Nursing Diagnosis Application to Clinical Practice* (Philadelphia: J. B. Lippincott, 1983), 508–11; Susan Martin Tucker, Mary Anne Breeding, Mary M. Canobbio, et al., *Patient Care Standards*, 3rd ed. (St. Louis: C. V. Mosby, 1984), 6; Karen Creason Sorensen and Joan Luckman, *Basic Nursing*, 2nd ed. (Philadelphia: W. B. Saunders and Co., 1986), 636–43; and Patricia A. Potter and Anne G. Perry, *Basic Nursing* (St. Louis: C. V. Mosby, 1987), 611–13.

25. For early references to restraint in nursing journals, see Florence Hale Abbot, MD, "Feeding and the Use of Restraint in Caring for the Insane," *American Journal of Nursing* 3 (November 1903): 85 (hereafter cited as *AJN*); and Emma A. Hawley, "Manifestations of Delirium in the Night-Time," *AJN* 8 (July 1908): 758, 760. After 1940, Mabel G. Weeks, "Falling Out of Bed is a Needless Hazard," *The Trained Nurse and Hospital Review* CX (January 1943): 111; Edith L. Marsh, "Stabilization Instead of Restraint in the Care of Elderly Patients," *AJN* 44 (November 1944): 1050; Helen Marie Blackman and Isabel Cook Seeley, "Use of Restraints in Care of Medical and Surgical Patients," *AJN* 45 (August 1945): 632–33; Emma Marie Pascente, "The Geri-Chair," *AJN* 58 (December 1958): 1703; Frances Gold Brown, "Protective Vest," *AJN* 59 (September 1959): 1261.

26. Advertisements with pictures of restraining devices manufactured by the J. T. Posey Co. appear in many issues of *Nursing Outlook*; see especially the issues for June 1955, page 511; June 1962, page 434; and September 1963, page 628. Preoccupation with concerns over liability become evident in James E. Ludlam, "Bedrails Up or Down?" *AJN* 57 (November 1957): 1439–40; Grace C. Barbee, "More About Bedrails and the Nurse," *AJN* 57 (November 1957): 1441–42; and Marjorie Gould, "Nursing Care of the Patient with a Fractured Hip," *AJN* 58 (November 1958): 1561–63. The quote is from Alice R. Meehan, "Accident Prevention in a Geriatric Setting," *Journal of Psychiatric Nursing* (May 1963): 214.

From the 1950s onward, fear of malpractice intensified, with increasing recommendations for use of physical restraint, as described in Evans and Strumpf, "Tying Down the Elderly: A Review of the Literature on Physical Restraint," 69–70 (see note 2, above). A counterargument to this trend began to occur in the 1980s, with

H. Rubenstein, F. H. Miller, S. Postel, and H. B. Evans, "Standards of Medical Care Based on Concensus Rather Than Evidence: The Case of Routine Bedrail Use for the Elderly," *Law, Medicine & Health Care* 11 (No. 6, 1983): 271–76; Sandra H. Johnson, "The Fear of Liability and the Use of Restraints in Nursing Homes," *Law, Medicine & Health Care* (Fall 1990): 263–73; and Marshall B. Kapp's report for The Commonwealth Fund of New York in 1991, *Nursing Home Restraints and Legal Liability: Merging the Standard of Care and Industry Practice.*

27. Calls from nurses included Irene Burnside, "Are Nurses Taught to Tie People Down?" *Journal of Gerontological Nursing* 10 (May 1984): 6; Doris Schwartz, "Call for Help," *Geriatric Nursing* 4 (January 1985): 9; and Jill Blakeslee, "Untie the Elderly," *AJN* 88 (June 1988): 833–34. Consumer advocacy came especially from the National Citizens' Coalition for Nursing Home Reform, Washington, D.C., and also from social work and medicine. For the latter see Carter Catlett Williams, "Liberation: Alternative to Physical Restraints," *The Gerontologist* 29 (May 1989): 585–86; and T. Franklin Williams, who at the time was the director of the National Institute on Aging, "Research and Care: Essential Partners in Aging," *The Gerontologist* 28 (May 1988): 579–85.

28. In the *New York Times*, see "Legal Group Says Bellevue Abuses Its Prison Patients," 9 October 1987; "Where the Sick Lie in Chains," 1 November 1987; "Unshackle Nursing Home Patients," 8 April 1991; and "Free Nursing Home Patients," 7 March 1992. A lengthy article by Tamar Lewin beginning on the front page and entitled "Nursing Homes Rethink Merits of Tying the Aged" appeared on 28 December 1989.

29. Conditions at Byberry were described by the *Philadelphia Inquirer* in "Report Cites Violations at Byberry," 6 February 1988, and in its magazine section, "The Shame That Was Byberry," 10 July 1988. In another vein, see "Choosing to Die: The New Option," 15 January 1989.

30. In the *Washington Post*, see "Restrained Patient Died of Burns From Cigarette Fire in Bed," 5 February 1989; and "Modern Epidemic Threatens New York's Hospital System," 11 February 1990.

31. See "Committed Youth," *Newsweek*, 31 July 1989; "Safeguards That Kill," *Minneapolis Star Tribune*, 2–5 December 1990; and "Nursing Home is Liable in Restraint Case," *Wall Street Journal*, 26 March 1990.

32. For details on acceptance of a "therapeutic milieu," see Paul H. Soloff, "Behavioral Precipitant of Restraint in the Modern Milieu," *Comprehensive Psychiatry* 19 (February 1978): 179–84; "Physical Restraint and the Non-Psychotic Patient: Clinical and Legal Perspectives," *Journal of Clinical Psychiatry* 40 (July 1979): 302–5; and "Historical Notes on Seclusion and Restraint." For continued debate on use of restraints with psychiatric patients, see B. Bursten, "Using Mechanical Restraints on Acutely Disturbed Psychiatric Patients," *Hospital and Community Psychiatry* 26 (November 1975): 757–59; E. Guirguis, "Management of Disturbed Patients: An Alternative to the Use of Mechanical Restraints," *Journal of Clinical Psychiatry* 39 (April 1978): 295–303; and E. F. Morrison, "The Tradition of Toughness: A Study of Nonprofessional Nursing Care in Psychiatric Settings," *Image: Journal of Nursing Scholarship* 22 (Spring 1990): 32–38 and "Violent Psychiatric Inpatients in a Public Hospital," *Scholarly Inquiry for Nursing Practice* 4 (Spring 1990): 65–82.

33. Lois K. Evans and Neville E. Strumpf, "Myths About Elder Restraint," *Image: Journal of Nursing Scholarship* 22 (Spring 1990): 124–28.

34. Lois K. Evans and Neville E. Strumpf, "Patterns of Restraint: A Cross-Cultural View" (Paper presented at the Gerontological Society of America, Washington, D.C., November 22, 1987).

35. "Untie the Elderly: Quality Care Without Restraints," Symposium before the Special Committee on Aging, United States Senate, Washington, D.C., 4 December 1989. Available from the Superintendent of Documents, Congressional Sales Office, U.S. Government Printing Office, Washington, D.C. 20402, ser. no. 101–H.

36. *Omnibus Budget Reconciliation Act, Subtitle C, Nursing Home Reform* (Washington, D.C.: U.S. Government Printing Office, 1987), Publ. No. PL 100–203.

37. For background on these multifaceted issues, see *Quality Care Advocate*, the newsletter of the National Citizens' Coalition for Nursing Home Reform, July/August 1990 and January/February 1992; proposed rules in the *Federal Register*, 57 (5 February 1992); and "Potential Hazards With Protective Restraint Devices," *FDA Medical Bulletin* 21 (December 1991): 3–4.

38. Annie Warburton Goodrich, "University Schools of Nursing," in *The Social and Ethical Significance of Nursing*, a series of addresses reprinted on the occasion of the 50th anniversary of the Yale School of Nursing, June 1973, 334.

"Dearest Friend"

The Correspondence of Colleagues Florence Nightingale and Mary Jones

JoAnn G. Widerquist
Department of Nursing
Saint Mary's College

Florence Nightingale, superintendent of nurses at Scutari, Turkey, during the Crimean War, and Mary Jones, superintendent of St. John's House, London, began a formal and rather cool exchange of letters over Nightingale's treatment of St. John's House nurses in Scutari. Florence Nightingale termed four of them "flibbidity gibbets" and arranged to have them sent home. Mary Jones defended her nurses and so gained Florence Nightingale's respect.[1] In 1860, when the Nightingale Fund began the Nightingale Training School at St. Thomas Hospital, Nightingale wrote to Mary Jones for advice on numerous matters—even the cost of tea and sugar connected with the training.[2]

That the collegial relationship became a friendship was reflected in their change of salutations to "Dearest friend" and "Very dearest friend." Jones also referred to Florence Nightingale as "Dearest Mistress," even though Nightingale relied heavily on Jones's expert advice about all manner of nursing issues. Some of those issues were: the training of midwives at King's College Hospital; hospital construction and management; workhouse and district nursing in Liverpool and other cities; Indian nursing; sanitary measures; military nursing, including the tragic allegation of manslaughter against Jane Catherine Shaw Stewart;[3] cholera epidemics; and statistical papers and conferences. Many more letters were preserved between Florence Nightingale and Mary Jones than between Nightingale and some of her other correspondents. Nightingale often asked correspondents to burn her letters, but Mary Jones did not.

Themes of the Nightingale and Jones Correspondence

The Nightingale–Jones correspondence spanned thirty years of their lives and the beginning of modern nursing in the Victorian era. The private

Nursing History Review 1 (1993): 25–42.

sharing of their deep concerns, professional and personal, illuminates their struggles as early nurses dealing with societal constraints, some of which continue to affect nursing today. The letters provide a rich mine for exploration into the early throes of professionalization.

Several themes emerge from the correspondence. One is the religious motivation or calling shared by Nightingale and Jones. A sense of "calling" or vocation was a common characteristic of many Victorians. Religious belief and experience gave added meaning in a time when the roles of both men and women were undergoing a shift from a rural to industrial urban society. Christian calling became a source of strength for Nightingale and Jones as they pioneered roles for single women in a society that made no place for them.[4] Another theme that emerges is their difference over strategy for nursing—individual and secular as opposed to collective and religious. A third theme is the issue of authority in nursing. Examination of these themes helps us clarify the mindset of Victorian nurses while illustrating some ongoing issues still inherent in nursing.

Religious Motivation

Many Victorian women of the upper class were drawn to the aesthetic forms of worship and call to service of the Oxford movement, an Anglican (Church of England) high church spiritual renewal group. The charitable work encouraged by the Oxford movement gave a meaning to these women's lives that went beyond house and drawing room. Nightingale, although from a wealthy Unitarian family, was baptized Anglican and was somewhat influenced by the movement. Mary Jones, however, was an ardent follower of this group. In fact, she was referred to as a Tractarian, an early term given to those who both formed and followed the Oxford movement.[5]

The movement originated with Anglican churchmen at Oxford University who desired spiritual renewal for the state church within an intellectual framework. They wished to capture some of the zeal of the evangelicals, such as the Wesleyan Methodists, as well as the ascetic, mystical nature of Catholicism. Men such as John Keble, John Henry Newman (later cardinal), and Henry Edward Manning (later cardinal) were its leaders. The latter two left the Anglicans to join the Roman Catholic church, as did many high-born English women, such as Mary Stanley, who led the second group of nurses to Scutari, and Nightingale's friend Elizabeth Herbert, wife of Sir Sidney Herbert, the secretary at war, who requested Nightingale to supervise nursing at Scutari. Because of these "secessions," as they were called, the Oxford movement was often suspect among other Anglicans.

One of the results of the Oxford movement was the formation of religious communities (of both men and women) in the Church of England for the first time since the Reformation. Most of the women's groups were formed to provide an opportunity for religious life and service, by home visiting and/or nursing. The earliest attempt (1825) to establish a nursing order was fashioned after the Sisters of Charity in France but did not succeed. The order was taken over by Elizabeth Fry, a philanthropic Quaker, and eventually provided the nursing for Guy's Hospital. The order was first known as the Society of Protestant Sisters of Charity and later as the Institution of Nursing Sisters. Tension over theology and proselytizing among Anglicans, Roman Catholics, Evangelicals, and others who dissented from the Church of England was always a backdrop for events in the development of Victorian nursing.[6]

Nightingale, born in 1820, was not part of these very early attempts to reform nursing. At the age of sixteen she perceived a call from God to service and eventually decided that the call was to nursing. As a mature single woman in 1851, she went to Kaiserswerth in Germany, to the dismay of her mother and sister. Her reason for selecting Kaiserswerth for training rather than Fry's group or any other in England is unknown. When the request came in October 1854 for her to organize female nurses to go to the military hospitals of the Crimean War, a few nursing sisterhoods were in existence; Nightingale immediately looked to these for nurses.

St. John's House

One of the first such institutions to respond, indeed one of the few places where experienced nurses could be found, was St. John's House. The sisterhood formed in 1848 at the request of a group of physicians who wanted to raise the caliber of nursing by improving the character and quality of nurses in London hospitals. Mary Jones was the second superintendent, appointed in 1853, possibly after some conflict with the governing council. Conflict between the sisters of St. John's House and the council was an ongoing problem, as we will later see. When Jones became superintendent, only one sister remained. After only one year with the order, however, Jones supplied six nurses for the original party going to Scutari and more nurses later in the war.[7]

The early records from St. John's House are very brief and do not include much information about Mary Jones and her background. She was probably in her mid-thirties when she joined the order and from an upper-class family. She, too, was single and dedicated to service because of a commitment to Christ. She chose to join with other women of like commitment rather than to remain independent, as Nightingale had elected to do.

The St. John's sisters that Mary Jones joined were the first of three levels of members or "Inmates of the House," as the women of St. John's House were sometimes called. The sisters were unpaid gentlewomen of the upper class who practiced nursing as part of their religious life. They were expected to be well educated and able to instruct and supervise the nurses. The nurses comprised the second level of members. They were employed to do the major portion of the nursing undertaken by the order in hospitals and homes. For this work they received wages, a certificate of competence after five years, and a pension after twelve to fifteen years' service.[8] The third level of members, the probationers, were expected to serve two years and then become nurses. All members had to be adherents of the Church of England and were required to follow the regulations and responsibilities spelled out in their Book of Order.[9]

In 1856, St. John's House, under the guidance of Mary Jones, assumed the nursing at King's College Hospital, a secular institution, and expanded training for nurses there. Nightingale, engrossed in the battle for reform of military medical care and recovering from the physical and emotional strain of the war years, did not keep in contact with Mary Jones. However, Nightingale knew of Jones's reputation for training nurses. She had even considered King's College Hospital as a possible place for the Nightingale training school. Even though Nightingale ultimately chose St. Thomas Hospital, probably for reasons of size, location, and finances, she sought expert guidance from Mary Jones in developing the training. The relationship provided both parties with much more than professional information.[10]

Spiritual and Personal Friendship

Some clues to a spiritual friendship between Florence Nightingale and Mary Jones can be found. For example, on 2 February 1865, Florence Nightingale wrote: "Do you remember coming to me February 7th last year—I remember it well."[11] The date 7 February 1837 marks Nightingale's "call." She kept 7 February as a day for contemplation and reflection. Perhaps Mary Jones joined her. Florence Nightingale's letters also offered spiritual succor to Mary Jones: Nightingale often quoted the French mystics, her favorites. Jones, in turn, responded with words of affection and blessing.

Not only did Nightingale try to provide spiritual support for those dear to her; she also gave attention to their physical comfort. A generous friend, Nightingale often sent a variety of gifts to Mary Jones and the sisters: wild game, honey, pictures, Christmas greens from Embley, books, money, and even a bedstead, when Mary Jones complained of back pain. Nightingale and Jones exchanged visits, and the Nightingale family homes were available for holiday visits.

Nightingale shared family concerns with Mary Jones, in particular Fanny Nightingale's senescence. Fanny Nightingale lived to age ninety-two, her last years marked by an incapacity that greatly distressed her daughters, Florence and Parthenope. Florence asked Mary Jones to recommend a nurse for her mother. Nightingale and Jones always included their own health problems in their letters. Sickness was seemingly an everyday occurrence, as was the necessity of bearing it with grace—as did Christ. Although these topics filled the correspondence of most Victorian women, they were not the meat of Nightingale and Jones's exchange.

The Professional Colleagues: Agreement and Disagreement

Nightingale and Jones were professional colleagues, as well as friends, engaged in discussing and debating the real work of modern nursing. They were strong women, personally and professionally, having had deep formative experiences as pioneers in nursing; they each, therefore, held firm convictions on many issues. Occasionally these convictions caused disagreement.[12] One such disagreement was over the role of nursing sisterhoods. Although Nightingale applauded the spiritual dedication and physical skill of Jones and the St. John's nurses, she believed that sisterhoods, in general, were simply not a practical solution to the vast need for nurses. Nightingale, therefore, advocated a committed but individualistic approach to nursing in a secular setting. Many letters passed between them referring to their differences. For example, in 1865, regarding nurses for India, Nightingale lauded Mary Jones thus:

> Here comes the difficulty, the material to be trained is almost nil. . . . decent women get married. . . . A religious society would be the only thing. And I am sure I would help them if I could. But there is only one person to do it and that is you.[13]

Jones, in a letter dated May 1866 from Lea Hurst, where she was on holiday to revise bylaws for the council, asked Florence Nightingale to reconsider her attitude toward nursing sisterhoods:

> My dearest friend
> . . . everyday convinces me more and more that "Sisterhoods" present the only *reliable* agency. . . . You know well that I do not say this lightly or without fully estimating the requirements of Hospital nursing. I mean only Sisterhoods only specially and thoroughly trained for this work—bodies of women who shall bring to the work all the annual skill-knowledge, common-sense of the best *Secular* nurses—and a great deal more besides. I know well that you do not quite agree with all my conclusions—and that you have some prejudice (in many respects well founded I know too) against Sisterhoods—but I feel *quite* sure Dearest friend that were you now actively employed—active enough, God knows,—I should rather have said personally engaged in actual nursing of Hospitals and you would, you must come to this conclusion.
>
> My motto is "make Sisterhoods for the work" not undertake the work as a pastime for ill (or non) understood Sisters. Forgive this long tirade between friends—but my very heart aches often and often at the difficulties and hindrances and misconceptions which so hinder our work—and wear away our strength.
>
> Yours ever most lovingly M[14]

Some of Nightingale's "prejudice" to sisterhoods stemmed from her experience with Roman Catholic and Protestant orders in the Crimea and other places.[15] She complained that the sisters were often poorly prepared to work and were more concerned with conversions and their own spiritual needs than with the physical needs of those entrusted to them. Nightingale, always the pragmatist, had also another reason for her disapproval of nursing sisterhoods, as expressed in a letter written to Sir John McNeill:

> As to the proposal concerning Protestant Nuns. . . . The material is doubtful and the numbers too few. And the best women do not choose to enter "Orders". . . . St. John's House of my dear friend and "pupil," Miss Jones is Superintendent. . . . But her system of nursing, which is first rate, has taken even less extension than ours has. The fact is that Orders in England (and this is quite as much the case with the Roman Catholics who are exactly in the same difficulty as we are) do not extend for this reason: —the best women, women fit to be heads, do not enter orders in England.[16]

She did not think enough sisters could be found in England to do the work of nursing, a strongly held belief that Nightingale repeated to Mary Jones and others:

> I have put it in print, that the highest average good nursing is secured by a religious society and a secular government in a Hospital. . . . I shall do everything in my power (which is little enough) to enable them to out-ride this storm. If they cannot, then I shall say Sisterhoods *are* impossible in the Church of England, not from the fault of the women, but from that of the priests. It *is* impossible for a priest of the Ch of Eng[d] [Church of England] to understand the sound principles of independence, of non-interference.[17]

Nightingale respected Jones for organizing nursing in a sisterhood within a secular institution, even though she preferred a somewhat different format. Nightingale wanted nursing to be done by women called to service because of their religious sentiment and commitment to service. She, perhaps because of her own personality, wanted nurses to do this individually and not as an organized group or "sisterhood." She was also suspect of religious administrative hierarchy. Jones, on the other hand, believed that nurses were strengthened by organization and formal commitment to a religious organization.

Control and Conflict

The idea that anyone other than a nurse could be responsible for nursing was unthinkable to Florence Nightingale. On this issue of authority Jones and Nightingale agreed. The heart of Mary Jones's conflict with the Anglican hierarchy concerned who had authority over the sisters and the nurses. In a long letter to Sir Harry Verney, her brother-in-law, Florence Nightingale exclaimed:

> Don't let the Chaplain want to make himself matron. Don't let Doctor make himself Head nurse. *There is no worse matron than a Chaplain.* It is so odd that practical Englishman cannot see this without being told. . . . Matrons don't want to be chaplains, why do chaplains want to be Matrons. But if a chaplain has ever tasted this, apparently to him, dear delight, he never can be put back in his place any more.[18]

Although Nightingale and Jones disagreed on the role of nursing sisterhoods, both believed nursing arose from a spiritual commitment and both strove to care for the poor and miserable. As Mary Jones mused, "I would rather train two midwives for the poor than build a Lying-in Hospital." Yet, despite her commitment, Mary Jones was becoming discontent. Fifteen years as superintendent and superior of the order had convinced her that the sisters needed to take religious vows and become more independent of the council and chaplain.

Originally the council from the parish of St. John the Evangelist used Pastor Fleidner's ideas and Kaiserswerth's structure as a model.[19] The title given to the group was the St. John's House and Sisterhood, a "training institution for Nurses, for Hospitals, Families and the Poor."[20] A master, an Anglican priest (at the grand salary £150 per year) and a lady superintendent (who brought £50 per year for her keep) were to administer the institution under a council composed of physicians from King's College Hospital and clergymen from the Church of England as appointed by the bishop of London.[21]

The sisters often carried heavy responsibilities for everyday operations without the autonomy to determine policy. When the group of sisters wanted to take vows and act more independently, it was clearly at odds with Anglican tradition and the antipapist spirit of its founders. Most nursing sisterhoods had developed because a particularly spiritual leader had developed the community and then sought church approval. St. John's House was different.

> No other Anglican religious community had such an unusual method of foundation; it seems that it was called forth from the heart of the church of England rather than by means of an individual founder or foundress . . . there would be no vows of poverty, monastic obedience, or celibacy, but a full, free, and willing devotion to the great cause of Christian charity.[22]

Those words, taken from the regulations of the order, formed part of the conflict that Jones and the sisters had with the council as they sought more control over their personal religious life and work as nurses.[23]

Mary Jones was not alone among Victorian women in having difficulties with male authorities who sought to control her activities. The men who governed the hospitals were usually physicians and clergymen; they wanted the work or care that was provided by women but did not want to relinquish authority. Nightingale, set apart as a Crimean War heroine, had more autonomy and was somewhat more insulated than were her professional friends in frays over issues of control. Not insignificantly, she no longer practiced active nursing and so was out of the direct line of fire. Nevertheless she tried to aid her friend.

In 1867, the all-male council of physicians and clergymen would not approve the sisters' choice of priest to fill the chaplain's position. Nightingale penciled a quick note encouraging Mary Jones not to accept such a situation.

> Tell them what you want is not a Committee of inquisition but a simple chaplain. Principiois Obsta—oppose any such ecclesiastic domination.[24]

The council finally appointed the chaplain the sisters wanted. In 1867, however, the sisters requested to take vows and to display the elements of the Eucharist in Mary Jones's room. The council held firm against this. Thus the council maintained its original spirit of full, free, and willing devotion (i.e., without vows), and antipathy to anything "Romanish." Mary Jones's objections to this situation were not entirely obvious to Nightingale, but clearly Jones felt that her right to religious expression had been trampled.

Nightingale tried to stay the tide and heal the breach between Jones and the council. She wrote to Dr. Bowman, one of the original members of the council and a long time friend, for help. She contacted her brother-in-law, Sir Henry Verney, and others who she thought might help to ameliorate the conflict. On 7 December 1867 in a long letter, one of many to Mary Jones about the situation, Nightingale cajoled,

> And now dearest, I have let a day or two pass . . . I have laid the case before you—not from the side of your Council but from the side of my own life's experience—just as I have tried to lay the case before Mr. Bowman, [Dr. Bowman of the council] not from your side but from the side of life's experience of all countries. I should be a very unfair and unfaithful friend if I did not. . . . You said no one could understand the differences between you and the Council, that is just what I feel. I do not understand them. I do not at this moment know the real reasons why you resign. I don't understand your grievances against the Council—nor theirs against you. And as on a point which I do not exaggerate if call it one of vital importance to the Church of England, that is, to know whether your Sisterhood, the only one on a sound basis, can stand or not—it is surely worthwhile that there should at least be a clear understanding—what the point of the differences are. . . . You and the council should set down propositions and grievances . . . and see by each side giving up on any point could rub off the one angle and a little off another angle that the wheels could be made to move again . . . I don't want to give you advice but only take the case before you.
>
> God bless you Ever yours, F. Nightingale[25]

Mary Jones did not take her "dear Mistress's" advice for compromise. On 12 January 1868 Mary Jones, six sisters, and one associate left St. John's House to begin their own work. Nevertheless Florence Nightingale remained loyal to Mary Jones and offered to give her a home at Embley.[26]

Midwifery and Puerperal Sepsis

This issue alone, however, did not compel Mary Jones to leave St. John's House. At the same time as the crisis with the council, an outbreak of puerperal sepsis at the Nightingale Lying-in Ward at King's College Hospital peaked. The outbreak added to the strain affecting Jones in 1867 and also disturbed Nightingale. Although Nightingale did not place her school of nursing under Jones, in 1861 she had begun to use the Nightingale Fund to support the training of midwives at King's College Hospital under Mary Jones. Both women were closely involved in the selection of wards to be used for training, the length of training, and other administrative concerns. When numerous deaths occurred in the lying-in ward from sepsis, Nightingale and Jones were consumed with determining the cause.

On 14 June 1867 Mary Jones penned an anxious note to Florence Nightingale.

> Knowing as I well do, how heavily you are taxed, I could not justify myself in asking to see you for any good or pleasure for myself and because I do so love and long for a word or a sight I the more strictly refrain from asking one unnecessary interview.
>
> But it is really important that I should see you about this matter, so please—as you leave me liberty I will say Sunday at 4 p.m. God willing.
>
> Yours in truth, M[27]

Jones writes again on 18 June 1867, in reply to Nightingale's request for statistics:

> Here are the lists of admissions, deaths and cause of deaths. They look bad enough altogether. The mischief lies at the door of either the abstract fact of the Mid Ward being in a General Hospital or the special one of the P.M. [Post Mortem] Theater proximity which is it? Perhaps somewhat of both. I am half afraid to acknowledge even to myself of the dread I have of that P.M. on account of my poor ward—and now what is to be done? . . . 23 June I ought to have insisted more strongly on that P.M. Theatre which has always haunted me. . . . The ward is never out of my mind.[28]

The wards were eventually closed, repainted, and refurbished. Florence Nightingale and Mary Jones followed the situation closely in their letters.[29] In the end, after Mary Jones's resignation, the Nightingale Fund ceased support of midwifery at King's College Hospital.

While Jones was worrying over the puerperal sepsis outbreak and struggling with the council conflict, she continued to have direct oversight of St. John's House nursing at Galignani Hospital in Paris and of nursing at Charing Cross Hospital. Many years of this administrative responsibility, in particular for the maternal deaths, weighed heavily on Mary Jones's conscience, as on Nightingale's. Nightingale, however, was able to perceive some good from their efforts, as is evidenced in letters in 1872.

> Dearest, very dearest friend: Feb. 9/72
> I am almost glad of something which compels me to write a letter I like—namely to you—when year after year I postpone to the thousands of letters which I *don't* like to have to write. . . . I can scarcely help alluding to what you once said as to your regret at ever having had Lying-In wards at King's College Hospital. If there was fault, it was mine—because I was supposed to know more about Hospital Statistics—and bitterly have I repented it. Had I known then M. Hussion's General Lying-In Ward Statistics at Paris I never would have done it. But these very Statistics were only brought out at our request. And so with a great many others I believe it is morbid, now the thing is done, (tho of course evil should never be done knowingly that good might come) not to see the good that has come. Thousands of lives of poor Lying-In Women will be saved by the attention that has been aroused.[30]

Mary Jones replied to her dear friend,

> Alas about the poor Midwifery wards, Dearest Mistress—I can never think of that attempt without mourning over the disappointed and anxiety it brought upon you—through my failure—and I did so long to have carried out your desire and plans successfully—it is most kind of you ever to think of it without reproaching me.[31]

Still, the issue of control of the order plus the strain of worry over puerperal sepsis may not wholly explain Mary Jones's reasons for resigning from St. John's House at the end of 1867. Perhaps she was simply tired: careful reading of her letters as early as 1861 provides some such clues, such as, "I am going to Hempstead for a day to be lazy until Thursday."

The demands on Jones to take ever increasing nursing responsibility were extremely harsh because Jones was a careful planner and meticulous in administrative detail. Little diagrams of pipe fittings, lanterns for night nurses, and dining arrangements dotted her letters—sometimes to the consternation of Florence Nightingale.[32] Mary Jones conducted a survey of many church parish priests and other leaders to ascertain whether or not they would accept trained women before agreeing to undertake the training of pupil midwives.[33] Jones not only wanted trained nurse midwives but also assurance of a place for them to practice. Writing on 9 May 1861, she expressed fear of turning an army of untrained nurses on the sick poor, a fear she held for King's College Hospital midwives and also for workhouse nurses in Liverpool.[34]

Mary Jones always insisted on thorough planning and preparation before beginning anything. Her reaction to William Rathbone's request for her to assist in preparing women for workhouse nursing was typical: "his railway speed is perplexing—he often appears to me to wish so soon as he has chosen his row to drive his engine at full speed along it without waiting to lay down the rails."[35]

The Strain of Commitment

Mary Jones maintained high standards for herself and those under her administration. Even though she expected to suffer illness and trial for her Christian commitment to service, the toll on her reserves became evident. Small wonder her complaints of illness and tiredness were expressed poignantly in a letter to Florence Nightingale (6 December 1865).

> . . . and [I] am very busy and I cannot say that my work is quite easy to me for some months past I have not felt quite well—yet I fear more of laziness than real illness—for I do so long really for rest very often now though I would fain not be weary or a laggard till my work is done but each month the necessity for constant unflagging work seems to increase and helpers in any part of the work more difficult to find—the need for nurses is pressing on every hand and the right sort of women are not to be found for even a thousandth part of the work waiting. Ladies, clergymen and others are wanting District and midwife nurses yet all suppose we can supply them at a minutes notice and these very people acknowledge themselves unable to find a woman fit to be trained.[36]

During her tenure as a nursing superintendent, Mary Jones had tried in numerous ways to begin convalescent nursing homes but was always thwarted. In spite of her claims of fatigue, she again expressed this desire 25 April 1867, saying, "I count the care of convalescents as part of the 'high art' of Nursing."[37]

Remorse over the midwifery ward, pressure of work from all sides, desire for a different kind of nursing, and longing for some relaxation piled like blocks on the tower of Mary Jones's anxiety over spiritual control of the order. Perhaps Jones could not just quit as superior of the order, superintendent of hospitals, and trainer of midwives, however, for she took on the conflict with the council as an opportunity to assume less strenuous work.

In an era when religious calling meant commitment to work until sickness or death intervened, she may have seen no other way of escape. So she left her position in the forefront of Victorian nursing practice. Nightingale, long retired from active practice, did not quite understand the situation and, although often advising rest, began suggesting new exacting work. For instance, in a letter dated 19 October 1868 Nightingale writes:

> Dearest very dearest friend,
>
> You say it is hard to forgive and be silent.
>
> I feel just as strongly as you do and just as I did last miserable Christmas—that it is hard to forgive and be silent. And this is not the less because, as you are aware, I venture to differ from you on some ecclesiastical points. I am glad you have taken parochial work. I do not feel surprised at your not feeling spirits or health for Hospital work at present . . . but Workhouse Infirmary needs to be done and so few (none like you) to do it. . . . I do not admit your plea (except for India) of "too old." . . . A real tried, experienced spirit, that is one who is used to work, does better work for God between 50 and 70 than during the whole of her previous life.[38]

After resigning, Mary Jones continued a variety of nursing activities with the sisters that were somewhat curtailed because of lowered financial resources and physical limitations from a carriage accident. Fulfilling her own hopes, Jones and the sisters eventually opened a home for incurables. She frequently wrote Nightingale long letters about the maternity ward; Nightingale used her letters liberally in writing *Notes on Lying-In Hospitals.* Their correspondence gradually tapered off as the two friends aged. Yet when Mary Jones died in June 1887, Nightingale wrote to her own sister, rather sentimentally as Victorians were wont to do, "she is my oldest friend in the Nursing cause."[39]

Conclusion

Nightingale found in Mary Jones a friend in service to the poor and miserable as she had in another Crimean War colleague, Mother Mary Clare Moore.[40] These two women fit Nightingale's description of true friendship, articulated in a religious essay to Benjamin Jowett, her spiritual advisor during her mature years, "There must be a third among them—a third in these 'twos' to make them real or ideal friends. And that third must be God."[41]

Nightingale and Jones probably found a meeting as both colleagues and friends because of this "Other"—a shared commitment to God. They viewed Jesus Christ, the suffering servant savior, as the author of their service. They envisioned nursing as a spiritual commitment and perhaps the nurse as a "hero (heroine) caretaker" who offers self-sacrifice for the benefit of others.

Their attitude may still permeate nursing today if a recent brochure from the National League for Nursing is any indication. The brochure contains a picture of Joan of Arc and the caption "Joan of Arc Saved France: Nurses of America Save Health Care Through Nursing Education." Apparently, nurses, like the French maiden, are to be martyrs for the cause. Such a perception makes it excusable to ignore the toll work takes on the caregiver and contributes to the exhaustion felt by even someone as committed as Jones. Jones and Nightingale were sustained by a sense of duty to God to continue for long periods. What is the sustaining force for women caregivers in today's secular society?

Although Nightingale and Jones held similar views about nursing, they differed in their approach to the issue of securing enough nurses with ability to carry out the work. Nightingale was a visionary who could see the possibilities for the future of nursing, but she was also a pragmatist who used the means available to reach as near her goal as possible.[42] Nightingale would have preferred that nursing, especially supervising and teaching, be conducted by a sisterhood in a secularly governed institution, but she believed this impossible and proposed secular nursing practiced by dedicated women. Jones, perhaps more idealistic, held to her conviction that nursing was best done by a group of women bound together by a commitment to God, to humanity, and to each other.

On the issue of authority over nursing care, both Nightingale and Jones held tenaciously to the same conviction—nursing must be controlled by a nurse, "a female head," they would say.[43] Both believed nursing an occupation for females, one that would especially give single women of their time a valued and respected place in society.[44] Nursing remains today primarily a woman's profession. A power struggle continues for autonomy, a power struggle clearly demonstrated in Mary Jones's life. Current issues and solutions may differ but the effects on nurses are unchanged.

Nightingale is the acknowledged founder of modern nursing, but in many ways Jones is more a prototype of modern nurses than Nightingale. Jones dealt with the great demand of active nursing practice and its often inadequate emotional, financial, and spiritual compensation. Nightingale, by virtue of her retirement from active nursing practice after the Crimean

War, did not experience the same kind of professional career that was Jones's life for fifteen to twenty years. Perhaps Nightingale's disappointment with Jones for leaving the fight for an Anglican nursing order can be explained by this difference.

Nursing again seems to be embracing caring as its essence—a return to its Victorian heritage. Still, the tension between the idealistic view of the "lady with the lamp" and the real situation of a modern nurse remains. Mary Jones appears to have been an excellent nurse, one sought by many in addition to Nightingale for expert advice and help. But Jones struggled with the problems confronting nurses today: responsibility without authority, overwork without adequate help, and lack of recognition of the special needs of the caregiver engaged in an activity on which society is slow to place high value. Nineteenth-century religious women engaged in nursing poured their money, their physical being, and their emotional and spiritual strength in providing care to the sick and help for the poor. They asked for and received little support in return. Their faith helped to sustain them. Caring carries with it a connotation of selflessness that cannot be denied. As Mary Jones found, the consequences of caring inevitably exact a price from the caregiver.

JoAnn G. Widerquist, DMin, MA, RN
Associate Professor and Chair
Department of Nursing
Saint Mary's College
Notre Dame, Ind. 46556
Phone: (219) 284-4680
Fax: (219) 284-4716

Acknowledgments

The research for this article was supported by grants from Saint Mary's College and the Nursing Research Consortium of North Central Indiana. I would like to thank the Florence Nightingale Museum Trust for permission to reproduce material from the Nightingale Collection at the Greater London Record Office; Alex Attewell, assistant curator, has been especially helpful. I also wish to thank C. M. Hall, high executive officer, Department of Manuscripts, for permission to quote from the Nightingale Collection at the British Library. And special thanks to my daughter, Kristine Widerquist Bosler, for critiquing the article during preparation.

Notes

1. Florence Nightingale to Miss Grippe, 5 December 1854, Greater London Record Office HI/ST/NC3/SU5 (hereafter cited as GLRO). Mary Jones to Florence Nightingale, 22 December 1854, GLRO HI/ST/NC3/SU17. Florence Nightingale to Council, 11 January 1855, GLRO HI/ST/NC3/SU18. Florence Nightingale to Council, 16 August 1855, GLRO HI/ST/NC/SU35. Martha Vicinus and Bea Negaard, *Ever Yours, Florence Nightingale* (Cambridge, Mass.: Harvard University Press, 1990), 7, 206, 226, 240, 322, 344.

2. GLRO Collection and British Library Nightingale Collection ADD MSS Vol. 47,743, and 47,744. The correspondence consists of well over 200 letters, those from Mary Jones in two volumes in the British Library and Nightingale's in the Greater London Record Office administered by the Florence Nightingale Museum Trust. (Hereafter British Library will be cited as BL.)

3. Jane Catherine Shaw Stuart was a superintendent of nurses in the Crimean War and later at the military hospital at Woolwich. In this incident, a patient died without an orderly present; Shaw Stuart was alleged to be responsible. Nightingale considered the accusation absurd. Florence Nightingale to Mary Jones, December 1864, GLRO HI/ST/NCI/64/24; Sir Edwin T. Cook, *The Life of Florence Nightingale* (London: Macmillan and Co., Ltd., 1914), I:330, 395; Francis Berry Smith, *Florence Nightingale's Reputation and Power* (London and Canberra: Croom Helm, 1982), 155–56.

4. Judith Moore, *A Zeal for Responsibility: The Struggle for Professional Nursing in Victorian England, 1868–1883* (Athens and London: The University of Georgia Press, 1988), 3–10, 12–24. Anna Brownell Jameson, *The Sisters of Charity, Protestant and Catholic Abroad and at Home* (London: Longmans, Brown, Green and Longman, 1855), 61. A. M. Allchin, *The Silent Rebellion: Anglican Religious Communities 1845–1900* (London: SCM Press, 1958), 38–39.

5. Allchin, 52–60. Allan T. Cameron, *The Religious Communities of the Church of England* (London: Faith Press, 1918), 20–23. GLRO HI/ST/SJ/Y 12/8: Frederick Cartwright, *The Story of Community of the Nursing Sisters of Saint John the Divine* (London: Faith Press, 1968). Cook, I:102–3. Jameson, 60–62. Sir Shane Leslie, *The Oxford Movement: 1833–1933* (London: Burns, Oates and Washbourne, Ltd., 1933), X–XIV, 4–12.

6. See Allchin, *The Silent Rebellion,* Cameron, *The Religious Communities,* and Jameson, *The Sisters of Charity* for detailed information on sisterhoods and deaconesses in England.

7. Zacharay Cope, *A Hundred Years of Nursing at Saint Mary's Hospital* (Paddington: Wm. Heinemann Medical Books, Ltd., 1955), 10–11, 132–46. Moore, 11–34. London, England, B. L. Saint John's House, *Tracts 1855–76 London III*, 2–13, St. John Council Records, GLRO HI/ST/SJ/Y12/8, 3.

8. Nightingale Collection BL ADD MSS 47,777 f47. GLRO HI/ST/SJ/Y10, 23.

9. London, England, B. L. *Rules in Tracts*, 11. GLRO HI/ST/SJ/Y10, 23.

10. Monica E. Baly, *Florence Nightingale and the Nursing Legacy* (London: Croom Helm, 1986), 30–39. Cook, 1:446–66. Smith, 157–58.

11. Florence Nightingale to Mary Jones, 2 February 1865, GLRO HI/ST/NCVI/64/4.

12. Smith, 155–78. Smith portrays Nightingale as a woman unable to sustain relationships with others, including Mary Jones, but the correspondence continued for many years in spite of disagreements.

13. Florence Nightingale to Mary Jones, 1865, GLRO HI/ST/NCI/65/3. Occasionally the Nightingale–Jones letters appear to be written hurriedly, making punctuation and some phrases difficult to discern.

14. Mary Jones to Florence Nightingale, 31 May 1866, Nightingale Collection BL ADD MSS 47,744 f90–ff91.

15. Nightingale Collection BL ADD MSS 45,794 f206.

16. Florence Nightingale to Sir John McNeill, GLRO HI/ST/NC/SU157.

17. Florence Nightingale to Henry Bonham Carter, 16 December 1866, GLRO. (See also Florence Nightingale to Mary Jones, 20 December 1866, GLRO HI/ST/NCI/66/25, about sisterhoods in the Church of England.)

18. Florence Nightingale to Sir Harry Verney, 15 February 1867, Nightingale Collection BL ADD MSS 45,791 f69.

19. The Protestant deaconess institution where Nightingale spent three months training.

20. GLRO HI/ST/SJ Index Book, 1–2.

21. Cameron, 20–23. The physicians from King's College Hospital wanted to improve the nursing care at the hospital and sought help from the bishop of London to form a nursing sisterhood.

22. Peter F. Anson, *The Call of the Cloister: Religious Communities and Kindred Bodies in the Anglican Communion* (London: S.P.C.K., 1955), 280.

23. GLRO HI/ST/SJ/H 1–2, and London, England B. L. *Rules of St. John's House*, 2.

24. Florence Nightingale to Mary Jones, August or September 1867, Nightingale Collection BL ADD MSS 47,744 f136.

25. Florence Nightingale to Mary Jones, 7 December 1867, GLRO HI/ST/NCI/67/8e.

26. Thus a pattern of interaction began between the St. John's House Council and the sisters. In the 1870s, a superior came into disagreement with the council and was bodily removed from King's College Hospital. Yet another conflict arose in 1883, at which time all the sisters, as well as many of the nurses, left the sisterhood and formed their own order as the Community of Nursing Sisters of St. John's. The original St. John's House continued without vows through several reorganizations until 1932, when vows were permitted. See Moore, *A Zeal for Responsibility,* Cartwright, *The Story of Community,* and St. John's Council Records for History of St. John's House.

27. Mary Jones to Florence Nightingale, 14 June 1867, Nightingale Collection BL ADD MSS 47,744 f121–ff121.

28. Mary Jones to Florence Nightingale, 18 June 1867, Nightingale Collection BL ADD MSS 47,744 f125.

29. For differing viewpoints on the puerperal sepsis outbreak see both Monica Baly, *Nursing and Social Change*, 2nd ed. (1973; reprint, London: Wm. Heinemann Medical Books, Ltd., 1980), 21–26, and Smith, 159–64.

30. Florence Nightingale to Mary Jones, 9 February 1872, GLRO HI/ST/NCI/72/2.

31. Mary Jones to Florence Nightingale, incomplete and no date, Nightingale Collection BL ADD MSS 47,744 f223.

32. Nightingale Collection BL ADD MSS 47,743 f37 to ff38.

33. Copy of printed letter, January 1861, Nightingale Collection BL ADD MSS 47,743 f57.

34. Mary Jones to Florence Nightingale, 9 May 1861, Nightingale Collection BL ADD MSS 47,743 f88–ff88.

35. Mary Jones to Florence Nightingale, 5 March 1864, Nightingale Collection BL ADD MSS 47,744 ff24.

36. Mary Jones to Florence Nightingale, 6 December 1865, Nightingale Collection BL ADD MSS 47,744.

37. Mary Jones to Florence Nightingale, 25 April 1867, Nightingale Collection BL ADD MSS 47,794 f115.

38. Florence Nightingale to Mary Jones, 19 October 1868, GLRO HI/ST/NCI/68/12.

39. Florence Nightingale to Parthenope Nightingale Verney, 3 June 1887, Nightingale Collection BL ADD MSS 52,427 f73.

40. JoAnn G. Widerquist, "Dearest Rev'd Mother," in *Florence Nightingale and Her Era*, ed. Vern Bullough, Bonnie Bullough, and Marietta Stanton (New York and London: Garland Press, 1990), 288–308.

41. Religious essay (no date), Nightingale Collection BL ADD MSS 45,843 f58.

42. The complexity of her personality and spiritual beliefs sometimes caused Nightingale severe problems when her means to achieve an end conflicted with her ideals. See JoAnn G. Widerquist, "Spirituality of Florence Nightingale," *Nursing Research* 41:1:49–55.

43. Their similar conceptions of an organizational hierarchy for nursing, involving a head or matron, better educated sisters, nurses, and probationers, deserves study. The structure for nursing that they espoused may have contributed to the different levels of present day nursing education and entry into practice issues.

44. Jameson, 61. This work describes succinctly the need for work for the "feminine element" in English society.

Old Nurses and New

Nursing in the London Teaching Hospitals Before and After the Mid-Nineteenth-Century Reforms

CAROL HELMSTADTER
Ontario Nurses' Association
Toronto, Canada

Introduction

The modern "trained nurse" emerged in the second half of the nineteenth century in the twelve London teaching hospitals.[1] Also called the "efficient nurse" or the "Nightingale nurse," this rigidly disciplined, unquestioning nurse became the standard throughout the English-speaking world for a hundred years. She personified a new professional model that has attracted much criticism and raised many questions in recent nursing history scholarship.

The rise of clinical medicine at the end of the eighteenth century made a more professional nurse necessary. A new, empirical medicine, based on teaching and research in hospitals, was replacing the old academic medicine, which was based on classical Greek and Latin texts. The new medicine placed increasingly heavy strains on hospital nursing systems. The old hospitals had been essentially social service agencies for the indigent, the lame, and the sick poor. As doctors gained more influence with hospital administrations, they began admitting patients increasingly for medical rather than social or economic reasons.[2] These much sicker patients required more intelligent and responsible nursing care than the great majority of old nurses could give. Doctors began demanding better nurses.

At the same time that doctors wanted better qualified nurses, the larger nursing staff that the new clinical medicine required forced hospital administrators to look for ways to train a more efficient nurse. The new nurse who emerged at the end of the nineteenth century was as much a product of the hospitals' need for the cheapest form of nursing work force as she was a product of the need for a higher standard of patient care. Christopher Maggs points out that the new trained nurse became subservient, dependent, and exploited. The formal training program contained a hierarchy of

Nursing History Review 1 (1993): 43–70.

duties and justified even the most menial duties such as sweeping, dusting, and polishing in the wards as an extension of the discipline and an essential part of the "art and science of nursing."

Discipline and supervision were all-pervasive in the new training schools, extending into the nurses' private lives in the nurses' home in their off-duty hours. The secret of good ward management was order and punctuality. The efficient nurse was always able to keep up with the clock.[3] A highly popular nursing manual of 1886 asserted, "The importance of getting work done up to time is quickly impressed on all newcomers, and there must be some defect in the way the work is arranged if all that is necessary is not accomplished in the allotted hours." Unquestioning obedience to orders and the denial of self were two of the new nurse's most fundamental claims to being called a trained nurse.[4] The atmosphere of obedience and conformity in which the Nightingale nurses were reared served to make the nurses themselves the greatest obstacle to change.[5]

In order to understand why the nursing reformers chose this harsh, repressive, paramilitary organization that crushed innovation and prevented the development of a true profession, we need to look at the structure of the old hospital and the society in which it functioned. When one sees the magnitude of the problems that the nursing reformers were trying to resolve, it is easier to comprehend why they chose the system of nurses' training with which we are all so familiar. They had to fashion an efficient but low paid nurse out of an ill educated and undisciplined work force. This nurse had to be able to function in the new world of scientific medicine, and she had to meet the new demands of Victorian respectability as well as the stricter, more orderly, time-oriented discipline of an industrialized society. Even more important, she had to be able to meet all these conditions in what was essentially an unpredictable environment, namely, a hospital ward of acutely ill, unstable patients.

The Inner World of the Nineteenth-Century Hospital

The eighteenth- and early nineteenth-century nurses served a very different patient population in a very different institution from the later nineteenth-century teaching hospital. In many ways these older hospitals were self-contained, almost self-sufficient institutions. The larger hospitals brewed their own beer, baked their own bread, and maintained an extensive staff. When Guy's Hospital pulled down one of their warehouses to build a new set of wards for one hundred patients in 1850, they unhoused a carpenter, a painter, a brewer, a bricklayer, a labourer, and seven sutlers, as well as a number of the standard hospital staff that we would expect today—nurses, porters, and so forth.[6] The staff was organized in much the same way as the staff of the larger landed estates, with a steward in charge of the male servants and patients and a matron or housekeeper in charge of the female servants and patients. The nurses, sisters,* and matron needed no nursing experience when they took up their jobs. They were simply the servants of the hospital, or of the house as we still often call it.[7]

Paternalism was the characteristic nature of the master-servant relationship in the nineteenth century with the employer, or lady of the house in the case of the female servants, exercising extensive moral and legal authority over the servants.[8] The matron, writes Benjamin Golding, a young St. Thomas's doctor, in 1819, "is the superior female of the establishment; she superintends those departments which could not be so well regulated by a person of the other sex. To her belongs the direction of all the female domestics. . . . She presides over their morals and good behavior, and sees that they execute the several duties of their stations with propriety."[9] Golding might more accurately have said that the matron attempted to establish good behavior and propriety among her staff. Above the matron, steward, and other hospital officers was the Board of Governors, which usually lumped the various members of the staff and the patients together as moral minors. Like the matron, the board members tried to enforce some kind of discipline within the hospital, also without notable success. The doctors and nurses fitted into the social structure of the hospitals as servants. "Doctors and nurses in our hospitals where the old system of nursing prevails are much in the position, with regard to each other, of head and underservants in a large household," a lady nurse wrote in 1880.[10]

The Patients

The Standing Orders of 1752 at St. Thomas's Hospital illustrate some of the problems the governors faced, as well as their major thrust to establish a more God-fearing community.

*The English use of the term "sister" to denote what North Americans call "head nurse" or "nursing unit manager" can be extremely confusing when one is also talking about Sisters of religious communities. It is all the more confusing because many of the religious Sisters were sisters in the nursing unit manager sense. I have used the lower case when referring to the nursing unit manager and upper case when referring to Sisters who belonged to Sisterhoods.

> Item, That the Patients shall not Swear or take God's Name in vain, nor revile nor miscall one another, nor strike nor beat one another, nor steal Meat or Drink, Apparel, or other thing, one from the other; nor abuse themselves by inordinate Drinking, nor incontinent Living, nor talk nor act Immodestly, upon pain of Expulsion; and that when they go to or return from their Meals and Beds, they crave God's Blessing, and return Thanks to God.

Patients were not to stay out later than 7 P.M. in the winter and 8 P.M. in the summer and were not to leave the hospital grounds on any account without the permission of the sister, matron, or steward; nor were they to smoke, play dice, or bring liquor into the house.[11]

Drink was the major problem of the patients, and hence it was a major responsibility of the hospital porters to see that patients did not go out or come back through the gates without passes from the matron or the steward. The porters marked the ticket and kept it until the patient returned. According to Dr. Golding,

> This obstruction to the natural disposition of the patients, who seize every opportunity to purchase strong drinks, is highly beneficial, because disregard to this particular, would be conniving at every kind of intemperance; and we know that one act of excess frequently renders abortive the skilful treatment of the medical officers for many months.
>
> Notwithstanding the utmost attention of the porters, we find the contiguity of several pot-houses to St. Thomas's affords the means of introducing spirits into the hospital, and the temptation too great to be resisted.[12]

Even so, the patients sometimes obtained leave of absence on false pretences, and "entered into those excesses from which it is so difficult for the lower classes to be weaned." On the annual visiting day of the governors in July, all patients were given leave of absence for the day, on which occasion many patients undid all the good medical treatment that they had received by heavy drinking.[13]

As late as the 1870s at St. Bartholomew's, the Standing Orders were essentially the same as those at St. Thomas's in 1752, except it was no longer necessary to enjoin the patients not to physically assault each other.[14] Despite this small improvement, however, maintenance of order in the wards proved difficult. For example, in 1857, University College Hospital had to extend the hours of the outpatient waiting room porter so that he could keep order there.[15] In November 1868, the treasurer at Guy's Hospital dismissed the sister of Samaritan Ward because she was unable to "exercise sufficient control over the patients within the ward."[16]

The Nurses

It was not only the patients who were disorderly. At St. Bartholomew's in 1771, Matron Susannah Robinson requested more help and a salary increase because of the expanded work that was being done in the hospital. She had upward of one hundred full-time sisters, nurses, watches (night nurses), and helpers under her direction. "The happiness and quiet of the patients," she said,

> depends upon the qualifications and dispositions of the Persons employed to attend them, that enquiring after their Characters, interposing in the several Disputes and Squabbles between the Sisters Nurses, Helpers and Patients, and removing the Sisters and Nurses into different Wards as their Tempers and Capacities best suit, takes up a great deal of the Matron's time.[17]

Indeed, the quarrels and disturbances in the wards with which the matron contended were numerous. In July 1771, a month after the matron's request for more help, Sister Dorcas Steward had to be discharged for drunkenness and misbehavior to her patients. A week later Sisters Hannah Seabrooke and Elizabeth Gray were reprimanded for misbehavior and creating disturbances in their wards at irregular hours.[18] The following January, nurse Elizabeth Starling was discharged both as a patient and a nurse. She had been admitted as a patient for a fever that turned out to be the Foul Disease, a common name for venereal disease.[19] In March of 1773, nurse Mary Ellison was discharged for misbehavior and Sister Susannah Careless was discharged for drunkenness, misbehavior, and neglect of duty.[20] In March 1775 Sister Hester Hill was discharged for selling "gin, etc." to the patients and giving away hospital provisions.[21]

This number of offenders is not a large proportion of the more than one hundred women for whom Robinson was responsible. One might therefore assume that the nurses did fairly well in terms of performing their duties. It seems much more likely, however, that these misdemeanors were the tip of the iceberg. For example, one hundred years later when general standards of behavior were much higher, the house physician reported that the sister of Hope Ward was drunk one evening. She appeared before the House Committee and did not deny the charge. The committee severely reprimanded her but did not discharge her because she had twenty years' service and had hitherto borne good character. Six months later, however, the committee did fire her after the husband of a patient who had died in her ward complained that his wife had been unkindly treated and that the

Sister was drunk more than once. The steward reported that when he had gone to see her the preceding Monday she had not been sober, all of which suggests that the House Committee had been simply unaware of her drinking habit in the preceding twenty years.[22]

Drinking was generally considered the outstanding problem of the old nurses as it was of the patients. Mary Stanley, who interviewed the nurses accompanying Florence Nightingale to the Crimea, and who later led a team of nurses to the East herself, commented, "They say they need the support of spirits under their harassing work." She believed that often the most skilled and able nurses were the worst in character.[23] In the 1870s it was still standard, even in the so-called reformed hospitals, for the sister to get the surgeon to order the nurse a glass of wine before she had to do an exceptionally unpleasant dressing, and the nurses often took beer "for comfort" before going on night duty.[24]

Hospital authorities took in stride the uncouth and sometimes unlawful behavior of the old nurses. For example, in March 1873 Sister Faith refused to allow the chimney sweeper to sweep her chimney and was defiant and rude to the steward about it. She had to appear before the committee and publicly apologize to him, after which the chairman expressed his displeasure about the way in which she had behaved.[25] The committee admonished a delinquent once; if the offense was repeated, it did so a second time more severely; and finally if there was a third offense, the individual was fired.[26]

Stealing or selling hospital property and provisions remained a standard problem throughout the nineteenth century. In May 1850 the Hospital Committee at University College Hospital reported that a night nurse who had been discharged for insobriety had taken hospital sheets and pawned them while in the hospital employ. She had been apprehended for theft elsewhere. In July 1854 night nurse Turner had to be discharged for stealing hospital sheets and other articles as well as selling morphine to the patients.[27] Indeed, whenever anything was missing the nurses were the first to be suspected. In May 1857 the resident medical officer reported the theft of the assistant medical officer's clothes; he believed the night nurses were responsible.[28]

Exceeding their leaves of absence was another characteristic failing of the old nurses.[29] Disrespectful and truculent behavior was also typical.[30] By the 1860s the reformation of manners and the insistence on a regular schedule, important characteristics of Victorian culture, were slowly beginning to penetrate into the hospital world. The new rules and regulations for the sisters at Charing Cross Hospital in 1865 specified obedience and respect toward the medical officers as well as toward the Board of Governors. The sisters were to offer kind and ready attention to the patients, administer medicines carefully, and maintain regular rest and meal hours. They were to behave with "gentleness and humanity" to both their nurses and patients, avoiding harshness of manner and language. If reproof was necessary, it was to be done with mildness, devoid of altercation and upbraiding.[31] Yet despite these new regulations, the sisters continued their disrespectful and unladylike behavior.[32] There were constant complaints from the doctors of not only poor discipline in the wards but of nursing incompetence. In fact, one of the duties of the resident medical officer was to report on the condition of the wards and the conduct of the sisters and nurses.[33] Expecting tips, or what were known as "vails," from guests to the house was a perquisite of the servant class in great houses, and one that administrators desperately tried to eliminate in the hospitals.[34]

The Medical Students and Staff

The less than decorous behavior of the nurses was hardly worse, however, than that of the medical students and doctors. Sir Henry Wentworth Acland, who came from a distinguished Devon family and later became Regius Professor of Medicine at Oxford, entered St. George's Hospital in 1840 immediately after finishing Oxford. The behavior of both the medical students and their instructors appalled him. He wrote that his heart well-nigh failed him in his new surroundings. "Everything wears the air of low men," he wrote a few days after arriving at the hospital.

> of low habits, such as I have never hitherto come in contact with. In consequence of my being treated uncivilly by my bookseller in Greenhill's presence, he (G.) made the pregnant remark: "You must be prepared for that wherever you are known to be a medical student."[35]

He told his mother that "low-bred" was too good a word by half for the medical students for they had no breeding at all, and he wrote in his diary:

> I am greatly horrified by the want of order and plans—the want of control and authority exercised among us students. The teachers truckle to us, joke; especially the evening lecturer, he will make any allusion or talk any folly to amuse the men.[36]

He found the comparison with Oxford, where he had associated with men "who from their age, piety and learning," were his superiors, very unfavorable.[37]

The want of order was quite striking. "As for the conduct of the medical students during operations," one of the *Lancet*'s writers exclaimed,

> keep me from witnessing such scenes. Who could fancy so much—we should not say inhumanity, but grown-up childishness, to exist among any class of persons. Whatever their behaviour over the carcasses of the dead might be they ought to have considered some for the living. To be sure they were awed to silence and decorum by the presence of the operators, but previous to their appearance such hideous yells were uttered as to make the rafters ring, and the poor patient.[38]

In 1837 a fight broke out among the students in the men's operating room at St. Thomas's. Mr. South, the senior surgeon, was unable to stop the brawl and had to call in the police to restore order. Nine Guy's students were arrested.[39]

This "moral disorder," as contemporaries called it, extended into the sexual realm as well. "What is the character of the young medical students in hospital wards?" Catherine Cappe, a lady visitor to Yorkshire hospitals, asked in 1816.

> Is it likely that they will all be remarkable for their good conduct, propriety and Christian morality, not seducing others or liable to be seduced themselves by licentious conversation, by the improper demeanour of a selfish unprincipled nurse, or by the opportunities sometimes unavoidably afforded in the course of their medical attendance.[40]

Florence Nightingale shared Cappe's apprehensions. In the 1840s Nightingale thought the only way women could work in a hospital without the surgeons trying to make love to them was by belonging to a religious order.[41] Again, one could give many illustrations of these difficulties. The treasurer at Guy's reported in 1880 that "familiar intercourse with, and admission of students into the Sister's private room, were matters of common occurrence." Two sisters had found husbands in that manner in the course of a year or eighteen months.[42] The fact that the sister lived in a small room adjoining the ward meant that such behavior was quite public.

The medical students could also be quite uncouth. Not only did the matron preside over the morals and good propriety of her own staff, as Golding had written, but she had to preside physically at the meals of the medical staff so that she could exercise a civilizing influence on them. Throughout the century there were constant problems with this policy. For example, at University College Hospital the "rude and unreasonably dissatisfied conduct" of the medical officers was a constant thorn in the matron's side.[43] In 1858 Sarah Robottom, who was then matron, tendered her resignation, giving Rule 136, the duty of having to preside at the dinner of the resident medical officers, as the principal reason.[44] She had appeared before the committee the preceding year asking for their support in dealing with the misbehavior of one house surgeon in particular, Tilbury Fox. The matter had been reported to the secretary and the dean of the Faculty of Medicine and both Fox and the matron had been interviewed by the dean.[45] Robottom had been a very successful matron: she had been matron of the Bermondsey Workhouse before coming to University College Hospital in 1853, and she was certainly not inexperienced as far as rude behavior was concerned.[46] The committee excused her from presiding at the table for six months while they made enquiries; they did persuade her to stay on.[47]

The Pervasiveness of These Problems in Contemporary Society

These problems were not unique to the hospital world. Drinking was a major problem among both sexes, and not only among the working classes, as Golding had pointed out, but in all social classes. Throughout the century, but particularly in the first half, drinking water was unsafe, especially in the cities. In the 1840s the public health inspectors were ridiculed for suggesting that city water could ever be safe to drink. Hospitals therefore provided alcoholic drinks for the patients and the staff because they were safer than water. Alcohol was also considered to be strengthening and to provide physical stamina. Not until the 1870s did the medical profession begin to effectively challenge the use of alcohol as a restorative, at about the same time that the major temperance movement began to take hold.[48]

Another major problem with these rather hard-drinking nurses was that they were extremely unreliable about getting to work at all, much less on time. As with the drinking, this problem was not unique to nurses. Regular attendance at work and the maintenance of an orderly workplace were central problems in the nineteenth-century work forces. For example, William Brown, a flax mill owner in Dundee at the beginning of the century, explained that the mill was a ticklish concern and "extremely liable to fall into disorder." He inspected all aspects of his mill every day, but only occasionally did he look into the number of workmen employed, their attendance, wages, and so forth.

Josiah Wedgwood's greatest problem in his china factories was the irregular attendance of his workers. In the first half of the century, cotton spinners frequently did not appear at the factories on Mondays and Tuesdays. In the South Wales mining and ironworks of the 1840s, the week after the workers received their monthly pay was usually completely lost. In one boot and shoe industry in Northampton, workers wandered in and out of the factory at will, and only became reconciled to regular attendance when their employers locked them out. The majority of the work force observed St. Monday.[49] Even at the end of the century, factory girls earning less than eleven shillings a week usually did so because they chose not to work one or two days a week.[50]

At the end of the century, in 1890, ten years after she had begun her iron rule at the London Hospital and despite her vastly improved record keeping, the formidable reforming matron Eva C. Lückes did not know how many nurses she had in the hospital.[51] The scheduled number of nurses often did not appear for work in the morning. In her manual for hospital sisters, Lückes suggested keeping the night nurses on duty for several more hours as a solution to this problem.[52]

This cavalier approach to work obtained not only in industry but throughout society. In 1870 only 68 percent of the children regularly attended those schools that the school inspectors visited.[53] The elementary teacher's most basic problem was getting the children to attend regularly, and elementary schools had a very high turnover in pupils as well. Punctuality presented yet another problem. As late as the 1870s, the teachers were often as unpunctual as the children.[54]

The Nature of Mid-Nineteenth-Century Nursing Reform

Nurses' Training and Moral Force

"The mid-nineteenth century hospital was a lower class institution in many ways," Charles E. Rosenberg writes, "organized in theory according to the moral assumptions of its lay trustees and administrators, but dominated in reality by values and behavior antithetical to those Nightingale saw as the only appropriate basis for a moral society."[55] All the nineteenth-century nursing reformers shared Nightingale's view of the unsuitability of the lower class morals and behavior of hospital nurses. Hence moral as well as technical training became the basis for the development of the new nurse.

In 1856 the Sisters of St. John's House, an Anglican lay sisterhood devoted entirely to nursing, took over the whole of the nursing and domestic services at King's College Hospital on a contract basis. The Sisters were ladies who trained in the hospital as nurses and worked without pay. These Sisters in turn trained working-class women, who were salaried, in the "moral and technical aspects of nursing." The technical aspects of nursing consisted of an apprenticeship training in the hospital. Doctors instructed the nurses in the new medical therapeutics while the upper-class Sisters provided the moral training. The doctors frequently called the moral training the "elevation of the character" of the nurse. St. John's House also provided the nurses with far better living and working conditions than those enjoyed by other nurses in London.[56]

The Sisters's system of hospital nursing was a novel practice in mid-nineteenth century England. There had never existed a formal system of apprenticeship for nurses, nor had ladies, in the sense of non-working-class women, worked as hospital nurses, paid or unpaid, in Protestant England. But the moral discipline and training that they sought to instill in the probationers was anything but a novel concept: it was one of the overarching concerns of the Victorian age. In discussing what the Victorians meant by moral training, I shall rely heavily on the intellectual framework established by Martin Wiener's *Reconstructing the Criminal: Culture, Law and Policy in England, 1830–1914*. Wiener's analysis illuminates the way Victorians viewed the disorderly, highly disreputable, and unrestrained working-class culture that flourished in the hospitals and helps to explain what the nursing reformers were trying to do with their moral training.

"For early Victorians," Wiener writes, "the need to build popular character permeated virtually every field of understanding of human nature, society and public policymaking."[57] Victorians saw the central problem of their time as a lack of moral restraint. This lack of control became the focus for middle- and upper-class fears of working-class insubordination and potential for riot and revolution. The moral disorder had particular application to women, for the growth of women's waged labor gave women a somewhat wider freedom of action that threatened patriarchal authority in all classes. Generational differences also formed part of the gender concerns. The increased birthrate in the eighteenth century produced a declining average age while the growth of industry and the market economy undermined the old social controls of apprenticeship and other forms of prolonged youth dependence. Early Victorians thought young people were especially given to uncontrolled passions, and they believed that unregulated female sexuality was an important cause of what they perceived to be an increase in illegitimacy and prostitution. These problems were major preoccupations of the age and were often attributed to the intermingling of the sexes in factories and other workplaces.[58] This was, of course, particularly applicable to nurses who worked not only with male patients but with porters, medical students, and house doctors.

Victorians characteristically identified moral restraint or discipline with civilization, while they considered giving rein to instincts or impulse savagery or barbarism. They recognized that these instincts were a natural part of all men and women, but they believed that the middle classes, in particular, had developed the moral powers and will to restrain them. The lower classes, on the other hand, were thought to have little or no moral discipline and were frequently described as brutal and as a "race apart." Their uncontrolled instincts and passions made them similar to the primitive peoples in the British Empire. Much of early Victorian social policy can be interpreted as a series of efforts to contain and master the unregulated passions and instincts of the lower classes.[59] "Nearly every respectable attribute of humanity is the result, not of instinct, but of victory over instinct," John Stuart Mill wrote in the 1850s.

The Victorian use of the term "moral" had a distinct meaning, somewhat different from its twentieth century association with right and wrong or ethical considerations. Changes in the field of psychiatry perhaps best illustrate this meaning. The concept of madness shifted from the eighteenth-century construct as a lack or a loss of reason that reduced the lunatic to a bestial state; in the nineteenth century, madness became a lack of self-control. A new moral treatment for lunatics was thus instituted. The new psychiatric nosology contained a diagnosis of "moral insanity" in which the restraints of religious feeling, prudence, and self-esteem were weakened by mental disease.[60] A benchmark law case, *Frere v. Peacock*, defined moral insanity as not involving delusions but as affecting "only the feelings and affections, or what are termed the moral powers of the mind, in contradistinction to the powers of the understanding or intellect."[61] Loss of control over feelings and affections caused individuals afflicted with moral insanity to become excitable, violent, and extravagant.[62]

Victorians frequently spoke of the working and the upper classes as the "two nations" that never intermingled or spoke with each other. Disraeli, the future prime minister, identified them as the rich and the poor in his novel *Sybil* (1845).[63] In 1851 Henry Mayhew defined them in *London Labour and the London Poor* as the wanderers and the settlers: the wanderers moved from place to place preying on the earnings of the settlers, who were the more industrious and prosperous portions of the community. The wanderers suffered from underdevelopment of the moral powers of the mind and were distinguished "for their use of slang language—for their lax ideas of property—for their general improvidence—their repugnance to continuous labour—their disregard of female honour—their pugnacity—and their utter want of religion."[64]

Mayhew's description of the wanderers details precisely the characteristics of the working-class nurses that the Sisters of St. John's House addressed with their moral training. Apprenticeship would bind the nurses to their jobs while the moral training would elevate and refine their characters. The Sisters believed such training could only be carried out by "Christian women of a higher grade whose example and influence should form the most essential elements in the success of the scheme."[65] In addition, if the wealthy classes practiced nursing themselves, they would give dignity to the profession of nursing. They would teach the nurses to respect themselves and make them respected by others.[66]

In no area did the teaching of moral restraint and character building or elevation have more importance than in the elementary education designed for the working classes. Elementary schoolteachers prepared their working-class students for an apprenticeship in the honest trades and taught them to cheerfully accept the station in life to which God had assigned them. The teachers approached their pupils in the same way as the missionaries approached the heathen in the empire—they wished to civilize them by teaching them Christian morality. The ultimate aim of what became a state-subsidized education was the preservation of social order. In England, the teachers aimed at increasing church attendance, decreasing crime, preventing strikes and riots, and implanting the virtues of self-help, thrift, sobriety, and cleanliness in their pupils. Above all, the poor were to learn the importance of submission to established authorities.[67]

The new trained nurse received this type of education. First, her social and moral character was elevated, and, second, she received technical training, or the standard apprenticeship type of education that had now become necessary with the increasing sophistication of nursing care.[68] Florence Nightingale's "Monthly State of Personal Character and Acquirements of the Nurse" perfectly illustrates this method of education. This monthly evaluation system for the probationers first lists three desirable characteristics, namely, sobriety, honesty (especially as to taking petty bribes from the patients), and truthfulness, stating, "No degree admissible; the first dereliction ensures her dismissal." The five qualities of punctuality, quietness, trustworthiness, personal neatness and cleanliness, and ward management or order are described next. Finally, the technical accomplishments such as applying dressings, applying leeches, bandaging, making beds, waiting on operations, keeping the ward fresh, keeping utensils clean, and so forth are listed.[69]

The overriding concern with the moral and social character of the pupil or the worker, with inculcating obedience, and with controlling the total environment was characteristic not only of elementary education but also of employers toward the nineteenth-century work force in general. It was much more practical than it appears to twentieth-century observers.[70] These moral qualities were all characteristics of the reliable, highly productive, and respectable worker who did not pose any threat of insubordination. Contemporary feminists place the origin of this definition of the ideal nurse in the "woman's sphere" construct of the ideal woman as highly moral, submissive, and secondary to her husband.[71] The moral qualities that nursing reformers sought in the nurse were, however, sought indiscriminately among workers of both sexes throughout the century.

Administrative Reorganization

Nurses' training was the first approach to creating a more efficient nurse; administrative reorganization was the second. Increasing patient acuity in the early nineteenth-century hospitals shifted the lines of authority in the nursing services and forced them to expand. In this process, the sister (in the sense of nurse manager), appropriated a large share of the matron's authority for she became responsible to the doctor of her ward for the nursing care. She was hired and could be fired only by the administrators, and by reporting to the administrators and doctor she became quite independent of the matron. This system, with the sister having dual accountability, was known as the "old system" or "ward system" of nursing.[72]

The matron hired and dismissed the ordinary nurses and was in charge of the linen and housekeeping, but she was no longer able to move the sisters and nurses from one ward to another as Robinson had done at St. Bartholomew's in the 1770s. She visited the women's wards daily, but her visit was only to ensure that the wards were clean and in order.[73] She did not generally have systematic communication with her staff nor did she consider it her duty to train them.[74] The sister was responsible for the nursing. Parts of this system, in which the matron had to ask the sister's permission to enter the ward when she made her daily rounds, lasted well into the twentieth century.[75] It was a highly decentralized and inefficient system.

Mass production and division of labor represent the essence of the Industrial Revolution. Contemporaries, however, considered the cleanliness, order, discipline, strong sense of economy, and the new industrial worker's strict adherence to a time schedule to be an even greater achievement of the successful industrialist.[76] The ward system of nursing did not provide the matron with the authority she needed to enforce this new kind of order and economy. Doctors and administrators complained that the patients had no fixed schedule and that the matron was unable to enforce the hospital regulations.[77]

The Sisters of St. John's House solved this problem by making the matron a powerful manager, whom they called the lady superintendent. Probationers, nurses, and Sisters all reported directly to her. She was able to give orders directly to the nurses without passing them through the sister; doctors and administrators could not interfere in this hierarchical chain of command.[78] Under the ward system, the nurses were permanently attached to one ward, but under the Sisters' new centralized system, they were rotated from ward to ward throughout the hospital, breaking the power of the old sister and the medical officer over the nursing staff in the individual wards. The Sisters also introduced a division of labor whereby charwomen and porters did the heavier work so that the nurses could become more specialized and spend more time on patient care.[79]

Introducing strict adherence to a time schedule posed a particularly difficult problem in the hospital setting. In domestic and village settings, time was organized by artisans or farmers who were in control of their own working lives; the rhythm of work tended to alternate between periods of intense labor and periods of more relaxed work or even idleness. The day lengthened or shortened according to what needed to be done, or conversely, what could be done given the weather conditions, the availability of materials, and so forth. In the nineteenth century, this situation was compounded by the fact that few of the workers could afford clocks or watches.[80]

Upper-class ladies such as the Sisters of St. John's House, however, were accustomed to dealing with servants who shared this older, agrarian view of time. Domestic service was a major channel for migration from the country to the city in the earlier nineteenth century, and most recruits to domestic service were no more acclimated to the highly organized life-style of the middle classes than hospital nurses were. The numerous domestic economy manuals that began appearing in the 1820s compared the housewife to the new managers whom the industrialists were introducing in their factories and shops. There was a marked similarity: these ladies directed large staffs of domestics with highly complicated divisions of labor, exercising the same kind of control and all-pervasive discipline over them. The manuals are filled with time schedules and stress orderliness, efficiency, and the necessity of closely superintending the work of the servants. As much as a third of the typical manual dealt with the use of time.[81] It was therefore not surprising that the new lady superintendents emphasized the importance of routine and punctuality. Indeed, punctuality was the first virtue on Florence Nightingale's character list.

In the industrial economy, workers were no longer self-employed. Like the domestic servants and the nurses, they were employees who were paid for their hours of work. As one might expect, it became very important to the employer that the time for which he was paying should be used efficiently.[82] Lushington, the administrator at Guy's Hospital, complained that the principles of good management and economy and the proper degree of subordination to higher authorities did not obtain when he started at Guy's in 1876. Discipline was lax and money was not always well spent.[83] The sisters had no fixed hours of work. "They came into the wards when they pleased, and practically they went out when they pleased, so long as they were there when the surgeons and medical staff went round," Lushington explained.[84] The Standing Orders established regular hours of work for the nurses—from 7 A.M. until 10 P.M.—but no one enforced them.[85]

It was difficult to implement a factory type of scheduling for nurses because their work environment was essentially unpredictable. Unlike the factory workers who worked with programmable machinery, nurses worked with critically ill, unstable patients. Nurses had to be prepared to deal with the unexpected, as a nursing manual of the 1880s put it.[86] Nevertheless, the Sisters of St. John's House used the household economy manual strategies of close superintendence and a time schedule. They developed a ward routine, insisting that certain things be done by a certain time. Their probationers spoke of the "order and punctuality pervading all the arrangements of St. John's, the thoroughness of the nursing in each individual case, and the refinement and perfect neatness to be traced throughout the Wards."[87]

Living In

The system of living in proved a third form of attack on the problem of acculturating the nurses to the new hospital. Control of the total environment was only possible if the nurses were in the hospital twenty-four hours a day where they could be constantly superintended. The Sisterhoods provided better food at regular hours in a common dining room and better sleeping accommodation in dormitories.[88] Other hospitals built nurses' homes.[89] These new arrangements gave the nurses safer and far more comfortable living quarters than their former quarters in tiny rooms off the wards or in the attics and cellars of the hospital.[90] Again, this was part of a larger phenomenon and reflected the Victorian move toward regularity, order, decency, propriety, and the segregation of the sexes. The Victorians built large servants' wings so they could move the domestic servants out of the attics and basements where they had been lodged previously.[91] Lückes considered housing one of the keys to a proper nursing service, both in terms of discipline and recruitment. The nurses were lodged in six different places in the hospital, she said in 1883, which was inconvenient both for the nurses and for the maintenance of order and discipline.[92]

From at least the eighteenth century on, hospital administrators had tried to insist that the nurses live in the hospital primarily so that they could be searched for and gotten out of bed when they didn't appear for work on time.[93] However, not until the advent of the new centralized system of nursing with its powerful lady superintendents did it become possible to enforce these rules.

The Spread of Nursing Reform to Other Hospitals

The immense success of St. John's House in improving the standard of nursing care was immediately apparent, and some, if not all, of their principles quickly spread to the other teaching hospitals. By 1866 three of the twelve hospitals were nursed by Sisterhoods, King's College and Charing Cross Hospitals by St. John's House, and University College Hospital by the All Saints Sisterhood. The Royal Free Hospital contracted its nursing out to a secular organization, the British Nursing Association, which was run by an unpaid lady superintendent.[94]

The reforms that Florence Nightingale introduced at St. Thomas Hospital were somewhat different. She did not approve of "lady" nurses as such, much preferring the experienced hospital nurses. Roberts, the retired surgical Sister who accompanied her to the Crimea, was her ideal. Roberts had been a Sister for twenty-three years at St. Thomas's and as a result, Nightingale wrote,

> her qualifications as a *nurse* were infinitely superior to any other of those with me. . . . Her total superiority to all the vices of a hospital nurse, her faithfulness to the work, her disinterested love of duty and vigilant care of her patients, her

> power of work equal to that of *ten*, have made her one of the most important persons of the expedition.[95]

Roberts was of course a rare exception among hospital nurses, as Nightingale suggested when she spoke of all the vices of the hospital nurse, but her capacity for doing the work of ten was a quality on which Nightingale set a high premium.

Nurses in pre-reform days essentially were a specialized type of charwoman, and the Nightingale Fund contract with St. Thomas's did not seek a different type of recruit.[96] The matron was to choose fifteen of the thirty-seven nurses then working at St. Thomas's; these fifteen women would be trained by selected St. Thomas's doctors and sisters. The old matron, Wardroper, was in charge of the instruction, and the Nightingale Fund paid the doctors, sisters and Wardroper for these teaching responsibilities and for any other additional costs that the probationers incurred. Most important, unlike the arrangements that the Sisterhoods and the British Nursing Association made with their hospitals, the Nightingale Fund Council agreed that the training was to be done solely by St. Thomas's staff, under the direction of St. Thomas's treasurer.[97] The Nightingale School was unique in attempting to introduce nursing reform without introducing a better educated manager to carry it out. Mrs. Wardroper was neither a lady—Florence Nightingale's friend, Mrs. Bracebridge, considered her uneducated—nor was she a nurse.[98]

Nightingale and the council were soon unhappy with the arrangements. They realized that the hospital was using the school not for training but as a cheap source of labor for the hospital, and that the probationers were being worked so hard that many broke down. They considered starting over again elsewhere; they also tried to replace Mrs. Wardroper with a "real" lady superintendent, but with no success. The St. Thomas Hospital administration stood firm. "What we call the Nightingale system," Monica Baly writes, "was a hotch potch of what the Fund could wring out of St. Thomas's—which was not much. St. Thomas's was interested in keeping down its costs."[99]

If this was true of St. Thomas's, one of the wealthier hospitals, it was even more true of the other hospitals that were running into severe financial difficulties by the 1860s, a situation made worse in the 1870s by the agricultural depression.[100] In the remaining seven hospitals, the initiative for reform came largely from the hospital administrators, but, as at St. Thomas's, in every case they took care to keep the costs as low as possible. They did not try to replace the old sisters and they did not contract out their nursing service to a separate organization but kept control of the nursing firmly in their own hands. Their idea of nursing reform was to hire a lady superintendent who was an experienced nurse, to improve the accommodations for the nurses and insist that they live in them, and to demand a more orderly and productive work force. Between 1867 when the Middlesex hired Catherine Martyr and 1887 when St. Thomas's became the last of the teaching hospitals to hire a trained nurse as lady superintendent, the remaining hospitals all followed this format for reorganizing their nursing services.

The introduction of "lady pupils" or paying probationers, which began in the later 1860s, dramatically improved the working and living conditions for this class of probationer. Arrangements for the lady probationers varied from hospital to hospital, but normally probationers paid a guinea a week and their training lasted only a year, while the ordinary probationers had to stay for two, three, or four years.[101] St. Thomas's was somewhat of an exception. The lady or "special" probationers trained for only a year, but they were not all ladies nor did they all pay. Although they were supposed to be trained as superintendents, Wardroper did everything she could to block a special program for them and insisted that they all work as hard on the wards as any one else.[102] At most of the other hospitals the situation was very different. For example, at St. Bartholomew's, one of the last hospitals to introduce lady pupils, probationers lived in completely separate quarters of a very superior standard. They were used rather as auxiliaries to augment the staff than as real probationers: their training, the House Committee said, would give them nursing experience while lessening the duties of the regular nursing staff.[103]

Other hospitals made similar arrangements, and ladies were thus introduced into hospitals that were not nursed by the Sisterhoods. Most lady pupils did not remain in nursing, but a few did. These exceptions were rapidly promoted. Eva C. E. Lückes and Ethel Gordon Manson had both been lady pupils with only one year of training. In 1880 Lückes became matron of London Hospital at age twenty-six and in 1881 Manson became matron of St. Bartholomew's at age twenty-four.[104]

Nevertheless, until the 1880s ladies who made a career of nursing were rare exceptions. "The class from which the main body of nurses is derived," Dr. Steele, the professional administrator at Guy's, explained in 1875, "is the industrial, women accustomed to labour in households, mothers and daughters of the poor."[105] By the 1890s, however, there had been a major shift in the work force. More middle-class women were working for salaries, making waged labor more respectable; new areas of work had opened up for women. The Nightingale Council and other nursing pioneers were successfully advertising nursing as a romantic and exciting career for young women; as a result, the prestigious London teaching hospitals began to attract more candidates than they could accept.[106]

In 1890 St. Bartholomew's boasted that it had daughters of all the leading new professions—architects, accountants, stockbrokers, and so on—as well as daughters of the old professions—naval and military officers, the Church, medicine, and the law—in its training school. More important, they claimed that these women were not simply taking a few months training but that they intended to make a career out of nursing.[107] Probably none of the other schools could have boasted such a number of socially acceptable probationers, although it is notable that there were no daughters of aristocrats. The social mix at the London Hospital was more typical. Mary Ellen Yatman, a lady nurse at the London, described her colleagues in the same year, 1890, as "nice, well-conducted people of good moral character. . . . Some were uneducated; of course there were all kinds of social degrees in the hospital, . . . but on the whole I should say they were nice women."[108] The change in the social standing of nursing recruits since the 1860s was quite dramatic.

Conclusion

Given the unbusinesslike arrangements of the old ward system of nursing, the new larger work force in the hospital, and the recalcitrant, often truculent, and insubordinate old nurses, it was simply impossible to deliver a high standard of nursing care to acutely ill patients. The techniques that the reformers used to develop a more efficient nurse were standard, if unimaginative, nineteenth-century methods of dealing with large, uneducated work forces. The highly disciplined and regimented so-called Nightingale system was understandable in the 1860s. This system, with its values of punctuality, trustworthiness, order, and, above all, unquestioning obedience was a reasonable solution when nursing recruits were ill educated, unaccustomed to a regular rhythm of work, and unacquainted with working to the clock.

The way the system was applied, however, tended to differ between hospitals that the Sisterhoods nursed and hospitals where administrators maintained control of nursing. In the case of the Sisterhoods, the strictly regimented system seemed to be tempered by kindness and generosity.[109] The Sisters originally undertook nursing as a work of Christian philanthropy. One of the primary aims of St. John's House was to train the nurses in a regular course to fit them for their professional calling, improve their qualifications, and offer them a prospect of a better social position. The Sisters were to minister as ordinary nurses themselves as opposed to merely overseeing the work.[110] Although religious zeal and enthusiasm were to be wisely controlled, all levels of nurses—lady superior, Sisters, and ordinary nurses—were to live together in a spiritual family, joined by ties of sisterly love.[111] The Sisters never lost sight of this goal. "A St. John's House nurse," the lady superior wrote in 1874, "is not regarded by her superiors as a drudge, who is to be worked for the convenience of others until she can work no longer, and then cast aside as useless; but as a member of a community, entitled to sympathy and consideration from those under whom she is placed."[112]

For complex reasons that lie beyond the scope of this paper, the Sisterhoods had left the teaching hospitals by the end of the century, leaving the nursing services completely in the hands of the hospital administrators. The administrators continued to treat the nurses as they had always done—as drudges, as the lady superior put it. "The fact is the supply of the raw material for making Nurses out of was diminishing rapidly in London during the last few years," Dr. Steele, the professional administrator at Guy's told the governors in 1880. Some of the new, younger, and more respectable women whom the hospital was able to recruit after the arrival of the new lady superintendent in 1879 did not have the same physical power as the old nurses. However, they came for the first month on trial without pay, so that if they broke down or the matron and Steele found them unfit for the work, they were asked to leave and nothing was lost.[113]

Hospital administrators were not cruel or unkind men, but servants were traditionally considered part of the lower orders of humanity, and hospital administrators were working with deficit budgets.[114] It was the function of servants to work for the convenience of others. Hospital administrators were far more interested in using moral discipline to develop a highly productive and trustworthy worker than in using it to develop the self-respect and professional quality of the nurses. While they wanted efficient nurses who were up-to-date with modern medical practice, the administrators provided little by way of technical education for nurses; strictly limited education was also the preference of the nursing leaders.

What education the first generation of the new nurses did get stressed obedience and conformity, and as a result, Monica Baly suggests, they remained rigid in their thinking and uninnovative.[115]

In 1888 the British Nursing Association, the newly formed professional society, put forward a curriculum for the trained nurse. The only theoretical content in this curriculum was "some knowledge" of elementary anatomy and physiology and "a practical knowledge" of the various systems of disinfecting patients' clothes and keeping utensils and instruments clean. The rest dealt with sweeping, dusting, bed-making, poulticing, fomentations, leeching, and so on.[116] The nurses did have written exams, but Sidney Holland, chairman of the London Hospital, explained in 1904 that "A nursing examination is so childishly simple that you cannot invent a difficult one"—the limit of nursing knowledge was so small. What counted in a nurse was her character. "You would not take a cook from a registry," he said. "You would want to know that she had a good character and you would apply to her late employer." It was no different with a nurse.[117]

By 1890 the labor pool from which nursing recruits were drawn was radically different from that of the 1850s and 1860s. Even the "uneducated" probationers, as Mary Ellen Yatman put it, were well conducted and of good moral character. The strict, all-pervasive discipline was no longer required or justified but it continued. Although some of the matrons such as Eva Lückes and Ethel Gordon Manson were highly competent, they did not change their management styles to fit the new conditions. When they no longer needed the strict schedules and severe discipline to see that the basic work got done, they continued to use the same method to do what they called "raising standards," which really meant increasing productivity without increasing the cost of the hospital. "*Everything that takes place in a ward should have a fixed time, and be done to the minute* [original emphasis]," a nursing textbook stated. The ward routine was inflexible. It was a hallmark of the new nurse that she always moved at a smart pace and she was expected to be on the go all of the time.[118] A probationer at the London Hospital in 1890 told how she was so used to "trotting" up and down the ward to get her work done that she found herself trotting on her time off.[119]

The same probationer described herself as "behaving exactly like a general servant" a large part of the time. The scrubbers, or ward maids, did only the scrubbing. The non-nursing jobs of the probationers consisted of sweeping, dusting, cleaning the lavatories and bathrooms, making the sisters' beds, sweeping and dusting their rooms, taking the sisters their bath water and emptying their baths, preparing and serving the sisters' breakfasts, washing the patients' dishes, cleaning the ward lamps and inkstands, and polishing the brass, copper, and tin in the ward. Hospital administrators and matrons found it difficult to let go of nursing's domestic service inheritance. "The glory of a nurse's life is purely moral," a visitor to the London Hospital explained. "Socially she is inferior to the meanest 'dresser' [medical student], and under a severe—if doubtless often benevolent—tyranny of matron, resident officers, visiting staff and committee, to say nothing of her immediate masters, the patients in her charge."[120] The London Hospital was not atypical.

The highly competent and experienced Clara Collet, one of the writers for Charles Booth's *Life and Labour of the People in London*, which was first published in 1889, interviewed a number of matrons for her chapters on women and work. She perceived the new training schools rather as factories that mass-produced nurses and where training had become a kind of trial as well as a training. "The majority of matrons whom we saw," she wrote, "testified to the fact that no women pass out of the hospital mill unchanged." By the time they had finished, they were either distinctly better or distinctly worse women.[121]

The nursing reformers successfully produced a cheap, highly disciplined, and efficient work force that delivered a level of nursing care superior to that of the early part of the century. But the reform had been accomplished by developing what *Frere v. Peacock* called the moral powers of the mind in contradistinction to the powers of understanding or intellect. The result was that, lacking an intellectual foundation and totally controlled by hospital administrators, nursing had no possibility of taking its place beside the newly established Victorian professions such as architecture or accountancy. Some of the new nurses were daughters of these other new professionals, and nursing was far more respectable than at the beginning of the century. Nevertheless, the strategies of the reformers ensured that nurses remained the servants of the hospital.

Carol Helmstadter
Government Relations Research Officer
Ontario Nurses' Association
85 Grenville Street, Suite 600
Toronto, Ontario M5S 3A2
Canada
Phone: (416) 964-8833
Fax: (416) 964-8864

Notes

1. These twelve hospitals were St. Bartholomew's and St. Thomas's, founded in the Middle Ages; the Westminster, Mr. Guy's, St. George's, the London, and the Middlesex, founded in the eighteenth century; and the Royal Free, Charing Cross, University College, King's College, and St. Mary's hospitals founded in the nineteenth century. Each had a different constitution and a different funding base, and by the end of the century each had a medical and a nursing school. *Parliamentary Papers*, 1892, XIII:viii–xxviii (hereafter referred to as *PP*).

2. Brian Abel-Smith, *The Hospitals 1800–1945: A Study in Social Administration in England and Wales* (London: Heinemann, 1964), 1–11, 16–18.

3. Christopher Maggs, *The Origins of General Nursing* (London: Croom Helm, 1983), 88–98, 105–9.

4. Eva C. E. Lückes, *Hospital Sisters and Their Duties* (London: J. and A. Churchill, 1886), 72, 108, 164.

5. Monica E. Baly, *Florence Nightingale and the Nursing Legacy* (London: Croom Helm, 1986), 222–23.

6. Sub-Committee on the Accommodation of Patients, 21 November 1849 and 31 January 1850, Greater London Record Office H9/GY/A17/1 (hereafter cited as GLRO).

7. Abel-Smith, 1–16.

8. Theresa McBride, *The Domestic Revolution: The Modernisation of Household Service in England and France* (London: Croom Helm, 1976), 19–26.

9. Benjamin Golding, *An Historical Account of St. Thomas's Hospital, Southwark* (London, no publisher noted, 1819), 204–6.

10. Margaret Lonsdale, "The Present Crisis at Guy's Hospital," *Nineteenth Century* (April 1880): 682.

11. F. G. Parson, *The History of St. Thomas' Hospital* (London: Methuen, 1934), 207–13. For another example see H. C. Cameron, *Mr. Guy's Hospital 1726–1948* (London: Longmans, Green, 1954), 74–78.

12. Golding, 201–2.

13. Ibid., 240.

14. Treasurer and Almoners Committee (1878–80), Insert: Poster of Rules for Patients, St. Bartholomew's Hospital Archives Ha3/13 (hereafter cited as SBH).

15. General Committee (1844–57), 20 May 1857, University College Hospital Archives/A1/2/1 (hereafter cited as UCH).

16. Court of Committees (1861–69), 13 January 1869, GLRO/H9/GY/A3/9.

17. Board of Governors/House Committee (1770–86), 27 June 1771, SBH/Ha1/14.

18. Ibid., 10 and 17 July 1771.

19. Ibid., 22 January 1772.

20. Ibid., 3 March 1773.

21. Ibid., 15 March 1775.

22. Treasurer's and Almoners' Minutes (1874–76), 4 February, 5 August 1875, SBH/Ha3/12.

23. Mary Stanley, *Hospitals and Sisterhoods* (London: no publisher noted, 1854), 8–9.

24. Two Lady Nurses, *Hospital Nursing without Alcoholic Drinks* (London, National Temperance Depot Tract, circa 1882).

25. Treasurer's and Almoners' Committee (1870–74), 27 March, 3 April 1873, SBH/Ha3/11.

26. Golding, 189–90.

27. Gen Cttee (1844–57), 8 May 1850, 5 July 1854, 24 January 1855, 8 April 1857, UCH/A1/2/1.

28. Ibid., 6 May 1857.

29. Bd of Govs (1856–65), 1 January 1865, Charing Cross Hospital Archives, pp. 14–15 (hereafter cited as CCH); General Committee and Weekly Board (1867–70), 3 September 1867, Middlesex Hospital Archives (hereafter cited as MH).

30. Mr. Lushington's Statement, 12 July 1880, GLRO/H9/GY/A224/3, pp. 11–12; General Court and Weekly Board (1867–70), 1 October 1867, MH.

31. Bd of Govs (1856–65), 1 January 1865, CCH, pp. 14–15.

32. Med Cttee (1863–67), 21 March 1865, CCH.

33. Med Cttee (1863–67), 22 and 29 December 1863, 26 January 1864, CCH; Med Cttee (1866–69), 12 January, 30 March, 28 December 1867, MH.

34. McBride, 57–60. Hse Cttee (1814–20), 28 November 1815, London Hospital Archives/A5/16 (hereafter cited as LH); Bd of Govs (1815–26), 3 July 1821, SBH Ha1/17; Gen Cttee (1844–57), 12 March 1845, 9, 15, 23 February 1848, UCH/A1/2/1; Med Cttee (1863–67), 29 March 1864, CCH; Treasurer's and Almoners' Cttee (1878–80), Insert: Poster of Rules for Patients, SBH/Ha3/13.

35. J. B. Atlay, *Sir Henry Wentworth Acland, Bart* (London: Smith Elder, 1903), 81–84.

36. Ibid.

37. Ibid.

38. *The Lancet* (20 July 1844): 541–42. Most articles in this medical journal are not signed and do not have a title.

39. *Guy's Hospital 250 Years*, ed. Clive E. Handler (London: Guy's Hospital Gazette, 1976), 22.

40. Catherine Cappe, *Thoughts on the Desirableness and Utility of Ladies Visiting the Female Wards of Hospitals and Lunatic Asylums* (London: pamphlet, no publisher noted, 1816).

41. Sir Edward Cook, *The Life of Florence Nightingale* (London: Macmillan, 1913) I:44, 63.

42. Mr. Lushington's Statement, 12 July 1880, GLRO/H9/GY/A224/1, pp. 8–10.

43. Gen Cttee (1844–57), 10, 25 May 1848, 5 June 1850, 1 January 1851, 16, 30 November 1853, 7 November 1855, UCH/A1/2/1.

44. Ibid., 24 March, 7 April 1858.

45. Ibid., 6 May 1857. For another illustration of this standard type of problem see House and Finance Committee (1883–90), 28 November 1883, St. Mary's Hospital Archives AD7/6.

46. Gen Cttee (1844–57), 21 May 1854, 18 April 1855, UCH/A1/2/1. Ibid., 29 June 1853.

47. Gen Cttee (1857–66), 7 April 1858, 9 April 1862, UCH/A1/2/2.

48. Brian Harrison, *Drink and the Victorians: The Temperance Question in England 1815–1872* (Pittsburgh: University of Pittsburgh Press, 1971), 37–39, 306–9.

49. Richard Price, *Labour in British Society* (Dover: Croom Helm, 1986), 34–39, 42–43, 109–10.

50. Charles Booth, *Life and Labour of the People in London* (reprint, London: Macmillan, 1902), first series, IV:321–26.

51. *PP*, 1890, XVI:368, 473–74.

52. Lückes, 70.

53. Gillian Sutherland, *Elementary Education in the 19th Century* (London: London Historical Association, 1971), 18–19.

54. Phillip McCann, ed., *Popular Education and Socialization in the 19th Century* (London: Methuen, 1979), 85–87, 182–83.

55. Charles E. Rosenberg, "Florence Nightingale on Contagion: The Hospital as Moral Universe," in *Healing and History: Essays for George Rosen*, ed. Charles E. Rosenberg (New York: William Dawson and Sons, 1979), 125.

56. "Training Institution for Nurses," 1848, GLRO/H1/ST/SJ/A17/1; *Lancet*, 10 September 1864:298–99; Lionel S. Beale, *Hospital Patients, Doctors and Nurses* (London: J. Churchill and Sons, 1874), 19–24.

57. Martin J. Wiener, *Reconstructing the Criminal: Culture, Law and Policy in England 1830–1914* (Cambridge: Cambridge University Press, 1990), 45.

58. Ibid., 16–18.

59. Ibid., 26, 32–33, 35–38.

60. Ibid., 26–27, 38.

61. David N. Weisstub, *Enquiry on Mental Competency* (Toronto: Queen's Printer for Ontario, 1990), 345–46.

62. Ibid.

63. Earl of Beaconsfield, *Sybil, or the Two Nations* (reprint, London: Longmans, Green, 1920), 76–77.

64. Wiener, 31.

65. "A Short Account of St. John's House and Sisterhood," c. 1867, GLRO/H1/ST/SJ/Y8, pp. 1–3.

66. "Hanover Square Meeting," 13 July 1848, *Records, etc.*, Archives of the Community of the Sisters of St. John the Divine, Birmingham, England, pp. 13–14 (hereafter cited as CSSJD).

67. McCann, 68–70, 93–104; James H. Rigg, *National Education in Its Social Conditions and Aspects, and Public Elementary School Education English and Foreign* (London: Strahan, 1873), 292–95; Asher Tropp, *The Schoolteachers: The Growth of the Teaching Profession in England and Wales from 1800 to the Present Day* (London: Heinemann, 1959), 5–9, 12.

68. *Lancet* (3 September 1864): 272.

69. Florence Nightingale, "Suggestions for the Improvement of the Nursing Service of Hospitals" (London, 1873), Archives of the Sisterhood of St. Mary, London, England.

70. Sidney Pollard, *The Genesis of Modern Management: The Industrial Revolution in Great Britain* (London: E. Arnold, 1965), 192–206.

71. For example, see Eva Gamarnikow, "Sexual Division of Labour: The Case of Nursing," in *Feminism and Materialism: Women and Modes of Production*, ed. Annette Kuhn and Ann Marie Wolpe (Boston: Routledge and Paul, 1978), 96–123.

72. Appendix to Memorial from Medical Staff, 8 December 1879, GLRO/H9/GY/A219/8; J. Braxton Hicks, "On Nursing Systems," *British Medical Journal* (3 January 1880): 11–12.

73. Charity Commissioners' Report 1837, GLRO/H9/GY/A71/1, p. 686.

74. Bd and Hse Cttee (1871–74), 12 November 1972, GLRO/H2/WH/A1/44, or General Court, 11 March 1880, GLRO/H9/GY/A225/2, pp. 196–97.

75. Mary A. Hodkinson, "Recollections of Nursing in the 1930s," *History of Nursing Society Journal* 3, no. 2 (1990): 34–35.

76. Pollard, 259–65.

77. Hse Cttee (1814–20), 9 December 1818 LH/A5/16; Standing Orders of the House Committee, London Hospital 1820, LH/A1/6.

78. General Court, 11 March 1880, GLRO/H9/GY/A225/2.

79. *Lancet* (10 September 1864): 298–99, (1 October 1864): 384–85; Bd of Govs (1865–68) 30 May 1865, CCH; Florence Nightingale to Mary Jones, 8 January 1867, GLRO/H1/ST/NC1/67/1; Hicks, 11–12; John E. Neale, "On Nursing Systems," *British Medical Journal* (17 January 1880): 90; A. L. Pringle, *A Study in Nursing* (London: Macmillan, 1905), 8–13.

80. E. P. Thompson, "Time, Work-Discipline and Industrial Capitalism," *Past and Present: A Journal of Historical Studies* (December 1967): 70–79.

81. McBride, 10, 14, 19–23.

82. Thompson, 70–79.

83. Mr. Lushington's Statement, GLRO/H9/GY/A224/3, pp. 1–2.

84. *PP*, 1890–91, XIII:3.

85. Standing Orders, 1874, GLRO/H9/GY/A53/1, pp. 97–101; General Court, 11 March 1880, GY/A225/2, pp. 196–97.

86. Lückes, 2–3, 183.

87. Judith Moore, *A Zeal for Responsibility: The Struggle for Professional Nursing in Victorian England 1868–83* (Athens: University of Georgia Press, 1988), 33.

88. *Lancet* (10 September 1864): 298–99.

89. *Lancet* (11 July 1868): 91–92.

90. For a typical description of the nurses' quarters in the hospital, see Bd and Hse Cttee (1871–74), 20 May 1873, GLRO/H1/WH/A1/44, or Hse Cttee (1874–76), 16 May 1876, LH/A5/37.

91. F. M. L. Thompson, *The Rise of Respectable Society* (London: Fontana, 1988), 156–57.

92. Miss Lückes' Report on Nursing Home Arrangements, October 1883, LH/A17/48.

93. Grand Cttee (1847–54), 27 December 1853, GLRO/H1/ST/A6/12, Charity Commissioners' Report 1864, GLRO/H1/ST/A44/2, pp. 77–80; Officer's Reports (1853–57), 5 Aug 1857, GLRO/H9/GY/A67/1.

94. Bd of Govs (1874–77), Report of Nursing Sub-Cttee, 9 June 1874, GLRO/H2/WH/A1/45.

95. Sir Edward Cook, *The Life of Florence Nightingale* (New York: Macmillan, 1942), 299–301.

96. Brian Abel-Smith, *A History of the Nursing Profession* (London: Heinemann, 1960), 1–10.

97. Grand Cttee (1854–62), 10 April 1860, GLRO/H1/ST/A6/13.

98. Baly, *Nightingale and the Nursing Legacy*, 56. Monica E. Baly, "The Nightingale Nurses: The Myth and the Reality," in *Nursing History: The State of the Art*, ed. Christopher Maggs (London: Croom Helm, 1987), 40.

99. Monica E. Baly, "Florence Nightingale and the Establishment of the First School at St. Thomas's," in *Florence Nightingale and Her Era: A Collection of New Scholarship*, ed. Vern Bullough, Bonnie Bullough, and Marietta P. Stanton (New York: Garland, 1990), 8–13.

100. F. B. Smith, *The People's Health 1830–1910* (New York: Holmes and Meier, 1979), 280–82.

101. Baly, *Nightingale and the Nursing Legacy*, 53; Maggs, *Origins*, 90–92.

102. Baly, "Establishment of the First School," 10–11 (see note 99, above).

103. Bd of Govs (1879–85), 22 April 1884, SBH Ha1/25.

104. Martha Vicinus, *Independent Women: Work and Community for Single Women 1850–1920* (Chicago: University of Chicago Press, 1985), 95–96.

105. Report on Trained Nursing for the Sick Poor 1875, GLRO/H1/ST/NC15/13b, pp. 12–14, 73–75.

106. Vicinus, 102.

107. *PP*, 1890, XVI:167.

108. Ibid., 302.

109. For example, see the letter from ten probationers describing the nursing system at King's College Hospital in 1874, quoted in Moore, 33.

110. "Training Institution for Nurses," c. 1848, GLRO/H1/ST/SJ/A17/1; "A Short Account of St. John's House and Sisterhood," c. 1867, GLRO/H1/ST/SJ/Y8, pp. 1–3.

111. *Reports, etc.* Annual General Mtg 1878, CSSJD.

112. Sister Caroline's Statement, 17 March 1874, GLRO/H1/ST/SJ/A39/20.

113. Gen Cttee, 11 March 1880, GLRO/H9/GY/A225/2, pp. 176–78.

114. McBride, 21–22.

115. Baly, "Nightingale Nurses," 39–45.

116. *Nursing Record* (18 October 1888): 398–401. The articles in this weekly nursing journal were frequently untitled and unsigned.

117. *PP*, 1904, VI:759, 762–63.

118. Maggs, *Origins*, 106–9.

119. *New York Herald*, 2 February 1890, LH26/5.

120. Ibid., Letter to Editor from Evelyn Dickinson, "Sweat or Sweaters? A Reply to the Assistant Matron of the London Hospital," *Pall Mall Gazette*, 25 September 1890, LH/A26/5.

121. Clara E. Collet, "Women's Work," in Booth, 2nd series, IV:102–3. See also V:197–98.

Grace Under Pressure

The Nursing Sisters of the Holy Cross, 1861–1865

BARBRA MANN WALL
Department of Nursing
Saint Mary's College

Introduction

The outstanding 1991 PBS television series on the Civil War made no mention of the nursing care provided by religious women on the battlefields and in hospitals in spite of the fact that over one fifth of all the women nurses were Catholic sisters.[1] Nursing's wartime history includes many references to secular heroines such as Florence Nightingale, Clara Barton, or Dorothea Dix. But for every famous nursing figure, thousands more worked every day in the hospitals and on the battlefields and are rarely mentioned. Some of these lesser-known women, the rank and file of nursing history, were the Sisters of the Holy Cross from Notre Dame, Indiana. Their activity during the Civil War and their encounters while engaged in nursing at that critical juncture in our nation's history helped change the conventional view of nursing, the general public's image of the sisters, and perhaps society's view of the Catholic Church.

The Sisters of the Holy Cross embodied the spiritual values of their religious order and were part of the developing role of women in that era. The responsibility of mid-nineteenth-century women was to bring "faith and religion to all [their] encounters," to be submissive and pious, and to practice domesticity to perfection.[2] Nursing was part of women's domestic duty, usually practiced in homes and limited to caring for immediate families, other relatives, and neighbors. Some women, called "natural-born" or "professed" nurses, used their skills to provide an income.[3]

Roman Catholics promulgated a similar domestic ideology for women; God's appointed sphere for women was the home. They were to take a deep interest in the poor and practice the virtues of "generosity, fidelity, devotedness, and self-sacrifice."[4] The Catholic woman who did not wish to be a wife or mother had another option—to enter a convent.[5] Many such women, including the Sisters of the Holy Cross, were sincerely interested in caring for the needy.[6] One sister described their mission as "God's instru-

Nursing History Review 1 (1993): 71–87.

ment of good . . . to spread the congregation of the Holy Cross wherever there [is] need of ministrations for the sick, care for the orphan, and training for youth."[7]

The Sisters of the Holy Cross had no formal training as nurses. In fact, no nurse training schools existed prior to the Civil War. But, as did other women of the day, the sisters learned their nursing skills from life experiences and work with the needy. Their development as nurses was enhanced by their traditions of obedience, discipline, and selflessness. Hence the sisters' life experiences and religious traditions made them ideal recruits as military nurses.[8]

Origins of the Sisters of the Holy Cross

To understand the sisters' ministry during the Civil War, one must go back to Father Edward Sorin, the founder of the University of Notre Dame, and Mother Angela Gillespie, the first directress of Saint Mary's Academy. The Sisters of the Holy Cross was founded in 1841 in LeMans, France, by Father Basil Moreau. Four sisters came to Notre Dame in the United States at the request of Father Sorin in 1843. In a letter to Father Moreau, dated 5 December 1842, Father Sorin stressed the need for sisters:

> Once the sisters arrive—and their presence is ardently desired—they must be prepared not merely to look after the laundry and the infirmary, but also to conduct a school, perhaps even a boarding school.[9]

In 1844 the sisters went to Bertrand, Michigan, and established Saint Mary's Academy. The school was moved to Notre Dame, Indiana, in 1855, its current motherhouse and the location of what became Saint Mary's College.

The period from the 1840s to the beginning of the Civil War was one of great growth in religious orders in the United States, including the Sisters of the Holy Cross. Millions of immigrants came to the United States from Europe seeking relief from the Irish potato famine, political refuge from Germany, and economic opportunities. The Church actively recruited help from Europe to meet the immigrants' needs.[10] Daughters of immigrants entered religious communities in large numbers.[11] By 1860, the Holy Cross community had grown to 184 sisters. Although the four original Sisters of the Holy Cross were French, the majority in 1860 were Irish.[12]

Mother Angela, baptized Eliza Maria Gillespie, became the first American directress of Saint Mary's Academy. She was born in Pennsylvania to a prominent family with relatives including statesmen and senators. Her brother was Father Neal Gillespie, the first graduate of Notre Dame; a cousin was Ellen Ewing, wife of General William T. Sherman. Eliza (Mother Angela) was vivacious and energetic, graduating from the Visitation Convent School in Georgetown, D.C. She taught in an Episcopal seminary for girls. She became proficient in business matters as she managed her stepfather's farm hands, tenants, and household workers. In 1853 she joined the Sisters of the Holy Cross.[13]

The Sisters' Call to Military Nursing Service

Although the Sisters of the Holy Cross were first established as a teaching order, they answered an appeal for Civil War nurses. On 21 October 1861 a messenger on horseback from Governor Oliver P. Morton of Indiana galloped up the road to Notre Dame. He requested of Father Sorin twelve sisters to care for the sick and wounded soldiers of the Army.[14] While some priest-superiors from other orders objected to sisters' involvement in the war, Father Sorin saw the sisters' nursing service as an opportunity. He hoped the sisters could not only help the wounded but also lessen the people's prejudice against the Catholic faith.[15] Mother Angela and five other sisters immediately volunteered and left the next morning for Cairo, Illinois. Besides Mother Angela, the group included Sisters Veronica Scholl, Magdalen Kiernan, Winnifred McGinn, Adela Moran, and Providence Daget.[16] Upon their arrival three days later, they were met by General Ulysses S. Grant who sent them to the regimental hospitals of General Lew Wallace's brigade in Paducah, Kentucky.[17] Eventually eighty Sisters of the Holy Cross served the sick and wounded—primarily in Illinois, Missouri, Kentucky, and Tennessee.

Immediately after the fall of Fort Sumpter in April 1861, the federal government sent forces, with General Grant in command, to Cairo, Illinois, to hold that strategic area for the Union. The Union forces attempted to gain control of the Mississippi River from this western front. While the happenings in Virginia made the biggest headlines, the Civil War actually moved into high gear in the West. Before George B. McClelland got his Army of the Potomac into action, battles of lasting consequence were fought in the Mississippi Valley.[18] Grant split the Confederacy in two by his victories in the West, but the price he paid was high. The battles of Fort Donelson,

Shiloh, and Vicksburg all brought heavy casualties.[19] It is precisely in this area where Mother Angela and the Sisters of the Holy Cross served.

The sisters' work in the Civil War met with many obstacles. Few hospitals existed in the United States when the Civil War began, and those that were in service were charity hospitals. Many of these early hospitals were developed by Catholic sisters.[20] Other hospitals of that era, however, were staffed with untrained personnel, many being disreputable women, and sanitation and hygiene practices were often ignored.[21] At the start of the war, most physicians perceived women as having delicate natures that rendered them unsuitable for the work as nurses. The following is a physician's view of women nurses early in the Civil War:

> Our women appear to have become almost wild on the subject of hospital nursing. . . . With the best intentions in the world, [they] are frequently a useless annoyance. . . . As a rule, [they] have not the physical strength necessary.[22]

In the early part of the war, hospital arrangements were grossly inadequate. The army had no hospitals, trained medical staff, sick-diet kitchens, or nurses. An entire medical system had to be assembled for the Union troops after the war began. Churches, hotels, warehouses, and other buildings were used as hospitals. Lack of ventilation and basic cleanliness contributed to a high rate of illness.[23]

At this time, outbreaks of measles were prominent, as were pneumonia, tuberculosis, smallpox, malaria, dysentery, and typhoid fever. Typhoid alone caused an estimated one fourth of all the disease-related deaths among those participating in the war.[24] War injuries resulted in massive numbers of amputations from gangrene. In 1889 Mary Livermore, a Civil War nurse, published a seven-hundred-page volume of her experiences with hospitals and relief work while traveling as a representative of the Chicago-based Western Sanitary Commission. She reported that, after the battle of Fort Donelson in February 1862, an unexpected snowstorm struck. Many who fell at the beginning of the battle, when the ground was soft, were "frozen into the earth" at the end. It was necessary to cut them out of the ground when help finally arrived.[25] She vividly described hospital life, quoting Union soldiers as saying,

> Our hospitals are so bad that the men fight against being sent to them. . . . In the hospital, the sick men lie on rotten straw. . . . The nurses are "convalescent soldiers," so nearly sick themselves that they ought to be in the wards. . . . We need . . . sick-diet, proper medicines . . . and good nurses.[26]

The Sisters of the Holy Cross helped change this image of hospital care. While some of the women who answered the call for Civil War nurses believed that "the saving grace of a loving and serene mother figure could counter the authority of male surgeons," they were met instead with disdain and abuse.[27] The Sisters of the Holy Cross, however, with their history of firm discipline, dispelled the physicians' suspicions of women as nurses. Father Neal Gillespie, Mother Angela's brother, wrote their mother on 13 December 1861, referring to this very subject.

> General Wallace and the officers of the Brigade . . . are delighted with the Sisters and at the great good they are doing in the hospitals in Paducah. . . . The Surgeons there . . . and the soldier-nurses are also much pleased with the way things go since the arrival of the Sisters; although there was great opposition . . . to their coming, the Surgeons and officers who really took an interest in the good management of the hospitals having been disgusted with the female nurses who had been in attendance and discharged, with the determination on the part of the officers never to have any females about the hospitals as nurses.[28]

Mother Angela's Organizational Activities

Mother Angela left Paducah to organize hospitals in Mound City and Cairo, Illinois, in November and December of 1861. Susan E. Wallace, wife of General Lew Wallace, wrote, "Mother Angela has orders from General Halleck to prepare a thousand beds at Cairo, which means battle."[29] Mother Angela's work in the organization of the convent, as well as her earlier farm management experiences, prepared her for this task.

In 1894 Mother Augusta Anderson, the first elected superior general of the Congregation of the Sisters of the Holy Cross, sent a questionnaire to all the Civil War nursing sisters still living.[30] Mother Augusta herself was a nurse during the Civil War. Excerpts from these memoirs give poignant evidence to the sisters' involvement in the war and its effect on them. Sister Magdalen referred to Mother Angela being in charge of the hospitals in Paducah and Mound City:

> Mother Angela got the Mound City Hospital from Gen. Grant while we were in Cairo. Col. Smith was stationed in Paducah with his Regiment, we had a great many sick there and we remained four months and then came to Mound City Hospital, and stayed there until the last day of Aug. '65. When Mother Angela left the Hospital Sister Conception had charge till the end of the War.[31]

Mother Angela placed a sister-nurse in charge of each hospital ward. Sister Mary of the Holy Cross, who worked in a Memphis hospital, stated, "After the Sisters went home for their Profession . . . I had Sister Odelia's Ward A and Sister Matilda had Ward B. [In] Ward A, there [were] 62 beds mostly always full with the very sick and dying."[32]

From his headquarters in Memphis, Tennessee, on 2 August 1862, General Sherman wrote the medical director at Louisville, Kentucky. He spoke about Mother Angela's energy and organizational skills:

> Sister Angela who bears this, has had charge of the Mound City hospital and now of Overton hospital and is now going to Louisville at your call. I have been acquainted with her since her childhood and know the great energy of her character and believe that . . . she may be made the instrument of infinite good in so organizing our general hospitals that a soldier may not be retained in them one hour after he convalesces.[33]

Not only did Mother Angela organize people and their activities, she also worked to get needed supplies for the hospital. Father Neal Gillespie wrote that Mother Angela went to Chicago in December 1861, at the invitation of a railroad executive. She accepted the invitation to go

> with a view to the good of her sick and succeeded admirably in engaging the good will of all, especially the President, who the next day busied himself in procuring things from the Sanitary Committee, Chicago, and at once had ten boxes of articles sent by his road, guaranteeing specially that he would see to the safe delivery of those boxes and everything sent thereafter for the hospitals.[34]

In a letter to a friend in Peoria, Illinois, on 4 December 1861, Mother Angela wrote,

> Can you not speak to the Ladies Relief Association in Peoria and have them send us a large supply of clothing such as shirts (flannel and cotton), drawers, socks and slippers;—canned fruits & jellies? We stand greatly in need of all such articles for the comfort of the poor, suffering Soldiers.[35]

The Sisters' Nursing Services

In Military Hospitals

In Mound City a large block of warehouses served as a hospital for the wounded. In responding to Mother Augusta's questionnaire, Sister Augustine Flannigan wrote,

> When the Sisters arrived in Mound City Mother Angela was in the Hospital with a little girl and the house filled with wounded Soldiers. Mother was more than glad to see the Sisters. We had many privations during the first year. . . . many a night the Sisters had not a bed to sleep in. Mother Angela very often slept on the floor. . . . It was nothing unusual to hear the alarm given at night that the Rebels were crossing the Ohio River. It was amusing to see the Sisters then. one of the Sisters could not find her shoes one night when the alarm was given.[36]

Mary Livermore's book highlights her recollections of the conditions of the sisters working in Cairo and Mound City. She stated that the Mound City Hospital became

> the best military hospital in the United States. . . . A Shaker-like cleanliness . . . pervaded the various wards. . . . The "Sisters of the Holy Cross" were employed as nurses, and by their skill, quietness, gentleness, and tenderness, were invaluable in the sick-wards. Every patient gave hearty testimony to the kindness and skill of the "Sisters."[37]

Sister Paula Casey, a young novice who had left her family in Ireland, entered the Congregation of the Sisters of the Holy Cross at age nineteen. She had only been in the convent three years in 1861 before she was sent to St. John's Hospital in Cairo. Out of the freshness of youth, she described the appalling conditions of the hospital upon her arrival:

> As we stepped in-to each room on the first-floor what a fearful sight stared us in the face. Every room was strewn with human legs and arms. . . . At this time the fighting was going on in good earnest. We were shown through the different wards by the genial Dr. Burke, but O! terrors. We could see nothing but human flesh everywhere around some of the wards on the first floor resembled a slaughter house the wals were so spattered with blood. . . . Sister M. Isidore and I cryed with horror until we were tired. to our heart-felt disappointment we met far more than we expected or ever thought of. of course we never knew what war was until that 7 day of Dec. 1861. Then we tasted it to the fullest extent.[38]

Mother Augusta was in charge of the hospital at Cairo. Sister Paula continued,

> Mother looked at us both a kind, pitying look, and said now stop, you are here and must put your heart and Soul to the work. Pin up your habits, we will get three brooms, three buckets of water and we will first begin by washing the walls and then the floors.[39]

Sister Paula reported that they succeeded in cleaning the hospital after "some days and nights of constant brooming and watering."[40]

Mary Livermore praised the hospital in Cairo for the nursing that was provided by the sisters. She stated, "Here the 'Sisters of the Holy Cross' were employed as nurses, one or more to each ward. Here was order, comfort, cleanliness, and good nursing."[41] After visiting Mound City and Cairo, she wrote, "It was . . . evident from preparations that another great battle was pending. . . . The battle came off at Shiloh."[42] More American lives were lost at Shiloh than in all previous American wars combined. The casualties from both sides were nearly 24,000, and the hospitals at both Mound City and Cairo were full after the battle. Another Sister of the Holy Cross, Sister Frances De Sales O'Neil, cared for a Dr. Frank Larimore, a casualty of Shiloh, at the Mound City Hospital. In 1916 Dr. Larimore wrote her, "I am captivated with joy in finding the only one living who knew me at sixteen years of age . . . who rendered me such kindly and efficient service."[43]

In the spring of 1862, the Ohio River flooded the countryside around Mound City, and flood waters surrounded the hospital. Sister Fidelis Lawlor became ill and died in April of that year. Her body had to be taken in a rowboat through flood waters to the railway station in Cairo while en route to Saint Mary's. Three months later Sister Elise O'Brien, still a novice, died of illness at the age of twenty-four in the Cairo hospital.[44]

While at Mound City, the novices working in the military hospitals were called back to Saint Mary's by a messenger from Father Moreau. Obedience to religious superiors was essential to the sisters, and they dutifully responded to this charge. Still, the sisters' feelings of compassion gave way to feelings of guilt because they could not stay with their sick patients. Sister Paula evokes a compelling image in her recollections.[45] She recalled that they left at night, but as they were preparing to leave, the mules that were to take them to the railroad station ran away. Sister Paula lamented,

> The poor mules understanding the situation of the whole affair talked the matter over between themselves and naturaly [*sic*] came to the conclusion. If we take those Sisters to meet the train it will surely be a great injustice to the poor sick and dying, and again it will stir up the wrath of Dr. Franklin which is always near at hand. No we will not take them we will break loose run away and hide in the woods until morning, and so they did. . . . The night was extremely warm. . . . neither moon nor stars were visible. They too seemed not pleased with our leaving the poor sick and dying as they refused their light and . . . hid behind a thick cloud which guarded them well.[46]

As the number of wounded multiplied, Mother Angela was sent to Memphis by the army in July of 1862 to organize military hospitals.[47] The sisters' service in these hospitals routinely included long hours of work with critically ill or injured men. Typically their hospital work included housekeeping, cooking, feeding the ill or wounded patients, changing bandages, supervising wards, and assisting with surgery.[48] Mother Augusta, who was Sister Augusta at the time, described the hospital working conditions in a letter written to Father Sorin from the Overton Hospital in Memphis in March 1863. She stated,

> Poor Sister Flavia has her own ward and Sister Helen's [who had been ill], which gives her but little time to rest, having about 120 patients to attend. . . . They are fitting up the lower rooms for wards, which will require another Sister. . . . It would be impossible for the Sisters that are here now, to undertake more than they already attend, as each one has from 60 to 80 sick patients.[49]

While serving on the battlefields, Mother Angela kept a notebook of the sisters' pay and expenses. They were paid $12.00 a month as army nurses.[50] Privates in the Union Army, however, only received $13.00 a month.[51] The most frequent items of expense appearing in Mother Angela's book were shoes for the sisters.[52] How many hours they must have spent on their feet!

Through all her experiences, Mother Angela maintained a keen sensitivity to the human agony of war. A single torn page contains her terse note, dated 10 April 1862, from Mound City:

> General Strong and staff visited the hospital today. It was a grand display and contrast of the pomp of war on one side and of its misery and horror on the other—as they passed through the different wards filled with the wounded, sick and the dying.[53]

On the Red Rover

In April 1862, while the sisters were serving in the army hospitals in Mound City and Cairo, a federal gunboat, the USS *Mound City*, captured the Confederate barracks ship, *Red Rover*, on the Mississippi River. After repair and outfitting for service, the *Red Rover* became the U.S. Navy's first hospital ship.[54] Wounded soldiers were treated and transported by the *Red Rover* to military hospitals along the Mississippi River. Mother Angela volunteered her sisters to serve on the ship and on 24 December 1862 Sisters Adela Moran, Veronica Scholl, and Callista Pointan stepped on board the *Red Rover*, with Sister St. John of the Cross joining them on 1 February

1863.[55] The sisters were paid $15.00 a month for their work as nurses, twenty percent more than army nurses received.[56] Two African-American nurses, Alice Kennedy and Sarah Kinno, worked under the direction of the sisters on the *Red Rover* when it was commissioned on 24 December 1862.[57] A sketch on board the *Red Rover*, entitled "The Sister," was drawn by Theodore R. Davis for *Harper's* in May 1863. It is believed to be the only known Civil War reproduction of a Sister of the Holy Cross.[58]

Sister Adela wrote,

> [I] went on board the U.S. Navy Hospital Boat red Rover [in 1862] and remained there until Oct. 65 at the close of the War. . . . I remained all the time and was at Vicksburg when [it was] taken . . . near enough to hear the firing, also to see the Boats running the Blockade.[59]

While Sister Adela was serving on the *Red Rover*, the ship was fired upon on 21 January 1863 with two shots entering the hospital.[60]

Ministerial Care

The sisters touched the spirits of many as they cared for the physical and spiritual needs of their patients in the military hospitals and on the hospital ship. A priest serving on the battlefields stated that hundreds of sick and wounded soldiers begged to be baptized as they neared death.[61] Sister Augustine, while in the Mound City Hospital, filled this pastoral role when no chaplain or priest was available. She wrote,

> After the battle of Fort Donelson we had fourteen hundred soldiers between sick and wounded, and there were more baptised after that Battle than any other time during the War. Nothing but dressing wounds from morning until night, about seven or eight died every day.[62]

Another sister cared for a dying man while on a hospital ship.[63] He insisted he would not die until he saw a priest. The sister stayed by his side all night until a priest could come. She "did all she could to console him, and while not keeping from him that the end was near, exhorted him to make acts of contrition and to have confidence in God."[64] She was awed by the man's confidence and questioned him about his spiritual strength. He then described his undying faith in Saint Joseph, the Patron Saint of a Happy Death. A priest arrived, and shortly after seeing him, the man died.[65]

The Sisters of the Holy Cross did not limit their care to Catholic or Union soldiers alone. In 1885, at the death of Sister Josephine, Mother

Angela recalled the following incident. While at the Mound City Hospital, Sister Josephine cared for a wounded Confederate soldier. When one hundred Union soldiers stationed themselves outside his hospital room, threatening to shoot the wounded Confederate, Sister Josephine was asked by the doctor to leave the room for her own safety. She protested to her sister in charge, who in turn told the doctor that she would take her twenty-seven other sisters and leave the hospital unless she and Sister Josephine could have charge of the wounded man's care. The nurses were allowed to stay. Sister Josephine quietly and gently spoke to the frightened man,

> moistening his parched lips with a cooling drink, giving what relief she could to his poor tortured body, and assuring him that she and the other Sister would not leave him: so he need not fear that the soldiers would fire while they remained.

Eventually, the armed crowd of soldiers dispersed, and the officer survived.[66]

Tributes to the Sisters

Many tributes were paid to the Sisters of the Holy Cross, even though this was a time characterized by sectarianism and religious prejudice. The country was emerging from a period of bitter conflict fueled by feelings of nativism and anti-Catholicism. Fear of the Catholic religion and hostility toward immigrants, especially Irish immigrants, were widespread.[67] The superintendent of women nurses of the Civil War, Dorothea Dix, was particularly hostile toward the several hundred religious sisters who worked as Army nurses, fearing they would proselytize the sick and wounded.[68] However, Mary Livermore, from a Unitarian background, stated, "If I had ever felt prejudice against these 'Sisters' as nurses, my experience with them during the war would have dissipated it entirely." An Army captain praised the Catholic sisterhoods, stating, "My friends, I am not a Catholic, but I stand ready at . . . all times to defend these . . . women even with my life, for I owe that life to them." In a written commendation, Dr. Pinkney, fleet surgeon of the Mississippi River flotilla, praised Mother Angela. General Sherman placed his military hospitals in Mother Angela's charge.[69] After the war, much regret was expressed by a large portion of the people of Memphis, mostly Protestant, when the sisters left in 1867.[70] Also, Dr. John Brinton replaced female lay nurses in the Mound City hospital with the

Sisters of the Holy Cross. He reported that the patients improved from the sisters care and grew to love and respect the sisters.[71] The wife of General Lew Wallace wrote,

> Mother Angela of St. Mary's Academy has come with thirty nurses—a flock of white doves—to nurse in the hospitals, where the stillness is like the silence of death. Nothing in our churches equals the devotion of these women. When Protestant sisters get tired, they go home, but the Sisters of the Holy Cross live among the patients without thought of avoiding contagion by flight.[72]

Another tribute to the sisters occurred after the war. Commodore Davis, commander of the western flotilla, gave Mother Angela two Civil War cannons, the "Lady Polk" and "Lady Davis."[73] They remained on the Saint Mary's campus until World War II. In response to the critical shortage of metal, the sisters donated the cannons to the government to be melted for scrap iron.

Conclusion

The Sisters of the Holy Cross were, of course, influenced by the roles society assigned to women in the nineteenth century. They dutifully obeyed military and medical orders and those of their religious superiors. They were willing, however, to step out of a submissive role and take risks when necessary. They revered one of their members, Sister Josephine, who refused to stand by idly as a mob mentality threatened to take a human life. They took charge of sick wards in the military hospitals and had the courage and compassion to care for those with smallpox and other contagious diseases. They worked in the battle areas, at times in the direct line of fire.

The Sisters of the Holy Cross contributed significantly to Civil War nursing in hospitals and on naval vessels.[74] They had a wide influence on the improvement of nursing in the 1860s and set standards for local nursing wherever the congregation served. A system of Holy Cross hospitals was started after the war, beginning with the opening of Saint Mary's Hospital in Cairo in 1867.[75]

These are personal histories of only a few of the sisters who contributed to nursing care in the Civil War. Over twenty religious communities, such as the Sisters of Mercy, Sisters of Charity, Dominican Sisters, and Franciscan Sisters of the Poor, worked in other settings.[76] The Civil War became an opportunity for the Catholic sisterhoods to improve their public image as well as to contribute to the development of modern nursing in the United States.

War holds a fascination throughout history, and war heroes are revered by their compatriots and readers of history. Yet war heroes are not limited to soldiers and their commanders; they include many others such as the nursing Sisters of the Holy Cross. As nursing looks to the future and the technological promises that lay in store, it also needs to look to its past and remember the legions of nursing pioneers who remind us that nursing is, first and last, a human service.

Barbra Mann Wall, RN, MS
Assistant Professor
Department of Nursing
Saint Mary's College
Havican Hall
Notre Dame, Ind. 46556
Phone: (219) 284-4687
Fax: (219) 284-4716

Acknowledgments

The research for this article was supported by a grant from Saint Mary's College. The primary sources were the memoirs of the Sisters of the Holy Cross housed in the Archives of the Congregation of the Sisters of the Holy Cross at Bertrand Hall, Saint Mary's College, Notre Dame, Indiana. The author gratefully acknowledges the permission to use the collection for reference. Special thanks to JoAnn G. Widerquist, Department of Nursing chair, Saint Mary's College, for her assistance during the article's preparation.

Notes

1. Dolores Liptak, RSM, review of *To Bind Up the Wounds: Catholic Sister Nurses in the U.S. Civil War*, by Sister M. Denis Maher, in *The Catholic Historical Review* (January 1991): 137–38.

2. Ellen Giarelli, "Nursing Ethics Education in Victorian America," in *Florence Nightingale and Her Era*, ed. Vern Bullough, Bonnie Bullough, and Marietta Stanton (New York: Garland Publishing, 1990), 207. For a more comprehensive description of the role of women in the nineteenth century, see Barbara Welter, "The Cult of True Womanhood, 1820–1860," in *Women and Womanhood in America*, ed. R. Hogeland (Lexington, Mass.: D. C. Heath and Co., 1973).

3. Susan M. Reverby, *Ordered to Care—The Dilemma of American Nursing, 1850–1945* (Cambridge: Cambridge University Press, 1987), 11–16.

4. Karen Kennelly, CSJ, "Ideals of American Catholic Womanhood," in *American Catholic Women—A Historical Exploration*, ed. Karen Kennelly, CSJ (New York: Macmillan Publishing Co., 1989), 3–4.

5. Mary Ewens, OP, "Women in the Convent," in *American Catholic Women—A Historical Exploration,* ed. Karen Kennelly, CSJ (New York: Macmillan Publishing Co., 1985), 17.

6. M. Patricia Donahue, *Nursing—The Finest Art* (St. Louis, Mo.: C. V. Mosby Co., 1985), 280.

7. Sister M. Eleanore Brosnahan, CSC, *On the King's Highway* (New York: D. Appleton and Co., 1931), 214.

8. Judith Metz, SC, "In Times of War," in *Pioneer Healers—The History of Women Religious in American Health Care*, ed. Ursula Stepsis, CSA, and Delores Liptak, RSM (New York: The Crossroad Publishing Co., 1989), 42.

9. Father Sorin to Father Moreau, 5 December 1842, *Circular Letters of Father Moreau* (Notre Dame, Ind.: Ave Maria Press, 1943), I:61.

10. Ewens, 25.

11. Dolores Liptak, RSM, *Immigrants and their Church* (New York: Macmillan Publishing Co., 1989), 79.

12. *Matriculation Book* of Sister Alma Louise Fitch, CSC, 1969, Archives of the Congregation of the Sisters of the Holy Cross, Bertrand Hall, Saint Mary's College, Notre Dame, Indiana (hereafter cited as CSC). Material is scant on the socio-economic and educational background of the sisters. The only references that were located describe their education as being "pretty good," "educated in reading and writing—little arithmetic" and "well-educated."

13. Sister M. Immaculate Creek, CSC, *A Panorama: 1847–1977* (Notre Dame, Ind.: Saint Mary's College, 1977), 17–19.

14. Mother M. Angela Gillespie to Annie Harmon, copy, 4 December 1861, CSC.

15. Metz, 44. *A Story of 50 Years*, in *Annals of the Congregation of the Sisters of the Holy Cross 1855–1905* (St. Louis, Mo.: Bechtold, n.d.), 91–92. Bishop Grant of Southwark, London, may have had similar reasons for sending the Sisters of Mercy (English), Bermondsey, Southwark to the Crimean War. JoAnn G. Widerquist, "Dearest Rev'd Mother," in *Florence Nightingale and Her Era*, ed. Vern Bullough, Bonnie Bullough, and Marietta Stanton (New York: Garland Publishing, 1990), 288–308.

16. Sister M. Adela Moran to Mother M. Augusta Anderson, 1894, CSC.

17. Creek, 30–32. General Lew Wallace was in charge of the 11th Indiana Volunteers and was attached to the command of General Grant in Paducah, Kentucky, in 1861.

18. Bruce Catton, *The American Heritage Picture History of the Civil War* (New York: American Heritage Publishing Co./Bonanza Books, 1982), 114.

19. Patrick R. Duffy, CSC, USN (retired), "The Navy Nurses' Hundredth Birthday," *Columbia* 42, 10 (1962): 34–35.

20. Sister Mary Denis Maher, *To Bind Up the Wounds: Catholic Sister Nurses in the U.S. Civil War* (New York: Greenwood Press, 1989), 27.

21. Philip Kalisch and Beatrice Kalisch, *The Advance of American Nursing* (Boston: Little, Brown and Company, 1986), 37–39.

22. *American Medical Times*, 18 July 1861, 25–26, 30, quoted in *America's Working Women*, ed. Rosalyn Baxandall, Linda Gordon, and Susan Reverby (New York: Random House, 1976), 75–76.

23. Metz, 40–41.

24. Bill I. Wiley, *The Common Soldier of the Civil War* (Gettysburg, Pa.: Historical Times, 1973), 55, quoted in *Pioneer Healers—The History of Women Religious in American Health Care*, ed. Ursula Stepsis, CSA, and Dolores Liptak, RSM (New York: The Crossroad Publishing Co., 1989), 40–41.

25. Mary Livermore, *My Story of the War* (1889; reprint, New York: Arno Press Inc., New York Times Co., 1972), 179.

26. Ibid., 126–27.

27. Reverby, 46.

28. Father Neal Gillespie to his mother, copy, 13 December 1861, CSC.

29. Mrs. Susan E. Wallace to her mother, copy, 18 December 1861, CSC.

30. Mother M. Augusta Anderson was born in Alexandria, Virginia, and entered the Holy Cross community in 1854 while the sisters were in Bertrand, Michigan. She was directress of Saint Mary's Academy from 1879–1882 and was elected the first superior general of the Holy Cross congregation in 1882. She held that position until 1895. Her questionnaire asked the sisters when and where they served during the war, with whom they served, who was in charge, and how long they stayed. She also asked them to recall any memorable incidents that occurred during their service in the Civil War.

31. Sister M. Magdalen Kiernan to Mother M. Augusta Anderson, 1894, CSC.

32. Sister M. of the Holy Cross to Mother M. Augusta Anderson, 1894, CSC.

33. Major General William T. Sherman, copy of letter to Surgeon Murray, 2 August 1862, CSC.

34. Father Neal Gillespie to his mother, copy, 13 December 1861, CSC.

35. Mother Angela Gillespie to Annie Harmon, copy, 4 December 1861, CSC.

36. Sister M. Augustine Flannigan to Mother M. Augusta Anderson, 1894, CSC.

37. Livermore, 218.

38. Sister M. Paula Casey to Mother M. Augusta Anderson, 1894, CSC.

39. Ibid.

40. Ibid.

41. Livermore, 204–5.

42. Ibid., 221.

43. Dr. Frank Larimore to Sister M. Frances De Sales O'Neill, 10 March 1916, CSC.

44. Sr. M. Paula Casey to Mother M. Augusta Anderson, 1894, CSC. *Matriculation Book* of Sister Alma Louise Fitch, 1969, CSC. In 1919 the government donated special U.S. Army markers for the graves of all the sisters who served in the Civil War. They are located in Our Lady of Peace Cemetery on the Saint Mary's campus.

45. Records in the sisters' Archives state that Sister Paula served as a military nurse from 1861 to 1862 in St. John's Hospital in Cairo and from 1862 to 1864 in Mound City Hospital. She left the battlefields to make her profession.

46. Sister M. Paula Casey to Mother M. Augusta Anderson, 1894, CSC.

47. Mother Angela returned to Saint Mary's Academy from the battlefields before the end of 1862. She destroyed most of her personal letters prior to her death in 1887 at the age of sixty-three.

48. Ellen Ryan Jolly, *Nuns of the Battlefield* (Providence, R.I.: The Providence Visitor Press, 1927), 133, 137; and Metz, 43.

49. Sister M. Augusta Anderson to Father Edward Sorin, 30 March 1863, CSC.

50. Mother M. Angela Gillespie, notebook, handwritten MS. CSC.

51. Mark Boatner, *Civil War Dictionary* (New York: David McKay Company, Inc., 1959). The army private received $16.00 per month by the middle of 1864 after the last raise was given by the government.

52. Mother M. Angela Gillespie, notebook, handwritten MS. CSC.

53. Ibid.

54. Emmet F. Pearson, "First Hospitals in Southern Illinois," *The Proceedings of the Institute of Medicine of Chicago* 35 (1982): 43–44.

55. Governor Oliver P. Morton to Mother M. Angela Gillespie, 6 May 1862, CSC. U.S. Navy Department, Office of Chief of Naval Operations, Division of Naval History, "History of U.S. Naval Hospital Ship Red Rover," Publication No. OP 09B9, Ships' History Section (Washington, D.C.: 1961), 7. For their services on the *Red Rover*, a 1962 Naval bulletin proclaimed the Sisters of the Holy Cross to be the first Navy nurses. This information is stated on a plaque erected by the Indiana Civil War Centennial Commission in 1965. The plaque is located on the grounds of St. Joseph Hospital in South Bend, Indiana.

56. Metz, 55. The sisters' salaries helped pay for a new building on Saint Mary's Campus, Bertrand Hall. Over a hundred years old, it currently houses the Archives and the Office of the General Administration of the Congregation of the Sisters of the Holy Cross.

57. U.S. Navy Department, 7.

58. Sister M. John Francis, CSC, "Holy Cross Sisters as U.S. Navy Nurses." Unpublished manuscript, 1961, CSC.

59. Sister M. Adela Moran to Mother M. Augusta Anderson, 1894, CSC.

60. U.S. Navy Department, 8.

61. George Barton, *Angels of the Battlefield* (Philadelphia, Pa.: The Catholic Art Publishing Co., 1897), 227.

62. Sister M. Augustine Flannigan to Mother M. Augusta Anderson, 1894, CSC.

63. The sister's name is unmentioned and it is unclear whether she served on the *Red Rover* or another hospital ship.

64. Sister Mary of the Annunciation to Mother M. Augusta Anderson, 1894, CSC.

65. Ibid.

66. "A Death That Recalls a Noble Deed," *The Ave Maria* 21 (1885): 678–81. Mother Angela wrote about this incident on the occasion of Sister Josephine's death. This story comes from a eulogy and is a rather hagiographic source.

67. James Hennesey, S.J., *American Catholics—A History of the Roman Catholic Community in the United States* (New York: Oxford University Press, 1981), 119–27.

68. Metz, 42.

69. Livermore, 218. Barton, 225. Dr. Ninian A. Pinkney to Sister St. John, 9 June 1866, CSC. Major General William T. Sherman, copy of letter to Surgeon Murray, 2 August 1862, CSC.

70. Patricia M. LaPointe, "The Disrupted Years: Memphis City Hospitals 1860–1867," *The West Tennessee Historical Society Papers* 37 (1983): 18–24.

71. John Brinton, *Personal Memoirs of John H. Brinton* (New York: The Neale Publishing Co., 1914), 44–45, quoted in *To Bind Up the Wounds: Catholic Sister Nurses in the U.S. Civil War*, by Sister Mary Denis Maher (New York: Greenwood Press, 1989), 126.

72. Mrs. Susan E. Wallace to her mother, copy, 18 December 1861, CSC.

73. *A Story of 50 Years*, 111.

74. A stained glass window in St. Bridget's Church, Lexington, Massachusetts, depicts the Sisters of the Holy Cross as Civil War nurses, not only for their contributions to nursing during the Civil War, but also for their work in early Catholic education in the United States.

75. The sisters eventually opened a School of Nursing at Mt. Carmel Hospital in Columbus, Ohio, in 1903. Other nursing schools were also started, both hospital and collegiate. Eight hospitals of the Holy Cross Health Care System are currently in operation across the United States. Sister Alma Louise Fitch, CSC, interview with author. Notre Dame, Indiana, 20 March 1992.

76. Donahue, 282; Metz, 53–57.

Medieval Nursing

Vern L. Bullough
Department of History and Social Studies
SUNY College, Buffalo

Bonnie Bullough
Department of Nursing
SUNY College, Buffalo

What was the role of nursing in medieval hospitals? Were nurses simply doing maid's tasks or were they really caring for the sick in the sense that the term *caring* is now used among nurses? Although historians are willing to admit that some actual nursing care took place in the medieval hospitals, they have generally held that the hospitals were primarily poorhouses, only incidentally providing care for the sick.[1] These historians assume that before the development of "scientific medicine," hospitals were primarily religious and charitable institutions and that the attendants had no need of any special knowledge.[2] Part of the problem with such a stance, however, is that it stems from hospital histories that focused on physicians, many of them using the American hospitals of the first half of the twentieth century as the norm. Traditionally, however, the physician's role in the pre-twentieth-century hospital was overshadowed by other health care workers. Medical ideology of the past differed from that of today, but it seems clear that, by the standards of science of the time, the hospital nurses were acquainted with medical theories.

Linda McCray Beier summed up traditional histories of medicine that tended to downplay the role of nurses and other health professionals:

> Until fairly recently traditional medical history satisfied the needs of both the medical profession and the general public. The pedigree provided for it by medical historians contributed to a necessary esprit de corps and allowed for a gradual inflation of its demands for respect and rewards. The general public, relieved from the age-old tyranny of infection and encouraged by a rise in living standards, gave its gratitude to the doctors who were the most visible agents of the improvements it perceived. Miracle medicine and miracle surgery heralded an irresistible combination of confidence in the future and relief from personal responsibility for the health and illness of themselves or their loved ones.[3]

Nursing History Review 1 (1993): 89–104.

Physician-oriented histories treated patients either as irrelevant or as the vehicles or beneficiaries of medical discoveries. Doctors were expected to be and were usually portrayed as being totally in control of the experience of illness. When health care is examined from a different view, however, a somewhat different picture emerges. What, for example, did people do when they became ill, were injured, or had babies? The answer to this question leads us to see that what we now call nursing care, as distinct from medical intervention, whether done by a physician or by others, was an essential part of the healing process. In fact, it was the major part.

The most commonly used kinds of medical therapy were self-treatment or treatment rendered by lay people, whether they were relatives, friends, or neighbors. For much of the early medieval period in the West this was about all there was; occasionally, certain individuals gained expertise if only because they were able to read the Latin or Greek medical writings. In the West these were few and far between in the early medieval period, and the wandering healers who were occasionally called on to intervene by locals developed their expertise primarily through experience. Later, beginning in the eleventh and twelfth centuries, more sophisticated medical practitioners emerged—ranging from university-educated physicians to apprentice-trained barbers, surgeons, or apothecaries. The title of physician was restricted to the university-educated physician who had read and studied the medical classics and was thereby believed to have a strong theoretical orientation. These physicians, however, were never numerous enough to care for all the sick, even if they wanted to do so. Their services were supplemented by barbers, surgeons, and apothecaries, most of whom could not read the Latin necessary to become a physician, and who in the larger cities began to organize into guilds at about the same time the universities appeared. Outside of the larger cities or university towns, however, health care in the medieval West remained primarily in the hands of the traveling healers or local community experts.[4]

Such local experts were not, however, necessarily different from those who belonged to the guilds of barbers, surgeons, or apothecaries even though they lacked the "sophistication" of the physician. Medical information based on Greco-Roman models was widely disseminated in the population, and women universally acted as amateur healers, regardless of their social status. Almost without exception, women midwives were the most frequent caretakers of women, and, in almost every community, one or two women gained significant enough reputations for their ability at healing to be called on in time of illness.

In general, although it is difficult to document, we can assume that the illnesses, births, and deaths in the medieval period were social occasions witnessed by crowds of primarily female family members, friends, and neighbors, as well as persons with special reputations for healing.[5] Common to both healer and patient was the belief that good health involved an equilibrium. If someone became ill, it was necessary first to determine what had thrown the body out of balance and then to act to restore it. This could be done by adjusting the diet of the ill person, prescribing exercise or rest, establishing the proper environmental conditions (perhaps by hanging a red curtain), or administering special remedies that had been handed down over the generations. The boundaries between food and medicine were unclear even for the educated physicians. Avicenna, in a much cited passage, declared that the formal distinction between the two was that food was assimilated by the body while medicine assimilated the body to itself.[6] Lettuce, for example, was both a food and a medicine, as were many other vegetables and spices.

Key to the concept of equilibrium were the four humors established by Hippocrates and Galen in the Greco-Roman period. The mixture of humors in the body determined a person's temperament and his or her permanent constitution: these were blood, phlegm, and yellow and black bile. Though the humors established the permanent constitution, there were cycles of dominance of each, with illness derived from the unnatural dominance of one humor over the other. According to this system, phlegm or mucus, the oldest constituent in the body, increases in the winter—as sputum and nasal discharges show. As the cold relaxes, the rains come on, bringing blood, which is moist and warm. This can be seen in the dysentery and nasal haemorrhage that comes in the spring and summer when people are hot and red. In summer blood is still strong, but yellow bile rises in the body and increases until autumn. As blood diminishes and bile increases, black bile also appears and for a brief time dominates, but then is gradually replaced by phlegm. These four humors vary seasonally in amount because of heat, cold, dryness, and moisture. When one humor is excessive beyond what is the normative course of change, treatment must be started to establish the proper equilibrium. Each individual also has a unique combination of humors, depending on the time of the year in which he or she was born. Thus people could be phlegmatic, sanguine, choleric, or melancholic in various degrees. Though it might take a literate physician specialist to give a very refined diagnosis, such as were sought by the rich and powerful in troublesome cases, simple diagnoses could be done by many who would treat individuals with wet, dry, cold, or hot treatments to get their body in balance. The healer who carried out this regime was, by today's definitions, both a nurse and a doctor, although most of the treatments were oriented toward care and observation.

Unfortunately, the sources do not fully reveal the details of care given. What is clear is that the early Christians gave an emphasis to caring that went beyond that of classical Greece and Rome. This seemed an area where women especially excelled.[7] Even the wife of an emperor might take care of the sick. For example, Flacilla, the wife of the Emperor Theodosius, was described in the fifth century as going

> about the guest chambers of the churches and ministering to the wants of the sick, herself handling pots and pans, and tasting the broth, now bringing in a dish and breaking bread and offering morsels, and washing out a cup and going through all the other duties which are supposed to be proper to servants and maids.[8]

The reference to servants and maids indicates who usually watched over the sick in the richer families, although the women in the house undoubtedly supervised the care.

Not everyone found themselves in a position to be cared for in their own home. Travelers, the poverty stricken without adequate lodgings (particularly in the cities), those without family ties, and, in the case of leprosy or the plague, those isolated into special dwellings served as the impetus for the emergence of the medieval hospital.

Hospitals, established first in the eastern part of the Roman Empire, came to the West very early. St. Jerome, who was often an intermediary for the introduction of Eastern ideas and institutions into Rome and the West, is a key figure. He attributed the introduction of the hospital in the West to one of his disciples, a woman named Fabiola. In a letter from about 399 of the modern era, he wrote:

> She was the first person to found a hospital, into which she might gather sufferers out of the streets and where she might nurse the unfortunate victims of sickness and want. Need I speak of noses slit, eyes put out, feet half burned, hands covered with sores? Or of limbs dropsical and atrophied? Or of diseased flesh alive with worms? Often did she carry on her own shoulders persons infected with jaundice or filth. Often too did she wash away the matter discharged from wounds which others, even though men, could not bear to look at. She gave food to her patients with her own hand, and moistened the scarce breathing lips of the dying with sips of liquid.[9]

Given the medical theories of the time, this is the best of care. That it met a real need is emphasized by the spread of hospitals. Each monastery and convent established a small hospital, known as an infirmary, to care for its own ill. Monasteries and convents located on pilgrimage and trade routes or near the larger cities also established special hospitals. Since the largest cities and the most travelers and pilgrims were found in the Eastern Roman Empire (usually called the Byzantine Empire) for much of the medieval period, the major hospitals were in the Byzantine Empire. Fortunately, we have considerable information on a number of these hospitals.[10]

Perhaps because so many of the Byzantine cities were large, nursing developed as a specialized occupation in the Byzantine state, something it did not do in the West until the nineteenth century. Instead of relying on caregivers in religious orders for nursing and health care, as did the West, the Byzantine hospitals hired paid assistants or nurses. These replaced volunteer ascetics—probably as early as the sixth century.[11] What challenges our traditional stereotypes, however, is that these paid attendants were, for the most part, male. This may have been because, as volunteers were replaced by paid employees, women dropped out—as so often has happened in the past. In the woman's wards, however, the nurses were women. Still, the Byzantine experience emphasizes that, in spite of the caring and nurturing image so usually associated with women, it was not necessarily inevitable that nursing develop as a woman's profession.

One of the hospitals for which we have the most information was in Constantinople. Known as the "Pantokrator" (Almighty), it was established by Emperor John II Comnenus early in the twelfth century. Its main purpose was to provide the many visitors to Constantinople, the capital of the empire, with more adequate care. The constitution of the hospital—known as *Typikon*—is extant, and indicates just how important the caregiving role for the ill and injured was. There were five main clinics in the hospital. The first included ten beds for illnesses requiring surgery; the second had eight beds for patients suffering from illnesses of the eyes and the intestines; the third had twelve beds set aside for ill women, although it is not clear whether this included obstetrics as well. The other clinics each had ten beds for general illnesses, plus an extra bed for emergency cases, and six additional beds for extreme illness or long-term bedridden patients.[12]

There were fourteen physicians to staff the hospital, two for each of the five clinics, only one of whom was there at any one time. Four other physicians, two specializing in surgery and two in internal medicine, were part of a rotation plan with other physicians in the city. None of the physicians were regular employees. The ten clinic physicians were private practitioners who were under contract for short terms, probably four months, after which they went back to their private practice. The four other physicians were more like consultants and changed frequently. A physician associated with Pantokrator in the Byzantine Empire achieved much the same recognition as contemporary physicians who have clinical appointments in medical schools in the United States. The difference between physicians and other health practitioners was the association to which they belonged and the requirements for entry. The physicians were better educated in traditional liberal arts and were regarded as learned individuals. They also had to pass an examination in order to be licensed.[13]

The more or less adjunct status of the physicians is important to emphasize since it means that the key to the effectiveness of the hospital was the full-time nursing staff. Each of the four clinics devoted to male patients had three "ordained" medical assistants (*hypourgoi embathmoi*), two "extra" medical assistants (*hypourgoi perissoi*), and two servants (*hyperetai*). In the women's ward, the two rotating male physicians were also joined by a female physician; there were also four "ordained" female assistants (*hyaourgissai embathmoi*), two "extra" female assistants (*hynourgissai aerissai*), and two female servants. There were also four "extra" medical assistants to staff an outpatient clinic, as well as five pharmacists, an usher, five laundresses, one keeper of the kettles, two cooks, one groom, one porter, one pursuer, two priests, two lectors (readers), two bakers, four pallbearers, one priest for funerals, one latrine cleaner, a miller, a craftsman to keep the surgical tools clean and sharp, and a part-time specialist in hernia surgery. The only "religious" were the priests, although the lectors and ushers were probably in training to be priests since both usher and lector are titles in the four minor orders of priesthood.

The terms *ordained* and *extra* set off in quotation marks in the above text are titles, implying that the assistants were members of a guild. To achieve such titles, they had to undergo basic education and professional training and to pass an examination.[14] In short, they were the equivalent of registered nurses, although how literate they were is not clear. The existence of a lector or reader would indicate that most of the attendants in the hospital were not particularly literate. Little is known of the training of these nurses, but the guild titles implied some sort of apprenticeship training, probably similar to that received by those who were barbers, barber surgeons, or apothecaries in the West. Interestingly, the female assistants also received the same salary and apparently belonged to the same guild as their male counterparts at the Pantokrator. Women physicians, who were contracted in the same way the men physicians were, received only half of the salary of their male counterparts even though they were on call all twelve months of the year while their male counterparts worked shorter terms. The salary differential might have been justified by the fact that the woman physician might not have had to be present for all examinations. The reasons are by no means clear, but it does not seem to be a difference simply because of sex since the male and female nurses were paid the same.[15]

Women were not always cared for by women nurses or women physicians. One Byzantine Hospital, a hospital for women established by the empress Theodora in the thirteenth century in conjunction with the Lips Monastery, was staffed entirely by men, including six male nurses.[16] It has been argued that this staffing policy was new and might have resulted from the fact that Constantinople was briefly under Western control in the thirteenth century as a result of its capture by the Crusaders.[17] Certainly the West did not develop secular guilds for hospital care but both religious men and women ended up as nurses. Since the West had guilds in other areas, there was apparently no perceived need or demand to develop one for hospitals.

In many ways these medieval Byzantine hospitals operated like modern ones in that the physician in charge made rounds each day, examining new patients and checking on progress of others. He may have given instructions to the nurses, although most procedures would have been undertaken without physician direction. Standard nursing procedures included bloodletting, bathing, applying salves and plasters, giving sitz baths, and overseeing the administration of a number of oral medications. Cautery, however, was done by the surgeons.[18] The Pantokrator and Lips were only two of the many hospitals found in the Byzantine Empire, but all seemed to use the same kind of assistants or nurses, with nurses providing much of the care and treatment.

As Western Europeans became familiar with the Byzantine model, they adopted its general concepts but kept nursing care in the hands of the religious. At first, hospitals were established primarily in male orders, probably because the Western groups most likely to establish hospitals on the Byzantine model were the Crusaders, who staffed them with various groups of religious. Italian merchants from Amalfi were given permission in the eleventh century by the Caliph of Egypt, who then controlled

Jerusalem, to build a hospital in that city to take care of the pilgrims and travelers who went there. A brother Girard was put in charge. When Jerusalem was captured in 1099 as a result of the First Crusade, the hospital was expanded. Its medical attendants were given official recognition by the pope in 1114 as the Knights of St. John, usually known as the Hospitalers.

The Knights of St. John were charged not only with the care of the sick but with the defense of the Holy Land as well. Saladin's capture of the city in 1187 forced the Hospitalers to flee to Acre. When Acre fell they moved to Rhodes, and when the Turks took Rhodes they ended up in Malta. The nursing activities of the Knights were not confined to the Holy Land or to their headquarters but spread into Western Europe where numerous hospitals were either established or taken over by them throughout Europe. Though their hospitals resembled the Byzantine hospitals in many ways, care was given by the Knights themselves and not by secular nurses.

The extant ruins of the hospital in Jerusalem can give only a sketchy idea of its original extent, but contemporary travelers often left accounts. Among these is one by John of Wurzburg, a German pilgrim who visited Jerusalem circa 1160. He recorded that there were

> an enormous multitude of sick people, both men and women, who are tended and restored to health daily at very great expense. When I was there I learned that the whole number of these sick people amounted to two thousand of whom sometimes in the course of one day and night more than fifty are carried out dead while many other fresh ones keep continually arriving. The same house supplies as many people outside it with victuals as it does those inside, in addition to the boundless charity which is daily bestowed upon poor people who beg their bread from door to door and do not lodge in the house.[19]

Every sick person who came to the hospital was bathed before being carried to a bed where the attendants were instructed to treat him or her as if he/she were a "Lord." Each patient in a Hospitaler hospital was given a cloak of sheepskin and a pair of boots for going to and coming from the latrines located outside of the hospital. The beds of the sick were constructed to be as broad as they were long; this was considered most convenient for repose for the individual patient. Each bed had its own coverlet and special sheet. It is not clear how many wards there were, but each ward had a brother in charge who was required to visit the sick both mornings and evenings. There was also a scribe for clerical duty. Each ward of the hospital had nine sergeants who washed the feet of the sick, changed their linen, made the beds, fed the weak, and in general took care of the sick according to medieval ideals of equilibrium. Just as Byzantine hospitals did, those of the Knights had physicians and surgeons associated with them. A physician was supposed to visit the hospital at least twice a day, accompanied by the nurse-brother, to look over the critically ill patients, and probably to give orders about change in diet or other treatments.

During epidemics a strict quarantine of forty days was imposed, although this probably developed as a procedure after the Knights had left Jerusalem. Many of the knightly hospitals had sisters attached for the benefit of women patients; some also handled maternity cases since the regulations provided that cradles be made for the babies of women pilgrims born in their hospitals. The Knights still exist but are now known as the Order of Malta or Knights of St. John.[20]

Coinciding with the appearance of Western hospitals sponsored by the various crusading groups was an increase in hospitals run by other orders to provide care for the growing numbers of pilgrims, travelers, and indigent poor. Many of the hospitals were administered by the Order of the Holy Spirit, a male order, a smaller number by the Hospitalers, and still others by religious groups such as the Antonines. Nuns staffed some hospitals, but the great expansion of the convent occurred in more modern times. The great majority of hospitals were more or less autonomous without any contact with the others unless the nurses belonged to the same order. There were, however, general guidelines for hospitals in order to ensure some uniformity, with specific policies spelled out in canon law, that is, church law. It is important to emphasize the male dominance in medieval nursing. Although religious women gained considerable influence in the nonknight hospitals, male nurses most likely remained dominant in the West as in the East. It probably was not until the time of St. Vincent de Paul in the seventeenth century that this male dominance was challenged.

Before entering any of the orders that had hospitals, the applicants, whether men or women, had to show that they were freeborn, celibate, free of debts, and not lepers or epileptics. After entering they served a novitiate of about a year where they learned both the care and service of the sick as well as their obligatory religious duties. If the would-be nurses passed the novitiate phase successfully, the chapter voted on whether they would enter fully into the order; each would-be nurse was examined by the bishop. As members of religious orders, they had to observe and perform certain religious duties, but canon law stipulated that these duties were not to interfere with the care of the patients.

The smaller rural hospitals had a master, one or two brothers, and perhaps one or two sisters. They were to attend to the land belonging to the hospital (the source of its income) as well as feed and take care of the pilgrims, the travelers, and the sick poor; the Western hospital served both as a hotel and a hospital. Urban hospitals were much more specialized than those in rural areas, although Western hospitals were never quite as specialized as those of the Byzantine Empire.

The beds in the hospitals varied in size depending on their purpose The so-called great beds (for more than one person) were given to the pilgrims, travelers, or the poor who needed lodging for the night. The truly sick person had a smaller bed of his own, at least this is what the canon law stipulated. Men and women were separated into different wards or rooms, with the seriously ill being put into special wards, designated as infirmaries, to receive special care.

Night nurses or guards were on duty in all wards, partly to assist the patients but also to see that they were properly dressed if they left their beds. In the Middle Ages, both men and women slept naked (but with a nightcap to prevent chills), and one of the duties of the night nurse was to give clothes to the persons leaving their beds, usually to use the latrines. Some hospitals, however, had a series of cisterns and sluices that enabled running water to remove sewage from the hospital so that the latrine might be indoors at one end of the hospital.

By canon law, patients were supposed to be fed before the brothers and sisters working in the hospital and were to eat at least as well as the staff did. If the patients could not feed themselves, the nurses were to do so. Most hospitals had the same meal system as the large Hôtel Dieu in Paris: a main meal at 11 A.M. and at 6 P.M.[21] Though few of the smaller hospitals had physicians attached to them permanently, some occasionally did, especially those with a nearby university. For example, the University at Montpellier, one of the major medieval medical universities, had a practice of sending students to nearby hospitals. Several other universities had similar policies.[22] By the fourteenth century, many of the hospital regulations called for visits by physicians when needed, including those at Paris, Argentan, Angers, Amiens, Dijon, Lyons, Nîmes, Grenoble, and Saint-Quentin in France, and Bruges in modern Belgium.[23] Italian hospitals also had physicians attached; records on English hospitals are not so complete.[24]

Physicians, however, were never as dominant in health care in the Middle Ages as they were to be during much of the twentieth century. Their numbers were limited, and their fees, except in the charitable institutions, high. They simply did not treat the ordinary person. Care in the hospital was given primarily by the attendants who were usually in religious orders; for them, nursing training was an integral part of their novitiate. The caregivers were more than simply servants to the ill and injured, although this aspect was not overlooked. They cared for the sick within the context of the medical theories of the time that emphasized diet, rest, and only occasionally drastic interventions such as bleeding.

The one place where women dominated in nursing was outside the hospital where they were regarded as important healers. Many, if not most, went beyond the simple nursing duties we associate with the aide of today and assumed responsibilities now associated with the modern nurse practitioner or the general medical practitioner. Nurses in the hospital and the folk healers outside the hospital knew the popular pharmacopeia and could distinguish between helpful and unhelpful herbs. Treatments for many of the diseases were standard, done according to a formula; nurses, whether men or women, could carry them out as well as physicians. Since both the religious nurse and the secular healer could purchase or grow the special herbs themselves, only rarely did they need to ask for more expert help. Minor surgery such as lancing boils or pulling teeth was also in their province, although a troublesome tooth might call for the intervention of a barber. Surgery involving amputations, however, did not usually form part of their task. Interestingly enough, in the West all matters dealing with gynecology and obstetrics were usually done outside of the hospital and were reserved for the midwife. Only in the most troublesome cases was a male physician consulted.[25]

Women whose healing knowledge was widely respected were often called "leech," "la Lèche," or "sage femme" (wise women), among other terms. The control that the guilds exercised over the male healing trades was absent among female healers. This meant that the status of the women healer was more informal, as was their education and training. The only kind of institutional education available to women healers was in the convent or in the Byzantine guilds.

What began to separate the healer and the nurse from the physician was the exclusion of women from the universities in the twelfth and thirteenth centuries. Physicians from universities alone had access to the learned treatises of the past, to which they then added their own knowledge. Though medical students were in minor orders, beginning in the twelfth century the church moved to prevent ordained priests from practicing medicine.[26] The exclusion was justified in order to prevent a priest from accidentally shedding blood. However, the church probably wanted to force priests to spend more time on their religious obligations instead of practicing medicine as a sideline as some had done in the past.[27]

Women were also further handicapped when the guilds for barbers, surgeons, and apothecaries developed in the West. Generally, only men could go through the appropriate apprenticeship. Women were occasionally allowed in; these were widows taking over their husband's business and they were aided by other members of the guild. No guild developed for hospital attendants—nor for midwives or women healers of any kind. Women who attempted to extend their practice beyond midwifery or special women's problems were often brought to court by the various guilds. This meant that, as nursing became more of a woman's occupation in the early modern period, women were handicapped by their inability to become members of a guild or to be formally educated. The folk knowledge they had did not grow with the times. Even the women in religious orders, who were often better educated, were prohibited from doing certain medical procedures that were carried out by their male counterparts.[28]

Nursing in the medieval period was far more sophisticated than it usually is given credit for. Also, men played a more prominent role than they do today or than has generally been recognized. In the Byzantine system, hospital nursing became part of the guild system and nurses had wide knowledge of health issues. Nursing was secularized and in a sense professionalized; unfortunately this model did not get translated to the West. In the West the religious nursing model emerged dominant, perhaps because even at the end of the Middle Ages no Western cities could match the Eastern ones in population and wealth.

But the difference between the models was not simply a factor of urbanization. Western monks and nuns, following St. Benedict, had always emphasized work as part of their religious obligations. No such requirement existed in the East and so organized religious orders did not enter into sick care to the same extent as those of the West. Moreover, in the West the disruptions, migrations, and ruralization taking place between the fourth and the eighth centuries cut down secular learning and led to the institutionalized learning confined to the monastery and convent.

When guilds did develop in the West in the eleventh and twelfth centuries, the hospital was already well established as an institution dominated by the religious orders. Though guilds developed for barbers, surgeons, and apothecaries in the West, these people were not necessarily associated with institutions. Physicians, for their part, turned to the university as their entry to practice, and, in their own drive for status, tried to limit the practice of others. As they moved into the hospital their drive for status worked against the nurses.

Complicating the issue in the West was the growing reluctance of the Church to allow clergy and the religious to shed blood, and so Western clerical and religious nursing, especially after the end of the medieval period, could not keep up with changing knowledge. This was especially unfortunate in Catholic areas because many of the new orders for women that appeared in early modern Europe were dedicated to the care of the sick. After the Reformation, the religious nun/nurse was replaced in hospitals in Protestant countries, but the caregivers who replaced them were neither as sophisticated nor as educated and lacked the guild status of the Byzantine caregivers. Nursing in the Protestant West dropped even further behind medicine than was true in the Catholic West. It was not really upgraded until the nineteenth century. Even then many of the reformers—such as Pastor Fliedner—used a religious model.

By that time the physician had become all powerful and dominant—so powerful that historians could simply overlook medieval nursing. In both the Byzantine model and the Western religious model men were extremely influential, but they became much less important in the early modern period. Outside of the hospitals, however, most nursing and, for that matter, most health care was done by women who apparently were regarded as "natural" caregivers and healers.

Men, by excluding women from higher education and from the guilds, maintained authority over health care. When educated women did enter the field again, as women nurses did in the nineteenth century, they were able to do so because they emphasized that women were "natural" caregivers and healers. Therefore, they argued, they were the most appropriate providers of nursing care. Medieval history, however, tends to suggest that this "natural" allocation of rules was not necessarily always the case.

VERN L. BULLOUGH, PhD, RN
SUNY Distinguished Professor
Department of History and Social Studies
SUNY College, Buffalo
1300 Elmwood Avenue
Buffalo, N.Y. 14222
Phone: (716) 878-5412

Bonnie Bullough, PhD, RN
Professor of Nursing
School of Nursing
SUNY College, Buffalo
1010 Stockton Kimball Tower
Buffalo, N.Y. 14214
Phone: (716) 831-3332

Notes

1. Henry Sigerist, "An Outline of the Development of the Hospital," *Bulletin of the History of Medicine* 5 (1936): 579.

2. Paul Starr, *The Social Transformation of American Medicine* (New York: Basic Books, 1982).

3. Lucinda McCray Beier, *Sufferers and Healers: The Experience of Illness in Seventeenth Century England* (New York: Routledge and Kegan Paul, 1987), 2.

4. For discussion of this in greater detail, see Vern L. Bullough, *The Development of Medicine as a Profession: The Contribution of the Medieval University of Modern Medicine* (Basel: Karger, 1966); Vern L. Bullough, "The Development of the Medical Guilds at Paris," *Medievalia et Humanistica* 11 (1958): 33–45; Vern L. Bullough, "Training of Non-University Educated Medical Practitioners in the Later Middle Ages," *Journal of the History of Medicine and Science* 14 (1959): 446–58; Vern L. Bullough, "Status and Medieval Medicine," *Journal of Health and Human Behavior* 2 (1961): 209–20; "Population and the Study and Practice of Medicine," *Bulletin of the History of Medicine* 36 (1962): 620–70.

5. This was true in the seventeenth century and there is little reason to think that that period was different from the Middle Ages. See Beier, *Sufferers and Healers*, passim.

6. See Avicenna, Canon, Book 1, fen 2, doctrina 2, summa 1, chap. 25, fols. 33–34, ed. and trans. by R. Cameron Gruner, *A Treatise on the Canon of Medicine* (London: Luzac and Co., 1930).

7. For an account of this with source documentation, see Vern L. Bullough and Bonnie Bullough, *The Care of the Sick: The Emergence of Modern Nursing* (New York: Neale Watson, Prodist Books, 1978), 28–31.

8. Theodoretos of Cyrrhus, *Ecclesiastical History*, V, 19, 314, ed. Leon Parmentier, under the title of *Theodoret Kirchengeschichte*, 2nd ed. (Berlin: Akademie-Verlag, 1954).

9. St. Jerome, *Select Letters*, LXXVII, par. 6, in *Select Letters of St. Jerome*, ed. and trans. F. A. Wright (London: W. Heinemann, 1933).

10. See Timothy S. Miller, *The Birth of the Hospital in the Byzantine Empire* (Baltimore: Johns Hopkins University Press, 1985). See also Demetrios J. Constantelos, *Byzantine Philanthropy and Social Welfare* (New Brunswick, N.J.: Rutgers University Press, 1968).

11. Miller, 156.

12. There is a vast literature on the Pantokrator, some of it in English. See Pan S. Codellas, "The Pantokrator, the Imperial Byzantine Medical Center of the XIIth Century A.D. in Constantinople," *Bulletin of the History of Medicine* 12 (1942): 391–410; Miller, especially 12–29, 141–66; S. Megaw, "Notes on Recent Work of the Byzantine Institute in Istanbul," *Dumbarton Oaks Papers* 17 (1963): 335–65. The *Typikon* has been edited by Paul Gautier, "Le typikon du Christ Sauveur Pantocrator," *Revue des Etudes Byzantines* 32 (1974): 1–145.

13. Venance Grumel, "La profession medicale à Byzance à l'époque des Commenèes," *Revue des Etudes Byzantines* 7 (1949): 43. For actual source see *The Book of the Eparch* 1.2–3, reprinted with an introduction by Ivan Dujcev (London: Variorum Reprints, 1970), as cited in Miller, 160.

14. Miller, 157–59.

15. Ibid., 215.

16. "Typicon du monastere de la Kosmosotira," ed. Louis Petit, *Bulletin de l'institut russe à Constantinople* 8 (1908): 19–75.

17. Miller, 214.

18. Ibid., 163–64.

19. Aubrey Stewart, "Description of the Holy Land by John of Wurzburg," *Palestine Pilgrims' Text Society* V (1896): 44, and quoted by Edgar Erskine Hume, *Medical Works of the Knights Hospitallers of Saint John of Jerusalem* (Baltimore, Md.: Johns Hopkins University Press, 1940), 14–15. Hume's book is invaluable for an account of the Order since he has collected together so many primary sources.

20. Ibid., passim.

21. For nursing regulations in canon law, see Jean Imbert, *Les Hôpiteau en Droit Canonique* (Paris: Librairie Philosophique J. Vrin, 1947), passim.

22. Vern L. Bullough, *The Development of Medicine as a Profession*, 60, 92; and Vern L. Bullough, "A Note on Medical Care in Medieval English Hospitals," *Bulletin of the History of Medicine* 35 (1961): 74–77. See also Nancy Siraisi, *Medieval and Early Renaissance Medicine* (Chicago: University of Chicago Press, 1990), 39, 180, 188, 191.

23. C. H. Talbot, *Medicine in Medieval England* (London: Oldbourne Book Co., 1967).

24. For a survey of English hospitals, see Rotha Mary Clay, *The Medieval Hospitals of England* (London: Methuen and Company, 1909). There are also studies of individual hospitals such as Norman Moore, *The History of St. Bartholomew's Hospitals*, 2 vols. (London: C. Arthur Pearson, Ltd., 1918).

25. See Siraisi, *Medieval and Renaissance Medicine*, pp. 39–41, for such an example.

26. The clerical influence even extended to teachers to a certain extent; to teach at Paris, the physician had to take a vow of celibacy even though he had never been ordained as a priest. That requirement was abolished in 1452. See *Chartularium Universitatis Parisiensis*, 4 vols., ed. and annotated by Henry Denifle and Aemelio Chatelain (Paris: Delalalin, 1889–97), IV, No. 2690, 723.

27. Such prohibitions were adopted at the Council of Rheims in 1131, the second Lateran in 1139, and the Council of Tours in 1163. See Joannes Dominicus Mansi et al., *Sarcorum conciliorum nova et amalissima collectio*, 31 vols. (Florence and Venice, 1759–98), XXL, 459, 528, 1179.

28. See Bullough, *Development of Medicine as a Profession*, passim.

Nursing on the Canadian Prairies, 1900–1930

Effects of Immigration

INA J. BRAMADAT
Faculty of Nursing
University of Manitoba

MARION I. SAYDAK
Faculty of Nursing
University of Manitoba

Nursing Supervisor
St. Boniface General Hospital

During the early 1900s, thousands of European immigrants settled in rapidly growing urban centers, in small farming communities, and on isolated prairie homesteads in Western Canada. The new immigrants differed in two ways from earlier settlers who came to the Prairies before the turn of the century: First, they arrived in substantially greater numbers, and second, they were of different ethnic origin from the earlier wave of predominantly Anglo-Saxon, English-speaking homesteaders from Eastern Canada, Great Britain, and the United States. Both the magnitude of immigration and the different ethnic origin of the new arrivals had an impact on the development and organization of nursing services in the Prairie Provinces.

Health care services on the Prairies in 1900 were limited to twenty hospitals and a few dozen nurses and physicians; many settlers relied on home remedies and lay caregivers. Since little provision had been made for the health care of new immigrants, the rapid growth in population after 1900 placed extraordinary demands on existing resources. Agencies and individuals responded to the urgent need for health care. By 1930 several hundred trained nurses were registered in the three Prairie Provinces.[1] More than three hundred new hospitals had been established and health care was provided through a variety of agencies, including the provincial governments, Victorian Order of Nurses for Canada, Canadian Red Cross Society, Women's Missionary Society, missions, hospitals, and clinics.

This study examined the interaction between the rapid influx of new

Nursing History Review 1 (1993): 105–17.

settlers and the growth and organization of nursing services on the Canadian Prairies. Sources included census reports, public health records, reports of private agencies, personal memoirs, letters and articles in early nursing journals, and archival photographs.

Immigration

In the final decades of the nineteenth century, the newly formed Dominion of Canada faced a major challenge. Between the western boundary of the Great Lakes and the Rocky Mountains more than 1,000 miles west lay millions of acres of arable prairie grasslands. This land was then under the control of the Hudson's Bay Company as part of its fur-trading empire.[2] Rapid westward expansion in the United States threatened to overflow into the Canadian prairies and to challenge ownership of this territory.[3] In 1870 the Canadian government purchased the Hudson's Bay Company land and began building a railway to link the western provinces with eastern Canada. Recognizing that the railway could succeed only if the lands were settled, the Canadian government passed the Dominion Land Act in 1872, which provided free homesteads to settlers locating in the West.

The first wave of homesteaders to the Canadian prairies (1872–1900) were predominantly English-speaking and of Anglo-Saxon origin. Toward the end of the century, however, this wave of immigration tapered off, and the large landholders—government, railways, land companies, and a few individuals—launched major campaigns to attract settlers from other countries. The campaigns targeted farm workers or peasants of Eastern Europe. The plains of Austria-Hungary, Russia, and other European countries were similar to the Canadian prairies, and it was expected that peasants from these areas would be well suited to the prairie farms.

The frontier, with its relatively open social and economic opportunities, was attractive to East Europeans. Immigration handbills emphasized the prospects for work, improved life-style, and ownership of land in a country where men were their own masters. In reality, by 1900 much of the most arable land already was occupied. New immigrants faced years of extreme hardship as they cleared their land, built their first homes, and made their farms viable. Many immigrants did not have the finances to purchase the animals, implements, and seed needed to start a farming operation; they worked instead in mining and lumber camps or on railway construction. Other families congregated in cities, often living in impoverished conditions.[4]

Thousands of settlers arrived each year. Between 1901 and 1931 the population of the Province of Manitoba increased from 255,211 to 700,139 inhabitants; Saskatchewan increased from 91,279 to 921,785; and Alberta increased from 73,022 to 731,605 inhabitants.[5] Within one generation, between 1897 and 1913, the ethnic composition of the West changed dramatically.[6] The southern half of the prairies therefore became a mosaic of distinct ethnic and linguistic communities.[7]

Health Care of Settlers

Immigrants who settled in ethnic communities tended to remain outside the mainstream Anglo-Saxon culture. They retained many of their own cultural values and beliefs, including traditional health care practices. Earlier European immigrants, such as the Mennonites from southern Russia, had migrated in self-sufficient groups, bringing their own midwives and lay healers.[8] Settlers who arrived in the West after 1900 did not follow this pattern.

The new wave of settlers were fortunately fairly healthy. Immigration officials had learned from earlier experiences with contagious diseases in the mid-nineteenth century to impose strict quarantine regulations and detain immigrants for examination before leaving Europe. Concerns rose, however, about the incidence of diseases such as tuberculosis among the foreign population as a result of their living conditions. Dr. David Stewart, medical superintendent of the Manitoba Sanatorium in Ninette, and brother of Isabel Maitland Stewart, wrote in a nursing journal:

> In Manitoba, the settlements in which tuberculosis is most prevalent are those in which living standards are lowest, where ignorance is general, houses small, sanitary conditions bad, overcrowding common, work hard, the average of wealth low; old settlements of ignorant and unmodern type; foreign uncanadian settlements, out of touch with modern movements; pioneer settlements, in which there is more or less privation.[9]

Since no provision was made for sanitation or clean water supplies in the rapidly growing frontier communities, outbreaks of infectious diseases were common.

These problems were exacerbated by the limited health care services in the new homeland. Few settlers could afford medical care, even when it was available. Some medical supervision was provided at the Immigration Building in Winnipeg (the "gateway to the West"), and federal grants were made to hospitals to cover costs of treating needy immigrants. No other provisions were made for medical or nursing care for the settlers, however, and the responsibility for health care was left to the communities where they settled.

Growth of Nursing Services

The response of nursing to this rapid influx of new settlers was evident, first, in the rapid increase in the number of nursing services and, second, in the type of services that developed during the early 1900s. As cities and towns grew along the rail lines, hospitals were established in small communities. The 1901 census recorded twenty hospitals in the prairie region with a total of 621 beds.[10] Most nursing care was provided in the home, occasionally by a private duty nurse, more often by family members or neighbors. One nurse wrote rather poignantly about the hardships of private duty nursing "here in the West, where the field is so wide, nurses so scarce, and facilities, especially in smaller towns, so meagre."[11] Even when available, the services of a trained nurse were beyond the means of most new Canadians. A common fee for trained nurses ranged from twenty to twenty-five dollars per week.[12]

Urban Care

In the early 1900s, social reform was a pressing issue in North America. The concerns of reformers focused on sanitation, hygiene, and maternal and infant mortality. In major cities in the West, as in other parts of Canada and the United States, health-related services were organized, including milk depots where mothers could purchase inspected milk, well baby clinics, and antepartum clinics.[13]

The Victorian Order of Nurses for Canada (VON) was one of the first services formed in response to the growing need for community-based care. Founded in 1897 under the leadership of Lady Aberdeen, the wife of the governor-general of Canada, the VON initially was conceived as a means of providing nursing care to women and children in isolated western settlements.[14] The first branch of the VON was established in the West in 1905. Nurses employed by the VON coped with epidemics of typhoid and influenza, home emergencies, and care of the chronically ill. They also assisted physicians with home deliveries and provided prenatal and postpartum care. The VON employed mothers' helpers who worked in the

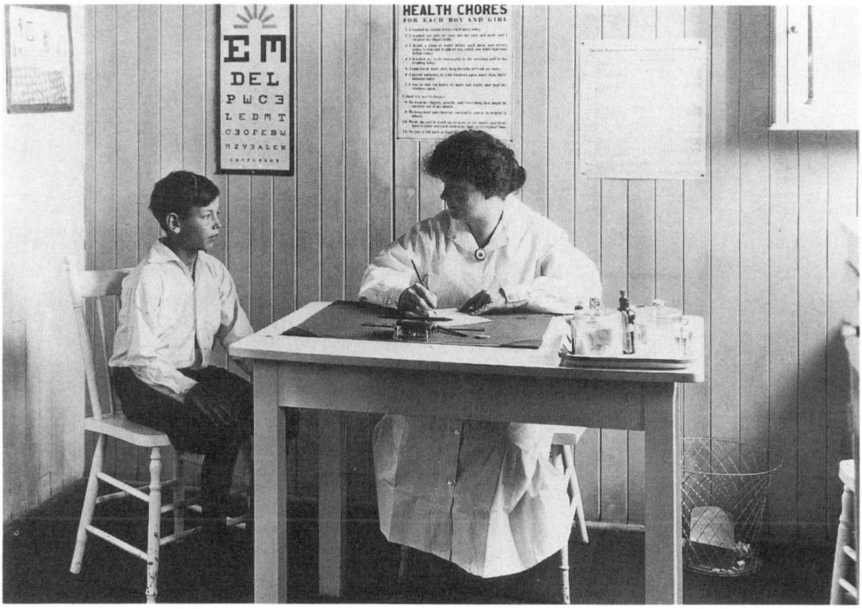

Health inspection of a schoolchild, Brooklands, 1923. (Provincial Archives of Manitoba, Public Health 63, N13039)

home under a nurse's supervision for a small fee. Some services were specific to immigrants. In the City of Winnipeg, for example, a clinic offered care for Ukrainian women.[15]

Poverty was endemic to urban areas; even though the VON based its fees on ability to pay, many could not afford home care. Missions took on the care of these families. The *First Annual Report* of the Margaret Scott Mission shows that nurses quickly had found ways to extend their care and to reach their non-English speaking clients: "We have now arranged that the assistants to the nurses shall do the chores in the homes of the sick, carry supplies, etc. . . . These helpers are, as a rule, foreigners, this being very useful among our cosmopolitan population."[16]

Rural Care

It was particularly difficult to deliver health care to rural areas in the early 1900s. After World War I, the Canadian Red Cross Society undertook a program of peacetime national involvement in health care. The Red Cross established outpost nursing stations in isolated regions and opened small hospitals in many rural communities.[17] The VON also established small, homelike "cottage" hospitals across Western Canada. The cottage hospitals initially were established to accommodate up to ten patients with quarters for two nurses and a maid.[18] The first VON hospital on the Prairies was established in Regina, Saskatchewan, in 1898.[19]

Missionaries also provided health care. As tides of immigration from Europe swept over the Prairies, religious denominations became aware of opportunities to spread their influence. Although many of the new settlers were Greek Orthodox or Greek Catholic, Protestant missionaries evangelized them in the belief that "assimilation would not be complete until 'Christianization' occurred," that is, conversion to evangelical Protestant values.[20] Catholic missions had long been present on the Prairies. Now Protestant missions undertook to "Canadianize" new immigrants by building hospitals, churches, and schools near ethnic settlements. Nurses and physicians served as medical missionaries in the communities.[21]

The impact of immigration on nursing was also evident in the development of public health services. Manitoba, in 1916, was the first prairie province to employ public health nurses; Saskatchewan followed in 1917 and Alberta in 1918. A public health report records that:

> At this period in our history, a great many deaths among the infant population, especially among our immigrants, were never reported—burials being made in the back yard. This was probably the underlying reasons for the employment of nurses, i.e. to investigate these deaths and to educate people as to what might be done to prevent them.[22]

Public health nurses detected "symptoms of disease and physical defects, unreported communicable diseases, unreported births, malpractice in midwifery, and unsanitary conditions, especially detrimental to the welfare of mothers and children."[23] It was noted that

> the attention of the government was repeatedly drawn to the fact that hundreds of thousands of dollars were expended annually out of the Public Exchequer to teach farmers how to raise colts, calves, and pigs, but not one dollar was devoted to teach the mother how to rear her young.[24]

The belief that "the health of the family is the health of the nation" provided the justification for many of the health-related services.[25] Nurses used a comprehensive, preventive approach, including instruction in personal and community hygiene; sanitation in the home, school, and community; care of infants and preschool children; simple home nursing; and first aid. Young girls thirteen years of age and older were encouraged to join the

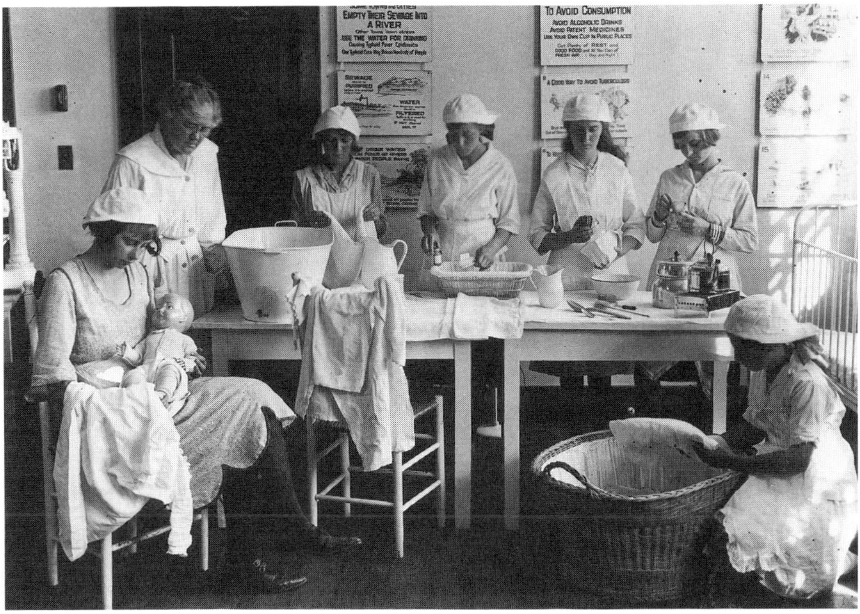

East Kildonan Little Mothers' League class, 1922. (Provincial Archives of Manitoba, Public Health 40, N14289)

Little Mothers' League where they learned home nursing and infant care. They were to share this teaching with their mothers, many of whom did not speak English. The targeted group were from "the underprivileged classes, and some from foreign homes, where old-time and old-country methods prevailed."[26]

Public health nurses also gave speeches to groups such as the Women's Institute and the Women Grain Growers. They taught short courses in home nursing, conducted child welfare conferences, arranged health exhibits at local fairs, examined school children, and provided teachers with health literature and teaching aids.[27] Initially, public health nurses provided a free demonstration of their services for the municipality; if the municipality then wanted to continue the service, it paid one third of the cost.[28]

Nurses in isolated rural areas faced a number of problems, including illiteracy, poverty, poor housing conditions, and inadequate transportation. They traveled on horseback, by railway handcars, by horse and buggy, or by sleigh in winter. Not until the late 1920s did automobiles and telephones begin to replace less effective means of travel and communication.

A director of public health nursing recalled that "the people were very kind, but the accommodations were very poor."[29] In one description of living conditions, it is noted that:

> Houses had no electric lighting, running water or central heating. In winter water froze in the wash basins overnight, and frost lined the windows. The joys of summer were diminished by black flies and mosquitoes. The nursing stations and hospitals lacked not only conveniences, but often necessities.[30]

The "Foreign Problem" in Health Care

The immigrants' traditional beliefs and their initial fear and distrust of the Anglo-Saxon dominated government and its institutions exacerbated the problems of new settlers by further alienating them from the Anglo-Saxon mainstream. British descendants, in turn, feared becoming a minority to European immigrants. Social Darwinism, or belief in survival of the fittest, was still a fashionable idea at that time. Proof of Anglo-Saxon superiority was considered self-evident in the ascendancy of the British Empire.[31] The Anglo-Saxon majority candidly expressed their attitude to "foreign" settlers and soon forgot the role of immigrants in securing the West for Canada.

In the early 1900s, nursing was one of the few respectable occupations for women, attracting Anglo-Saxons with mainstream attitudes and values, including the prevailing attitudes to new Canadians.[32] The "foreign problem" in health care was described by one nurse: "The Canadianizing of foreigners is the greatest problem that we have to deal with [in public health] today."[33] Another public health nurse subscribed to the belief that, since the teachings of childhood persist for life, "does not that truth make our duty [to teach the children Canadian ways] the more plain . . . if we would have our future Canadian citizens a credit, not a blight, upon our nation?"[34] Nurses often approached their task with a patriotic spirit and a missionary zeal that was not unlike that of the medical missionaries.

One area of health care in which mainstream values were evident was in the stance Prairie nurses took on the issue of midwifery. In contrast to their active and creative role in developing new services, Western nurses voiced their opposition to initiatives expanding "old country" practices such as midwifery. Many newcomers to the Prairies came from countries where midwifery was an established tradition. In 1921, when maternal/infant mortality first appeared as a separate item in the records of the Dominion Bureau of Statistics, it became evident that Canada had a mortality rate higher than most "civilized" nations.[35] The National Council of

Women took up this concern, attributing the high mortality rates to lack of care in isolated areas of the West. Sharply divided opinions were expressed about possible solutions to the problem. One solution was to train and license midwives; an alternative was to extend existing nursing services.

Western Canadian nurses soundly rejected the introduction of trained midwives. Suzanne Buckley, writing in 1976 from a feminist perspective, was appalled that health professionals blocked plans to bring midwives to Canada: "Most nurses were too unwilling to threaten their economic well-being and their professionalism to do much to mitigate the problems of infant and maternal mortality."[36] Instead, she argued, nurses deferred to physicians and fought to retain their status by refusing to perform obstetrical work since it involved the domestic labor associated with the old working-class image of nurses.[37] Buckley argued, in other words, that nurses abandoned other women in their drive for professionalization of nursing.

The writings of nurses from this time suggest a less severe interpretation. Their expressed motive for discouraging midwifery was not to professionalize nursing but to ensure provision of professional care. Prairie nurses shared the national concern for high maternal and infant mortality, but they refused to accept what they viewed as a second-class, "foreign" approach to maternity care. Western nurses informed the National Council of Women in Toronto (the "Easterners") that:

> The Canadian mother does not want a midwife, and you cannot make her want one. When you have midwives for yourselves and your daughters, then the prairies wife may begin to think there is something in it. I know the Prairie woman well. . . . She wants the best Canada has to offer and she gets it when the crops are good.[38]

Western nurses believed that they had developed a superior approach to meeting the needs of women and children in isolated settlements and outposts. In this approach preventive services were provided from birth through the childbearing years.[39] One nurse explained:

> While people have been talking for years and years of the perils to Mothers on the Prairies, the Canadian Red Cross Society has been quietly working out a solution. . . . Outposts have been established in outlying and sparsely settled districts. . . . A registered nurse is in charge. . . . A Doctor is always called for a case of labor, but if he cannot get there, the nurse delivers the case. . . . In Saskatchewan, of 400 cases delivered, there has not been a single death.[40]

Nurses recommended that the government fund the training of more nurses rather than restructure the system to provide for the training and licensing of midwives.

Conclusions

The influx of large numbers of immigrants to Western Canada during the early 1900s led to the development of a wide range of new nursing services on the Prairies. Rapid expansion of services and innovative approaches were needed to meet the challenge of providing health care for the wave of newcomers who settled in urban areas, small towns, and rural ethnic communities. Nurses developed services where few existed. Immigrant poverty, language barriers, traditional beliefs and health care practices, isolation, and difficult travel conditions challenged the resources of early nurses. Within a span of thirty years, many new health care services were developed. In addition to hospital and private-duty nursing, clinics, home visiting, outpost nursing, and public health nursing became available. Services were offered through a variety of agencies and institutions including the provincial governments, Canadian Red Cross Society, Victorian Order of Nurses for Canada, Women's Missionary Society, missions, and hospitals. Immigration thus provided the impetus for development of nursing and shaped the focus and direction of care. Nursing services, as they developed on the prairie frontier, reflected the values and biases of the Western Canadian Anglo-Saxon mainstream. Provision of nursing care to new immigrants represented a "cause" based on idealistic beliefs about service and the need to "Canadianize" foreigners to ensure the health of future Canadians. This bias also was evident in the vocal opposition of Western nurses to "foreign" practices such as midwifery.

In the present decade, the health care system in Canada is being challenged by the influx of new waves of immigrants from Asia and other countries with non-Caucasian populations. In contrast with the early 1900s, these immigrants are coming to already populated areas with a well-developed health care system. In addition, nurses now profess a strong commitment to multicultural sensitivity. It will be interesting to observe whether the interaction between the new wave of immigrants and contemporary nursing services differs substantially from that of the early 1900s.

Ina J. Bramadat, RN, PhD
Assistant Professor and Associate Dean
Faculty of Nursing
University of Manitoba
224 Bison Building
Winnipeg, Manitoba
Canada
R3T 2N2
Phone: (204) 474-6222
Fax: (204) 275-5464

Marion I. Saydak, RN, MN
Nursing Supervisor
St. Boniface General Hospital
Lecturer
Faculty of Nursing
University of Manitoba
224 Bison Building
Winnipeg, Manitoba
Canada
R3T 2N2
Phone: (204) 474-9132

Acknowledgment

The authors of this paper wish to acknowledge the editorial assistance of Glennis Zilm.

Notes

1. G. M. Weir, *Survey of Nursing Education in Canada* (Toronto: University of Toronto Press, 1932), 19. In 1930 the Provincial Registrars listed a total of 1,559 active registered nurses in the three Prairie Provinces. This number does not include inactive registered nurses, those working in occupations other than nursing, or untrained "practical" nurses.

2. The boundaries of the Territories and the Province of Manitoba subsequently were extended, and the "Prairie Provinces" now include three provinces: Manitoba, Saskatchewan, and Alberta.

3. Paul F. Sharp, *The Agrarian Revolt in Western Canada* (Minneapolis: University of Minnesota Press, 1948), points out that "American immigration had a marked impact on Western Canada. Year after year the national group making the

most homestead entries was the Americans. The keys were the differences in land prices—Dakota land was fifty dollars an acre in 1909 and the same type of land in Saskatchewan was two dollars an acre—and the fact that Canada promised the opportunity for continued ethnic and religious cohesion within settlement colonies" (p. 7). In Alberta, for example, 3,200 Mormons settled in the towns of Cardston and McGrath.

4. Harry Piniuta, *Land of Pain: Land of Promise—First Person Accounts by Ukrainian Pioneers 1891–1914* (Saskatoon: Western Producer Prairies Books, 1978), 167–68.

5. F. H. Leacy, *Historical Statistics of Canada*, 2nd ed. (Ottawa: Statistics Canada, 1983), ser. A2-14.

6. Gerald Friesen, *The Canadian Prairies: A History* (Toronto: University of Toronto Press, 1984), 244. Classification by ethnic origin and country of origin varies in early census reports. Detailed statistics are compiled for some Eastern European groups, for example, William Darcovich and Paul Yuzyk, eds., *A Statistical Compendium on the Ukrainians in Canada, 1891–1976* (Ottawa: University of Ottawa Press, 1980). For general information see, for example, Canadian Citizenship Branch, *The Canadian Family Tree* (Ottawa: Queen's Printer, 1967), which describes major settlement areas of ethnic groups.

7. Craig Brown, *The Illustrated History of Canada* (Toronto: Lester and Orpen Dennys Limited, 1987), 391.

8. Carl A. Dawson, *Group Settlement: Ethnic Communities in Western Canada* (Toronto: Ethnic Communities in Western Canada, 1936).

9. David A. Stewart, "Tuberculosis Problems of Today," *The Canadian Nurse* (May 1919): 1732 (hereafter cited as *CN*).

10. *Fourth Census of Canada 1901 D* 4 (Ottawa: Dawson, 1906). By the 1930s the number of hospitals in the Prairie provinces had increased dramatically. The *Second Annual Report of Hospitals in Canada for the Year 1933* (Ottawa: Dominion Bureau of Statistics—Canada, 1935) reported the following: Manitoba—48 hospitals, 4,243 beds; Saskatchewan—140 hospitals, 4,424 beds; Alberta—135 hospitals, 4,706 beds.

11. Lucy Hatch, "Private Duty Nursing in Alberta," *CN* (April 1920): 200–201.

12. Mrs. George Cran, *A Woman in Canada* (London: John Milne, 1910). Mrs. Cran, an Englishwoman, toured Western Canada in 1908. She promoted the importation of trained British midwives since midwives would charge only ten dollars per week for maternity services.

13. "Child Welfare Work in the City of Winnipeg," *CN* (January 1918): 811–14.

14. John M. Gibbon, *The Victorian Order of Nurses for Canada* (Montreal: Southam Press, 1947).

15. Annie P. Smith, *Twenty-third Annual Report of the Victorian Order of Nurses (Winnipeg Branch)* (Winnipeg: Victorian Order of Nurses, 1924), 6.

16. The Margaret Scott Nursing Mission of Winnipeg, *First Annual Report* (Winnipeg: Margaret Scott Nursing Mission, 1905), 6.

17. F. C. Middleton, "Report of Committee on Rural Communities, Nursing and Social," *The Public Health Journal* (June 1921): 254–58 (hereafter cited as *PHJ*).

18. John M. Gibbon, *Three Centuries of Canadian Nursing* (Toronto: Macmillan Company of Canada Limited, 1947).

19. Gibbon, *Victorian Order of Nurses*, 69.

20. Michael Owen, "Keeping Canada God's Country: Presbyterian Schoolhomes for Ruthenian Children," in *Prairie Spirit*, ed. D. Butcher, C. McPherson, A. Smith, and A. M. Watts (Winnipeg: University of Manitoba Press, 1985), 190.

21. Raymond Smith, "A Heritage of Healing: Church Work and Medical Work in Manitoba," in *Prairie Spirit*, ed. D. Butcher, C. McPherson, A. Smith, and A. M. Watts (Winnipeg: University of Manitoba Press, 1985), 265–82.

22. Public Health Nursing Division, *Public Health Nursing in Manitoba 1916–1936* (Winnipeg: Department of Health and Public Welfare, 1936), 6.

23. Ibid., 7.

24. Ibid., 4.

25. Annah L. Pritchard, "The Victorian Order of Nurses for Canada—Maternity," *PHJ* (July 1923): 323.

26. J. Stothart, "The Big Sister at School," *CN* (September 1928): 485. See C. Peers, "Home Nursing and Child Welfare in the Rural Districts," *CN* (December 1923): 722–24 for an account of district nursing activities in Saskatchewan, and Elizabeth Russell, "Provincial Public Health Nursing in Manitoba," *PHJ* (August 1921): 360–67 for roles and responsibilities of PHN in Manitoba.

27. F. C. Middleton, "Report of Committee on Rural Communities, Nursing and Social," *PHJ* (June 1921): 254–58.

28. Public Health Nursing Division, 6.

29. Elizabeth Russell, interview with Beatrice Fines, 1975, quoted in Beatrice Fines, *History of the Manitoba Association of Registered Nurses* (Winnipeg: 1978), 119.

30. Fines, 119.

31. Vaughan Cornish, "The Geographical Aspects of Eugenics," *PHJ* (July 1925): 317–19.

32. During this period names of students enrolled in nursing programs and contributors to nursing journals are of Anglo-Saxon origin.

33. Christine Smith, "Public Health Nursing," *CN* (August 1919): 1910.

34. Jean Crosbie, "The Foreign Problem as Related to Health," *CN* (March 1920): 137.

35. Helen McMurchy, "On Maternal Mortality in Canada," *PHJ* (September 1925): 410–16.

36. Suzanne Buckley, "Ladies or Midwives? Efforts to Reduce Infant and Maternal Mortality," in *A Not Unreasonable Claim: Women and Reform in Canada 1880s–1920s*, ed. Linda Keatley (Toronto: Women's Press, 1979), 149.

37. Ibid., 149.

38. Kate Mathieson, First Vice-President of Canadian Nurses Association, address to a meeting of the National Council of Women, Toronto, 1925, reported in Ethel Johns, "The Practice of Midwifery in Canada," *CN* (January 1925): 13.

39. Esther M. Beith, "Prenatal Nursing Supervision," *Canadian Public Health Journal* (October 1937): 595.

40. Kate Mathieson, 13.

Brilliance and Bureaucracy

Nursing and Changes in the Rockefeller Foundation, 1915–1930

SARAH E. ABRAMS
School of Nursing
University of California, San Francisco

"Are foundations showing the imagination and resourcefulness on social issues that their founders showed in business and that modern society so desperately needs?" Edwin R. Embree, former officer of the Rockefeller Foundation and president of the Rosenwald Fund, rhetorically posed the question to readers of *Harpers Magazine* in 1949.[1] It was not the first time he had raised the question; his letters to a close friend and his earlier publications had time and again described the nature, opportunities, and pitfalls of foundation giving.[2] Yet, after more than thirty years in corporate philanthropy, Embree still appeared uneasy about the gains achieved through foundation giving. He characterized the architects of foundations as men of noble intentions and creative thought, but continually reiterated his concern that these same foundations entrenched, bureaucratized, and professionalized their activities. Rather than search for new but possibly risky projects, foundations for the first time possessed an interest in perpetuating the status quo; this limited the role they might have played in improving society.[3]

Throughout most of the 1920s, Embree directed the foundation's nursing investments; during this period, the Rockefeller Foundation underwrote a program to reform nursing education and supported other selected nursing projects. The relationship between organizational developments within the foundation and its program of giving is part of the contextual background of a turbulent period in which the professional territories of medicine, public health, nursing, education, and social work were redefined.

Nursing in the Rockefeller Foundation Before 1930

Between 1918 and 1930, various divisions of the Rockefeller Foundation contributed approximately $2.3 million to nursing education, practice, and

Nursing History Review 1 (1993): 119–37.

professional development in the United States.[4] Foundation monies helped develop two university schools of nursing; supported the National Organization for Public Health Nursing through formative and financially precarious years; funded the Goldmark Report, a study of nursing education sometimes considered the counterpart of the Flexner report on medical education; enabled nurse leaders to travel the country and the world sharing ideas; and paid for nursing care in established and experimental projects of urban and rural public health. Although dwarfed by Rockefeller donations to medical science and public health during the same period, the commitment of these funds nonetheless symbolized social and professional legitimacy for those nurses who sought foundation support. The fact that nursing as an occupational field had, by the early 1920s, found patrons among the senior officers of the foundation and a place on the agendas of the board of trustees gave a small cadre of nurse reformers the leverage needed to accomplish objectives they had formulated at least a decade prior.

Given its program in health, the Rockefeller Foundation had an obvious stake in developing nursing. Reformed medical education required the support of nurses adequately prepared to provide and manage patient care in hospitals where medical students would be taught. Foundation activities in domestic and international public health were at their zenith between 1910 and 1930. Just as the hospital or private duty nurse might be considered "the physician's hand," public health nurses were the hands and feet of public health officers. Nurses were the field-workers in the campaign for improved public health; in this country they were considered the most effective agents of social acculturation for the masses of new immigrants and the lower classes in a rapidly changing New South.[5]

Documents recording official policies in the Rockefeller Foundation between 1915 and 1930 illustrate shifts in the foundation's approach to nursing. From a beginning posture of cautious and even skeptical inquiry about the nature of nursing and nurse training, the appeal of the profession reached its zenith in the early 1920s with publication of Goldmark's comprehensive report on nursing education and subsequent development of what were considered great educational experiments. The ensuing years saw the foundation retreat from demonstration to concentrate on dissemination of information through its fellowship program. Throughout the period, the foundation contributed small amounts directly supporting the work of nurses.[6] By the end of the decade, though, the foundation believed that it had laid the groundwork for widespread reform through its earlier activities. Coinciding with its move away from education and social services, the foundation gradually withdrew from new commitments to American nursing, even though appropriations to U.S. nursing education or practice did not end in the 1920s. Indeed, the endowment of the Vanderbilt University School of Nursing did not actually occur until the 1930s.

Origin of the Modern Foundation

The great foundations were created by applying the principles of trusteeship and corporate methods to scientific philanthropy.[7] During the late nineteenth century, scientific philanthropy emerged as a corrective for the supposed sentimentality and disorganization of private charity. Almsgiving became unfashionable "counterfeit philanthropy" by the 1870s and 1880s; charity, it was feared, would result in the pauperization of its beneficiaries. Replacing simple almsgiving were the reputedly scientific principles of organization and dissemination of information designed to aid those who would help themselves. Late nineteenth-century ideas of political economy and natural science, particularly social Darwinism and eugenics, informed the organization of charitable movements; by the 1890s the doctrines of scientific philanthropy were being promulgated throughout the country by the very powerful National Conference of Charities and Correction.[8]

Concurrently, a handful of geniuses in capitalist enterprise succeeded in amassing fortunes previously unknown in America. These men, at the peak of their careers, were faced with a problem: the possession of so much wealth that there seemed to be no way to spend it. Perhaps because of guilt about acquiring so much at the expense of so many, a sense of moral responsibility, or self-interest in improving public relations, several of the great "robber barons" of the nineteenth century turned to philanthropy as they grew older.[9] Reared according to his mother's values, John D. Rockefeller, Sr., had donated a portion of his earnings to charity since youth; true to Calvinist dogma, he claimed trusteeship as a spiritual duty—the obligation of the man who had been given the gift of making money by God.

The irony of the partnership did not escape one economist who noted, "Mammon made the money and then God decided how to spend it."[10] Andrew Carnegie's 1889 essay, "Wealth," made famous his perspective that a wealthy man became so because he was the fittest to survive and triumph in the corporate struggle. Carnegie believed that the wealthy individual should give, not because God had entrusted him with the obligation, but because trusteeship devolved on the man fittest to exercise it.[11] Carnegie may have been singularly secular in his perspective, but to one extent or another the major benefactors at the turn of the century adhered to a common understanding of their role as trustees.

Although the founders of the major philanthropies were guided by differing beliefs about the origin of trusteeship, most organized their foundations on sound corporate principles. Principles that worked well in business, they reasoned, could be imposed on philanthropic activity so that investments in health, education, or welfare would achieve for society results that investments in oil, steel, and railroads had produced for them. To this end, benefactors such as John D. Rockefeller, Sr., hired organizational expertise for their foundations just as they would in industry. Frederick T. Gates, chief architect of the Rockefeller philanthropies, was one such organizer. A Baptist minister by training, Gates had shown more talent as a planner and financier than he had demonstrated as a spiritual leader. His value to Rockefeller was that he was a rare blend of visionary and organizational genius.[12] Something of his power to inspire must have survived this turn in his career; Embree repeatedly stated how much he admired Gates's intelligence and "exuberant imagination," noting that Gates "attempted deliberately to find things that might be of fundamental benefit to society."[13]

Managing Corporate Philanthropy

Even with visionary leadership, foundations did not and do not operate strictly from ideological perspectives. While a policy may indeed be formulated and officially adopted by trustees, actual funding decisions may often be matters of political or financial expediency. Corporate philanthropy in the second and third decades of this century was highly reactive to social pressures and organizational politics. The officers and trustees of the Rockefeller Foundation reacted to allegations that their motives arose from self-interest and corporate greed. They frequently took pains to articulate broad social goals and to disavow any interest in controlling how projects were actually implemented. Direct philanthropy, such as that of the Rockefeller Sanitary Commission (1909–1914) or the foundation's later postwar reconstruction activities, for instance, helped reverse the foundation's negative public image. Nonetheless, the role and responsibilities of foundations were debated throughout the era in which industrial magnates created and defined these new philanthropic institutions. Perceptions of the social value of funded programs generated discussion among the emerging class of philanthropic managers and influenced the actions of trustees.

Foundations built on an amalgam of scientific principles and commercial practices, administered by paid executive staff with some expertise in specific fields of interest, became businesses in their own right. The initial goals were broadly sketched, but the directions taken were largely based on the interests and needs of the moment. The funds of foundations have been described as "the venture capital of philanthropy, best invested in activities requiring risk and foresight that are not likely to be supported either by government or private individuals."[14] Risk and lack of appropriate alternative support were common denominators in developing programs of giving for many early trustees and officers of the modern foundations. Carnegie, for example, refused to fund hospitals, seeing them as being appropriately supported by cities, just like prisons.[15]

John D. Rockefeller, Sr., had initially engaged in what Gates termed "retail giving," contributing funds as an individual in a random fashion to those presenting worthy causes. Gates was convinced that this enterprise was inconsistent with Rockefeller's dynamic approach to business. After successfully directing the establishment of the University of Chicago, Gates turned his attention instead to a plan for "wholesale philanthropy," suggesting a number of funds Rockefeller might establish: higher education, medical research, promotion of the arts, and scientific agriculture.[16]

Even before the establishment of the Rockefeller Foundation in 1913, Gates, with John D. Rockefeller, Jr., wrote strict guidelines for the distribution of the Rockefeller wealth using principles of scientific philanthropy. Money was to be given to proven organizations able to continue their work after gifts had been exhausted. Gifts should constitute "seed money" only—to stimulate support from other sources and develop independence in beneficiaries. Money would not be given to individuals or to local institutions except those that were established as models for the development of like institutions. Research institutions were preferred to organizations that treated individual problems since Gates and Rockefeller believed research could more effectively cut to the root of such problems.[17]

Paid staff gradually assumed responsibility for the daily functioning of the organizations encompassed within the Rockefeller philanthropies. The Rockefeller Institute (1901), the General Education Board (1903), and the Rockefeller Sanitary Commission (1909) all preceded incorporation of the foundation in 1913. The early officers and staff of the foundation frequently were ministers or educators who came to Rockefeller's attention through contact with influential members of his or Gates's circle of advisors or as a result of Rockefeller activities in public health and social hygiene.

Applications for aid were evaluated on the basis of their "goodness of fit" with the criteria of scientific philanthropy as outlined by Gates and the junior Rockefeller, but the personal and professional credentials of applicants were also weighed, particularly with regard to potential for leadership. More often than not, foundation officers told those who had been denied assistance that their proposals were worthy but that the specifics were not within the present fields of interest of the foundation. Sometimes they would refer applicants to other sources. Occasionally, staff provided specific reasons about why the Rockefeller Foundation was not interested, citing projects that, for example, should be supported by the community or by the government, organizations unlikely to become self-sustaining within a short period of time, and proposals that duplicated services already established were common reasons for denial of funds.

The initial chartered purpose of the Rockefeller Foundation was to promote "the well-being of mankind throughout the world."[18] The agenda, in the early years, can be characterized as an experiment for social betterment. Embree, who held various offices in the foundation for ten years, later noted, however, that it was difficult for some to reconcile to the fact that not every worthy cause would be funded. "A characteristic of the successful funds is that they are not charitable organizations in the regularly accepted sense; they are constructive forces, initiating or stimulating activity in a definite province."[19] Indeed, the trustees envisioned that their gifts to specific institutions and professional groups would have far-ranging impact, a view consistent with the guidelines established by Gates and Rockefeller, Jr. Officers of the foundation occasionally tried to explain this broader agenda of the organization or the rationale behind its policy decisions. George E. Vincent, who assumed the presidency in 1918 and was described by later president Raymond B. Fosdick as the foremost interpreter of foundation actions to America, explained the organization's 1921 world health goals.[20] Demonstrations were financed to convince authorities of the efficacy of certain policies and procedures: "hookworm" control was not only an end in itself but a vehicle for the transmission of public health education to rural communities; fieldwork had the purpose of investigation of conditions and extension of research; fellowships allowed for the training of health officers and leaders of professions and for the dissemination of knowledge; work in China aided the spread of Western technology and practice and helped support missionary efforts in Asia. In short, the worldwide efforts of the Rockefeller in linking people and information would serve as the advance guard for international interdependence.[21]

Perpetuity and Plutocracy

When, between 1910 and 1912, the Rockefeller Foundation sought a charter under U.S. law, leading newspapers and journals gave the proposals and progress of legislation extensive coverage—some favorable, others voicing popular sentiment that was concerned about leadership and the use of wealth. The leading social work journal, *Survey*, praised the concept because of its breadth, scope, and systematic approach to alleviating social ills.[22]

Concern about the potential for perpetuity provided the conceptual framework for Embree's criticisms regarding the entrenchment and bureaucratization of philanthropy. Julius Rosenwald, a trustee of the Rockefeller Foundation and founder of his own philanthropic organization, opposed bequests in perpetuity because they resulted in anachronisms and maintained the status quo in the face of altered social circumstances.[23] Indeed, Rosenwald felt so strongly about the matter that, in 1928, when he hired Embree to direct his giving, the philanthropist instructed him to spend the fortune within one generation.

Rosenwald's narrow construction of the perpetuity issue was only a secondary social concern. More broadly interpreted, wealth bequeathed in perpetuity had the potential to grow. Opponents of foundations feared that wealth sheltered under congressional charter would legitimize a plutocracy. By exercising stewardship over an ever-growing fortune, trustees of a foundation would, the argument went, ultimately wield power in all facets of life. Despite a willingness to make seemingly enormous concessions limiting its power, the Rockefeller Foundation did not succeed in gaining a U.S. charter. Although two radically different bills were introduced in Congress between 1910 and 1912, both failed. Instead, the foundation received a charter in 1913, with no restrictions, in the State of New York, and the business of philanthropy proceeded.

The rapid growth of monopolies during the latter decades of the nineteenth century spawned a host of labor and political grievances climaxing in the formation of a congressional investigatory commission under the direction of Missouri Democrat Senator Frank P. Walsh. While corporate philanthropies were not the focus of the investigations of the Commission on Industrial Relations, the rationale for their establishment and the nature of their operations came under scrutiny at least partly because of Rockefeller actions. Trying to avert a publicity disaster resulting from John D. Rockefeller, Jr.'s mishandling of the so-called Ludlow massacre at the Colorado Fuel and Iron Company, the foundation hired Canadian industrial relations expert Mackenzie King to conduct an independent study under its auspices. Use of the foundation to resolve an industrial problem was not only a tactical blunder opening the Rockefeller Foundation to scrutiny, but it rekindled the debate about the legitimacy of organized philanthropy in general.

The links among corporate, foundation, and institutional leaders were prime targets for critics. Jerome Greene, secretary of the foundation, acknowledged the interlocking directorates but argued (rather implausibly) that there was no real conflict of interest since no individual profit could be made from the sale of a product or service.[24] Morris Hillquit, leader of the Socialist Labor Party, observed that the growth of philanthropic foundations was analogous to the development of corporate monopolies and complained that the real beneficiaries of aid were capitalists who guaranteed labor pools at home and created new markets for American products abroad.[25] American Federation of Labor President Samuel Gompers was even more concerned about the foundations' attempts to create an "all-pervading machinery for the molding of the minds of the people."[26] The Reverend John Haynes Holmes summed up the situation saying that the American foundation as a social institution was "essentially repugnant to the whole idea of a democratic society."[27]

Some prominent nurses, of course, attended the Walsh hearings and probably engaged in debate about the relationship of laissez-faire capitalism to democracy and the role of wealthy industrialists in social welfare. Though they held politically different views from industrialists, these women, in positions of authority themselves, understood how wealth could help their own organizations. Lillian Wald and Mary Adelaide Nutting had secured the support of wealthy benefactors, including Rockefeller, for a number of projects over the years and were inclined to regard foundation interests as benign, if not always congruent with their own. In fact, following one particularly vitriolic hearing, Wald wrote indignantly to Jerome Greene that Chairman Frank Walsh had placed the commission "in an indefensible position" in stepping beyond its mandate to inquire into the causes of industrial unrest.[28] Greene acknowledged that dealing with the public relations disaster had drained energy and resources from projects of social benefit.[29]

Despite continued goodwill on the part of many professionals who were potential beneficiaries of foundation giving, the Commission on Industrial Relations had a negative impact on public opinion about foundations. The result, Fosdick remembered, was "discouraging, but in the long run it proved to be salutary." The trustees identified a "narrow range of noncontroversial subjects, notably public health, medicine and agriculture," and became convinced that the foundation must operate strictly as a fund-dispensing rather than an operating agency.[30]

Refined organizational policy was to choose the best qualified recipients for funding and leave programmatic decisions to them. But even when officers and trustees believed their decisions were without bias, selection of those who were "best qualified" meant making value and program judgments that influenced beneficiaries and set the course for future foundation actions.

Information and Internationalization

The magnitude and scope of Rockefeller activity, although still seen by its critics as inherently dangerous, was viewed in the postwar years by officers and staff of the Rockefeller Foundation as necessary for the stabilization and prosperity of society. President Vincent's apology for Rockefeller activities in world health might be dismissed simply as capitalist propaganda except that concurrent efforts in the nursing profession, in women's organizations, and in other voluntary and professional associations were directed toward establishing worldwide cooperation. American progressives were optimistic about the possibilities in postwar reconstruction, and social reformers felt they were riding a worldwide tide.[31] As Agnes Nestor, a social worker from Chicago, put it, "We were living in a time of great dreams—dreams of co-operation between the working peoples of the world, dreams of dignity and plenty for all, dreams of lasting international peace."[32]

Naturally, convincing beneficiaries, either here or abroad, of the "rightness" of the Rockefeller approach was not necessarily successful. Professionals and foundation executives did not always appreciate each other's viewpoints. The issues for American nurse leaders were not the same as for the officers of the foundation. Embree asked Gladys Adams in 1923 to explain why nursing leaders in the United States took so little account of the public health nursing and educational work in Europe supervised by F. Elisabeth Crowell and promoted by the Rockefeller Foundation.[33] Since Adams was in a delicate position as the newly appointed assistant to Crowell in the foundation's Paris office, she deferred response. She wrote immediately to Annie W. Goodrich, the new dean of the Yale School of Nursing, however, posing Embree's question. Goodrich's answer was lengthy and filled with innuendo (making analysis beyond the scope of this article); however, it is apparent that she had little respect for Crowell as a nurse, educator, or leader. According to Goodrich, Crowell was ashamed of being a nurse and did her best to dissociate herself from the profession and its formal organizations. She took, in Goodrich's view, the wrong side in nursing's effort to raise standards and was allowing herself to promote a "scheme of health education" for the foundation rather than concentrating on improving nursing conditions in France.[34]

The question provides a first clue related to an ongoing frustration of the Rockefeller Foundation, or at least of Embree, that nurses in the United States were willing to teach but not to learn from their counterparts in other countries. After the new program at the Yale School of Nursing had started, Goodrich was asked to accommodate visitors on Rockefeller fellowships. She did, of course, even though she occasionally complained that these visitors complicated the business of getting the new school off on a sound educational footing and cost money from the school's budget.[35] The Rockefeller Foundation soon remedied the money issue, but the 116 foundation-sponsored students and an untotaled number of other visitors that flowed through the Yale School of Nursing during those trial years would have put even an established program to the test.[36] At the beginning of 1925, only a year after the first class was admitted, Goodrich was asked to tour Europe with Crowell. In Embree's words, "much might be gained by more intimate acquaintance between the leaders of nursing. . . . you would discover new methods of work or fresh points of view."[37] Even though Goodrich was enthused about the prospect of traveling with her friend S. Lillian Clayton, the tour with Crowell wasn't necessarily something Goodrich was eager to do. But Yale President James R. Angell may have advised Goodrich, as he did a few years later, that relations with the Rockefeller Foundation would be strengthened by her acceptance of the invitation.[38] She responded cordially to the foundation, agreeing to make the trip and acknowledging the opportunity to compare and confer with nurses in Europe.[39]

Initially, all of the progress made through corporate philanthropy was exciting. Building on advances in medical knowledge and a faith in the reforming power of science in nearly all aspects of life, philanthropoids (a named coined by those who made their living giving away other people's money) embarked on a program of reform characteristic of liberal and optimistic progressivism. Nursing was one of the beneficiaries of this pioneering spirit. The National Organization for Public Health Nursing was stabilized by limited foundation contributions. A question that had been plaguing the health care community seemed at least partially resolved by the creation and 1923 report of the Committee to Study Nursing and Nursing Education in the United States. The report established a blueprint for progress in nursing education that certain of the Rockefeller Foundation officers were able to endorse. Vital services to the poor of New York City were aided by foundation donations. Nurses in prominent positions throughout the nation were able to learn from one another and were encouraged to exchange information with their counterparts overseas through fellowships from the foundation's Division of Studies.

Internal Dissension: Brilliance to Bureaucracy

Within a few years, however, the fields had been tilled and the social landscape looked different. Despite its munificent contributions to medicine, science, and agriculture, as well as its support of smaller and riskier ventures, the Rockefeller Foundation was not the driving force in this altered environment. Political, economic, and cultural conditions had changed. Republican administrations spanned the 1920s. The "return to normalcy" platform of Harding and the conservatism of the Coolidge years gave way to managerial liberalism represented by Herbert Hoover.[40] By the mid-1920s, the American economy was dominated by large corporations; before the end of the decade, capitalist planning supplanted the rough and tumble of earlier competitive industrialism.[41] Barons of business were now widely perceived as benefactors and middle-class Americans were more interested in the new consumerism than in political foment and social reform. Professional expertise replaced family and religious authority; gender roles shifted with increased prosperity and working women accommodated to the corporation-oriented social order. The society of the mid- to late-1920s was one of increasing specialization and management; universities that were frequent beneficiaries of foundation support also reflected this trend.

The foundation began to adjust its goals to perceived social realities and to deal with internal strife related to competing goals and personal ambitions. First-generation leaders in the Rockefeller Foundation were aging. Their broad social visions had created boards and programs that required technical and administrative expertise beyond what they could provide. Concurrently, the Rockefeller boards were losing some of their most able younger officers to universities.[42] Until 1928 most Rockefeller philanthropy was devoted to educational reform and social welfare, but even before 1925 a change in the foundation's mode of operations had begun to take place. Research gradually took priority over the application of knowledge and education. Organizational structure and politics made the mediation of conflicting interests difficult. Embree's analysis in a late 1927 letter to a friend relating why he had been unhappy at the foundation for the previous few years was that "the very brilliance of the initial successes seemed . . . blinding as to new opportunities."[43]

By 1925 the problems created by self-perpetuating programs, stagnation of ideas, and vested interests among the officers of various boards were well recognized. Money kept pouring into the same kind of projects throughout the United States, and there was pressure to standardize the foundation's policies here and abroad. According to Embree, "Policies have got confused and timid; foundation giving, instead of concentrating on the social frontiers, is losing its leadership and becoming conventional and stereotyped."[44] Among those fields of interest Embree had begun by 1927 to see as fashionable rather than pioneering were medicine and public health. His perspective was not inconsistent with his experiences mediating conflicts between the International Health Board and the General Education Board related to the joint public health nursing course at Peabody College and Vanderbilt University. Remaining an idealist and a self-styled progressive reformer in the tradition of men like Gates and Rose, Embree was frustrated by the failure of the foundation to engage in new fields of applied science. As director of the Division of Studies, created in 1924 to explore new areas for foundation attention, he attempted, unsuccessfully, to promote a program of "human biology" encompassing anthropology, psychiatry, and physiology. Embree's interest in the possibilities of applied social research remained, however, throughout his career in philanthropy.

Concomitant with an inclination toward stagnancy was an increasingly large body of officers and paid staff who caused the foundation to develop "professional self-consciousness"—to become, according to Embree, "respectable and timid."[45] A dearth of enterprise was only one aspect of the problem. The desire of some philanthropoids to control the outcomes of spending was just as stifling to creative solution of social problems. Some of the strongest criticism of Rockefeller Foundation actions, for instance, came as a result of Abraham Flexner's insistence on controlling the details of medical school reorganizations.[46] Hans Zinsser's public attack on the General Education Board's (GEB) handling of medical education asserted that the autonomy of the university in setting policies and in determining the details of medical curricula had been usurped by the GEB, "however benevolent in its autocracy."[47] Medicine presented, perhaps, the clearest example of one model dominating all others in the foundation's giving program; it was not, however, the only instance in which foundation preference tried to direct the institutional choices of its beneficiaries.

Despite his own abhorrence of Flexnerian manipulation, Embree exercised a significant amount of personal control in the planning and early decision-making of the Yale School of Nursing. On the other hand, bucking the trend to impose a single vision on the developing profession, Embree at least on one occasion advised those interested in public health nursing in Cleveland not to implement a model that was in too close concordance with the plan for the Yale School of Nursing because of the benefit of having more than one type of experience.[48]

Competition between the Rockefeller boards already hindered the work of the foundation by the mid-1920s, and the central administrative staff enjoyed only nominal control of the organization. Raymond Fosdick, who had been associated with the Rockefeller philanthropies since 1913 and served as the foundation president from 1936 to 1948, recalled that because the boards had been established at different times and for different purposes, difficulties were inevitable. The almost fortuitous distribution of programs created confusion not only in the offices of the foundation but in the public mind as well.[49] Anxious to redefine their roles and to meet the demands of a new environment partially created by the foundation itself, a lengthy and conceptually difficult program of restructuring its philanthropies ensued, spearheaded by Fosdick.[50] Embree left the foundation at the close of 1927, lured by Julius Rosenwald's offer to direct his program of giving along lines more in keeping with Embree's own interests. A year later Vincent retired, but those who survived the turmoil of the 1920s formed an alliance that ultimately resulted in overhaul of the foundation's mission.[51]

Although the younger officers of the foundation may not have been overtly cognizant of them, they too had interests to advance or protect as the organization changed. President Vincent, who was not young but who identified with less entrenched personalities in the organization, responded to criticisms by Rosenwald in mid-1929, admitting that his bias toward educational endowments was traceable to his years of university administration.[52] Vincent and Beardsley Ruml, head of the Laura Spelman Rockefeller Memorial Fund, attempted to promote the advance of the social sciences at a time when there was a great deal of skepticism about their value. Embree, grandson of a famous abolitionist, possibly envisioned himself as successor to Rose or Flexner, as one author has suggested.[53] Embree's personal correspondence with close friends and colleagues, however, is hardly self-aggrandizing and reflects his lifelong commitment to social innovation.[54] Among his special interests during the 1920s and later were higher education in the South, creation of opportunities for the education of Southern African-Americans, and the fostering of intercultural relations. His lengthy personal correspondence with Goodrich indicates an ongoing interest in nursing as well as a shared admiration for certain ideas, particularly those of John Dewey.

Conflicts among boards and personalities troubled the joint public health nursing program at the George Peabody College for Teachers and Vanderbilt University. Ruml and Embree were close friends, and their vision for rectifying social and health problems in the rural South, although not ultimately those that prevailed, fueled some of the conflict between the schools. They had visited Nashville in early 1924 and were impressed with the progress that Peabody College personnel had made in promoting public health and public health nursing in the city. Peabody President Bruce Payne believed that sickness was at the heart of Southern social problems and that the best way to effect changes in health behavior was through education at the public school level.[55] To accomplish this, Payne asserted that public health nurses, teachers, and social workers ought to be trained together and coordinate their work in practice. The Department of Public Health Nursing served not only graduate nurses who wanted preparation for public health work but all students in the college. Ruml's desire to move the memorial into the training of social workers at Peabody combined with Embree's profound commitment to public education in the South. Both men, who considered themselves Young Turks in the New York office, were eager to try new methods to solve seemingly intractable problems. Their desire to engage in social engineering pitted them against more powerful figures on the Rockefeller boards, namely, Abraham Flexner and F. F. Russell.

The General Education Board had invested several million dollars in the reorganization of the Vanderbilt University School of Medicine; a nurse training program was essential to the functioning of the university's teaching hospital. Foundation money, therefore, according to Flexner's line of reasoning, should be invested in what would be beneficial to the GEB project. Waller S. Leathers, who was associated with Rockefeller philanthropy in the Sanitary Commission and the International Health Board, was disinterested in public school education and opposed joint efforts of social work and public health nursing. When he joined the Vanderbilt medical faculty in 1925, his influence helped tip the balance toward Vanderbilt where he hoped to build a separate department of hygiene that would encompass public health nursing. Embree conceded to a joint program that fit the mission of neither school. After a year or so of trying by foundation edict to bring the two institutions closer together, Embree effectively withdrew, leaving Mary Beard, his assistant in the Division of Studies, to monitor the results.

Between 1927 and 1930, the joint program got scant attention from the Rockefeller Foundation. After the foundation had been reorganized, the program fell to the Division of Medical Education, where Beard reported to Richard M. Pearce. The joint program limped along without making any appreciable change in the education of public health nurses because it lacked ideological support from Peabody College, Vanderbilt, and the foundation. Funding was withdrawn in 1930 and the money turned over to Vanderbilt for its School of Nursing. The internal turmoil of the Rockefeller Foundation manifested itself in ambivalence about the nature of commitments in nursing during the latter part of the decade. Plans for the immediate development of comprehensive nursing education for public health and educational leadership were thwarted not only by institutional rivalry in Nashville, but by the eclipsing of nursing during the reorganizational period within the foundation.

Conclusion

By the close of the 1920s, the nature of Rockefeller philanthropy had changed. During the decade, foundations had indeed become bureaucratized in the strictest interpretation of the word, and a cadre of professional managers emerged both in the foundations and in academia. Embree's ideal of "untrammeled freedom" for experimentation was never again achieved, but the Rockefeller Foundation gradually implemented policies geared to the advancement and dissemination of scientific knowledge. In the process of reorganization, it focused attention away from social services, with which it associated nursing, and toward research.

The impact of the changed philanthropic environment and the particular organizational development of the Rockefeller Foundation was quickly felt by the nursing profession. As individuals involved in research became legitimate beneficiaries of Rockefeller funding, the shift funneled money away from nursing education and service activities. Cooperative ventures among foundations became more common after the mid-1920s and a larger proportion of gifts was contingent on matching; that is, the beneficiary organizations or local communities would raise at least as much money as had been given. The lack of money in nursing made this criterion difficult to guarantee and therefore weighed against funding. The subsequent difficulties experienced by the Vanderbilt School of Nursing in raising funds and the incremental way in which the Rockefeller Foundation finally endowed the school suggests that this was the case.

As the type of giving changed, so did the role of foundation trustees and staff. Trustees set more general policies for giving and were less involved in the specific details of any particular action; staff engaged in a more analytical dialogue with both institutional applicants and independent area experts regarding the benefits and costs of each prospective gift. The foundation officers' circle of advisors grew much wider as the sciences and the professions matured. These developments, too, may have worked against nursing because of its low place in organizational hierarchies and the relative weakness of its formal professional structures.

In an earlier nursing history, the author commented that Rockefeller support for nursing was secondary to its programs in medicine and public health.[56] This conclusion has, I believe, hindered study of other factors that made nursing of interest to the foundation or influenced its choice of people and programs to support. While evidence supports the writer's observation as a partial interpretation of events, the interests of one or more officers, the changing goals of the foundation, and the interdivisional rivalries of the 1920s also appear to have affected the foundation's program in nursing.

The fifteen year period 1915 to 1930 in Rockefeller Foundation history illustrates a waxing and waning of interest in nursing related to the definition of professional domains and to political and social developments. The foundation's self-defined mission changed with these currents and with the personalities of key decision-makers. Edwin Embree's 1949 critique highlights a problem for those who study the influence of philanthropy on professions. Although there can be little doubt that individual nurses and institutions benefited from Rockefeller Foundation funding for nursing during this period, the long-term effect on the profession is still open for discussion. As a result of its restrictive policies for giving and vested interests, the foundation ignored a wider range of educational and practice models being discussed at the time. In so doing it may have prematurely foreclosed on options that could have helped to shape differently the course of modern American nursing.

SARAH E. ABRAMS, RN, MS
Doctoral Candidate
School of Nursing
University of California, San Francisco

428 Westcliffe Circle
Walnut Creek, Calif. 94596
Phone: (510) 932-8430

Acknowledgments

The research for this paper was conducted while the author was the 1990 American Council of Nurse Researchers "Teresa Christy Fund" Scholar. I would like to acknowledge the American Nurses Foundation, the Alpha Eta *chapter of* Sigma Theta Tau, *and the Department of the History of Health Sciences at the University of California, San Francisco, for partial support of my research.*

Notes

1. Edwin R. Embree, "Timid Billions: Are the Foundations Doing Their Job?" *Harpers Magazine* 180 (March 1949): 28–37.

2. Embree to Clarence Day, 1 December 1927 and others, Embree Papers, HM 167, ser. I, box 1, folder 14, Sterling Memorial Library, Yale University (hereafter cited as SML); and Edwin R. Embree, "The Business of Giving Away Money," *Harpers Magazine* 161 (August 1930): 320–29.

3. Embree, "Timid Billions," 30–33.

4. "Rockefeller Foundation Nursing Activities, 1915–1955," RF1.1-100C-38-341, Rockefeller Foundation Archives (hereafter cited as RFA).

5. For instance, see Michael M. Davis and Linda James, "Industrial Medicine and the Immigrant," *Journal of Industrial Hygiene* 2 (March 1921): 397–422; Editorial, "Are You to be Counted a Friend?" *Modern Medicine* 3 (February 1921): 117–18; George Martinson, "Industrial Nurses in Metal Mining Communities," *Modern Medicine* 3 (March 1921): 186–87.

6. Minutes of the Rockefeller Foundation, 1917–1929, RF3.1-906-2-15, RFA.

7. Robert H. Bremner, *American Philanthropy*, 2nd ed. (Chicago: University of Chicago Press, 1988), 100–115.

8. Bremner, 91.

9. Waldemar Neilsen, *Golden Donors: A New Anatomy of the Great Foundations* (New York: Truman Talley Books/E. P. Dutton, 1985), 84.

10. Attributed to J. A. Hobson, English economist, in Peter Collier and David Horowitz, *The Rockefellers—An American Dynasty* (New York: Holt, Rinehart and Winston, 1976), 48.

11. Bremner, 101.

12. Meyer Kutz, *Rockefeller Power: America's Chosen Family* (New York: Simon and Shuster, 1974), 22.

13. Embree to Day, 11 November 1936, Embree Papers, HM 167, ser. I, box 2, folder 17, SML.

14. F. Emerson Andrews, "Foundations," in *International Encyclopedia of the Social Sciences*, ed. David Sills (New York: Macmillan, 1968), 5:543.

15. Joseph F. Wall, *Andrew Carnegie* (Pittsburgh: University of Pittsburgh Press, 1989), 832.

16. Kutz, 26.

17. Ibid., 25.

18. Embree, "Timid Billions," 28.

19. Embree, "The Business of Giving Away Money," 323.

20. Raymond B. Fosdick, *The Story of the Rockefeller Foundation* (London: Odhams Press Ltd., 1952), 45.

21. George E. Vincent, "World Health and the Rockefeller Foundation," *The Nation's Health* 3 (May 1921): 270–72.

22. Edward T. Devine, "Editorial," *Survey* 23 (12 March 1910): 901–3, cited in Barbara Howe, "The Emergence of Scientific Philanthropy, 1900–1920: Origins, Issues and Outcomes," in *Philanthropy and Cultural Imperialism: The Foundations at Home and Abroad*, ed. Robert F. Arnove (Bloomington: Indiana University Press, 1982), 25–54.

23. Julius Rosenwald, "Principles of Public Giving," *Atlantic Monthly* 143 (May 1929): 599–606.

24. Howe, 37–39.

25. Ibid., 41.

26. Ibid., 43.

27. Ibid., 44.

28. Wald to Greene, 2 February 1915, RF1.1-200C-121-1498, RFA.

29. Greene to Wald, 1 February 1915, RF1.1-200C-121-1498, RFA.

30. Fosdick, 43.

31. Alan Dawley, *Struggles for Justice: Social Responsibility and the Liberal State* (Cambridge, Mass.: The Belknap Press, 1991), 228.

32. Quoted in Dawley, 234.

33. Adams to Goodrich, 24 July 1923, Records of the Dean, School of Nursing, YRG 29, ser. V, box 254, folder 108, SML.

34. Goodrich to Adams, 8 August 1923, Records of the Dean, School of Nursing, YRG 29, ser. V, box 254, folder 108, SML.

35. Correspondence between Goodrich and Florence Read, RF Secretary, November-December 1924, Records of the Dean, School of Nursing, YRG 29, ser. V, box 254, folder 107, SML.

36. "Annual Report of the Yale School of Nursing, 1930," Records of the Dean, School of Nursing, YRG 29, ser. I, box 101, folder 1364, SML.

37. Embree to Goodrich, 19 January 1925, Records of the Dean, School of Nursing, YRG 29, ser. V, box 254, folder 107, SML.

38. Memo regarding telecon, 12 November 1929, Records of the Dean, School of Nursing, YRG 29, ser. V, box 245, folder 18, SML.

39. Goodrich to Embree, 28 January 1925, Records of the Dean, YRG 29, ser. V, box 254, folder 107, SML.

40. Dawley, 294.

41. Ibid., 299.

42. Robert E. Kohler, "A Policy for the Advancement of Science: The Rockefeller Foundation, 1924–29," *Minerva* 16 (1978): 480–515.

43. Embree to Day, 1 December 1927, Embree Papers, HM 167, ser. I, box 1, folder 14, SML.

44. Embree, "Timid Billions," 30.

45. Embree to Day, 1 December 1927, Embree Papers, HM 167, ser. I, box 1, folder 14, SML.

46. Steven C. Wheatley, *The Politics of Philanthropy: Abraham Flexner and Medical Education* (Madison: University of Madison Press, 1988), 141–45.

47. Hans Zinsser, "The Perils of Magnanimity: A Problem in American Education," *Atlantic Monthly* 139 (February 1927): 249.

48. Progress Report, Nursing Education, U.S. General, 1918–1926, RF1.1-100C-37-309, 11 (23 May 1923), RFA.

49. Fosdick, 155.

50. Kohler, 480–515.

51. Wheatley, 140–66.

52. Julius Rosenwald, "The Trend Away from Perpetuities," *Atlantic Monthly* 146 (1930): 741.

53. Kohler, 500.

54. Edwin R. Embree Papers, HM 167, SML.

55. Payne to Wickliffe Rose, 18 May 1925, RF1.1-200C-122-1513, RFA.

56. Dorothy Sheahan, "The Social Origins of American Nursing and Its Movement into the University: A Microscopic Approach" (Ph.D. diss., New York University, 1979), 239.

Guarded by Standards and Directed by Strangers

Charleston, South Carolina's Response to a National Health Care Agenda, 1920–1930

KAREN BUHLER-WILKERSON
School of Nursing
University of Pennsylvania

The year 1912 was a triumphal one for public health nurses who, declared their foremost leader, Lillian Wald, finally attained the position of their dreams. Wald's enthusiasm was for her own idea—the newly created Red Cross Rural Nursing Service, which promised to promote and actually establish "nursing for the people throughout the country." Her proposal called for the Red Cross to "standardize" public health nursing in towns and rural districts and to integrate the work of isolated nurses and nursing organizations under a "central body." In Wald's estimation it was a cause that "carried its own appeal."[1]

At its peak during the 1920s, nearly 3,000 Red Cross nursing services were launched across the country. For several years, combined overseas and home nursing programs made the Red Cross the largest single employer of nurses in the world. This success was short-lived, however, and within a few years local chapters were closing their nursing services at an alarming rate. By 1930, 2,323 of these services had been discontinued. At the outset, Wald presumed they would make some mistakes in the organization of this "great movement," but she never anticipated such a dramatic collapse. The enthusiastic beginning and precipitous decline of the Red Cross nursing service is one of the more interesting stories of our ongoing American aversion to nationally organized health care.[2]

This historical account is a case study with its focus in Charleston, South Carolina, where the Ladies Benevolent Society (LBS) had been caring for the sick poor in their homes since 1813—as they saw best. While this may be a "peculiarly" southern story, it illustrates how, in the absence of locally perceived need, national agendas for health care find little sustenance or support at home.[3]

Nursing History Review 1 (1993): 139–54.

"The Greatest Mother": The American Red Cross

Wald first proposed her "vast" scheme for country nursing to the Red Cross in 1908. Despite their initial lack of interest, Wald eventually secured the support of New York businessman and frequent sponsor Jacob Schiff. Even with Schiff's support, however, the Red Cross began to share Wald's zeal only when Schiff and Mrs. Whitelow Reid offered to provide the money necessary to begin the nursing service.[4]

A special committee was immediately appointed. It recommended approval of the project, suggesting a trial year conducted under the supervision of the Red Cross Committee on Rural Nursing. The committee members were well known to Wald and her nursing colleagues; most were strong supporters of nurses of "professional caliber." At their first meeting, held November 1912, the nurse members were given the task of making recommendations for the nursing service. Taking advantage of this opportunity, they immediately convinced the other members that, due to the nature of the rural nurse's work, she would have to possess the highest qualifications. Their suggestions included not only the requirement that all applicants complete a four-month course of training under the supervision of a recognized visiting nurse association, but also the development of scholarships and loan funds necessary to underwrite this requirement. The committee's rapid acceptance of the nurse members' recommendations suggested that, at least for the moment, the Rural Nursing Service would develop under the careful control and protection of the nursing leadership.[5]

Despite the hopes of many, the recently renamed Town and Country Nursing Service remained a modest undertaking. Beyond the rather fundamental problem of finding qualified nurses, few local groups had the funds needed to establish a nursing service. By 1917, eighty-five affiliations with a total of ninety-seven nurses had been established in twenty-one states. The earliest programs were in the eastern states, followed by those in the South and the West. Their work mirrored that of the public health nurse in most urban settings; nurses did bedside care of the sick, preventive services for children and mothers, and tuberculosis cases, plus a few "sanitary inspections." But unlike big cities where health department nurses did most of the preventive work and visiting nurse association nurses did the bedside care, in these smaller communities the Red Cross nurse cared for everyone—sick or well.[6]

World War I interrupted this experiment, but these developmental years provided the opportunity for the Red Cross to establish the parameters of its peacetime mission. By April 1919 the Red Cross had resumed its ambitious plans for a "new era of health" by sending thirty-one Red Cross nurses out on the Chatauqua Circuit as a "publicity stunt."[7] Expanding on Wald's original idea, the nursing service was now conceived as "the basis and backbone of the Red Cross endeavor." The Red Cross developed policies and procedures for adoption by local chapters and planned to provide properly qualified, guided, and supervised nurses. Each chapter was expected to promote popular interest and pay the nurse's salary. Thus, the Red Cross plan called for national direction but local financing.[8]

Controlling the local chapters' activities rapidly proved more difficult than stimulating their interest. Most had a residue of funds from their war efforts and a score of workers anxious to replace war duties with another big cause. The "great boom," as Mary Gardner, temporary director and frequent critic of the service dubbed it, was overwhelming; overnight hundreds of chapters with money in hand established Red Cross Public Health Nursing Services. Insiders, who took to calling the Red Cross the "greatest mother," would later admit that these were "alarming" years when events proceeded almost out of control.[9]

Hoping to establish some uniformity, at least in its nursing staff, the Red Cross remained committed to only hiring nurses with postgraduate training in public health nursing. But the demand for nurses speedily outran the supply. Beyond this obvious problem, sending young and inexperienced city-bred and city-trained nurses to the country to harmoniously adapt their services to local conditions was an arrangement fraught with difficulties. According to Red Cross historian Portia Kernodle, a "kind of friendly feud" developed between some chapters and the distant national Red Cross over standards and policies. The "autocratic rulings of the Red Cross so necessary in war" were increasingly unacceptable to the local chapters that wanted to run their nursing service in a manner suited to local conditions. They preferred to hire a nurse "they knew and liked" regardless of her training. By 1922, despite the efforts of the Red Cross to maintain high educational standards, only 48 percent of the nurses employed by local chapters had any postgraduate training.[10]

The Red Cross also failed to keep its commitment to provide the personal visits, national correspondence, and definite standards that conveyed to isolated nurses a sense of support and encouragement. With shrinking budgets, the number of divisional offices and field personnel were reduced and visits to local chapters dramatically curtailed. Managing only an annual visit, nursing field representatives provided little guidance, support, or supervision. Predictably, in their absence other new programs began to compete with nursing for increasingly limited chapter funds.[11]

The American Medical Association and the National Organization for Public Health Nursing, as well as local health departments and tuberculosis associations, questioned and even disapproved of the Red Cross's new enterprise. Critics claimed that chapters initiated nursing services with insufficient funds or staff, inadequate community support, and without cooperative agreements with existing agencies, health officers, or local physicians. Public Health Nursing leader Mary Gardner viewed the Red Cross plan for expansion from the top as of dubious virtue. Demand for nurses, Gardner suggested, should come from the community. Only then could programs develop slowly, fostering essential community support and understanding as they grew.[12]

As if external faultfinding was not enough, opposition and criticism of the nursing service began to come from within the Red Cross. Somewhat surprisingly, Mabel Boardman, a longtime supporter of the program, publicly accused the Red Cross of "exceeding its rights and endangering its proper obligations." She regarded the Red Cross as an organization for meeting emergencies and thought it was stretching the meaning of the Red Cross charter too far to think of disease as a disaster that the Red Cross must attempt to prevent. While Boardman's remarks caused a minor sensation in the Red Cross, as with the opinion of other assailants they were discussed and duly dismissed.[13]

By the latter part of 1921, the number of Red Cross nursing services in operation peaked at 1,243, and local chapters' devotion began to waver as war surplus funds were used up. During the three years between January 1921 and December 1923, Red Cross nursing services closed at an average rate of 410 a year. By January 1924, only 804 services and 967 nurses remained. Although the withdrawal rate of Red Cross chapters lessened, the end was not yet in sight. According to Kernodle, an "original understanding or misunderstanding" partially caused the failure of some chapters to find the means to continue their nursing services when war funds were gone. Chapters were expected only to "demonstrate" the value of their service for a year or two and then some other agency (e.g., health department) would take it over. In most communities (64 percent) this transfer of responsibility never materialized and the services were allowed to lapse.[14]

The Southern Dilemma

The gap between Red Cross standards and pressure to keep up with demand for nurses was most pronounced in the southern division. There, in the words of Red Cross Division Director Jane Van De Vrede, southern people were generally unwilling to accept the policies of any "national body." The rather slow development of this work in the South resulted, she claimed, from the combination of the regions "marked conservatism in accepting all innovation" and Red Cross adherence to its ideals and policies: insistence on highly trained nurses and centrally derived decisions. This combination made it nearly impossible to supply nurses from local resources because southern training school graduates did not meet the eligibility requirements for Red Cross enrollment or admission to post-graduate public health nursing programs. Even those who qualified for training and scholarships were, according to Van De Vrede, reluctant to leave the South to attend these programs.[15]

Beyond the disparity between supply and demand, Van De Vrede also claimed that "the great number of negroes forming a dependent population which must be carried outright in any welfare undertaking" was another deterrent to the development of this work in the South. Apparently, the implication was that if white southerners established a nursing service they would immediately be confronted with caring for the significant health care needs of the black population. They therefore simply chose to avoid these rather complex issues in segregated communities. Whatever the cause, by 1920, with 50 percent of the southern chapters anxious to begin nursing services, only 5 percent (twenty-four) had been supplied a nurse.[16]

"In Charleston, We Trust the People We Know"

The Charleston Red Cross story strikingly elucidates the local dilemmas created by this well-intentioned national agenda, even when methods and outcomes precisely match those anticipated by the Red Cross planners. Three months after the 1918 Armistice, the Charleston Red Cross Chapter launched its new nursing service with adequate funds ($26,000) and requisite "machinery and spirit" (9,427 members). Enamored with the Red Cross idea of "making a great contribution to the welfare" of their community, they immediately called a meeting of all (nineteen) organizations in the city interested in health matters to seek their endorsement. The participants unanimously voted to "back up" the program as outlined by the Red Cross and promised their cooperation.[17]

A memo from Red Cross national headquarters describing these developments mentioned that "the Benevolent Society, which has supported colored visiting nursing since 1902 will also coordinate their service with the chapter, but without merging identity." The memo concluded with the hope that Charleston's nursing agencies would soon "see the wisdom of standards set by the Red Cross and act accordingly." Clearly, the memo writer at national headquarters had no idea of this organization's standing in Charleston society. Founded in 1813 by the wives, sisters, and daughters of the city's most prominent families, the Ladies Benevolent Society (LBS) was not an organization to be ignored. Evidently, the Red Cross, unaware of "local conditions," chose to categorize the work of the LBS as "colored" visiting nursing, because both of their nurses were black. In fact the LBS cared for both black and white patients and had, after several years of experimentation, found black nurses to be the most acceptable caregivers within the homes of Charleston's sick poor, black or white. After contracting to care for sick Metropolitan Life Insurance policyholders in 1911, the LBS grew tremendously with nearly nine hundred patients being cared for in 1920.[18]

The LBS Board's initial response to the Red Cross plan was "to wait and see." While they perceived the Red Cross to be a potentially competitive organization, publicly they expressed great interest in any endeavor to make theirs a healthy city.[19]

The Red Cross plan was to divide Charleston into four districts, providing a nurse for each and a supervisor to oversee the whole program. As in so many chapters across the country, plans were completed six months before qualified staff became available and as a result the office was not fully operational until February 1920. Despite this slow start, at national headquarters they were "all very proud of this chapter's activities, and the fine way the Charleston Committee on Nursing Activities [had] gone about organizing a very difficult piece of work."[20]

By April the chair of the Nursing Activities Committee became concerned that, despite their good start, sufficient work had not been done to warrant the large amount being spent by the chapter on this program. She was also distressed by the "great deal of unrest among the nurses" caused, she discovered, by a supervisor "not fitted for her position." A month later, the supervisor had handed in her resignation and Marie Lebby had agreed to replace her.[21]

Despite the mismatched supervisor and a total turnover of the staff, the nursing service somehow continued at a reasonably productive level that first year. The chapter looked forward to the future, confident that Marie Lebby would know how to get their program under control because, remarkably, she was a southerner, a lady, and a nurse.

A Lady Is a Lady, Even If She's a Nurse!

Marie Lebby came from Charleston. After graduating from Rollins College and making her debut, she felt little enthusiasm for her expected role as a southern lady. Wanting to "do something useful," she decided to go to medical school, but her family would not "hear of it" and practically disowned her. Eventually they agreed to let her go to nursing school at St. Luke's Hospital in Richmond where she would be under the watchful eye of family friend and "gentleman" Dr. Stuart McGuire. Much to her relief, Lebby found that, unlike Charleston, "in Virginia women from some of the best families were nurses."[22]

After graduation, Marie Lebby joined Base Hospital 45, serving with Stuart McGuire in France. Returning to New York, she completed the post-graduate public health nursing course at Columbia University. Anxious to return to the South, Lebby was delighted when her teacher, the well-known nurse leader Adelaid Nutting, "commanded" her to return to Charleston to straighten out their problems. Nutting wanted Lebby to take over the Charleston Red Cross Service and show them what a real nurse—meaning a lady with the right education—could do. Lebby returned home in June of 1920, working intermittently and part-time as an acting-supervisor for the Red Cross that summer.[23]

While the LBS had greeted the Red Cross plans for a nursing service with ambivalence, they welcomed Marie Lebby's arrival. Much to their relief, they found that Lebby recognized "the unique position of the Ladies Benevolent Society." She was anxious to cooperate with them and confident that the domains of the two nursing services need not overlap. Reassured that she "understood," they appointed her to their board. While Charlestonians may not have approved of "Miss Marie" becoming a nurse, local lore has it that, at least in this case, "a lady is a lady, even if she's a nurse."[24]

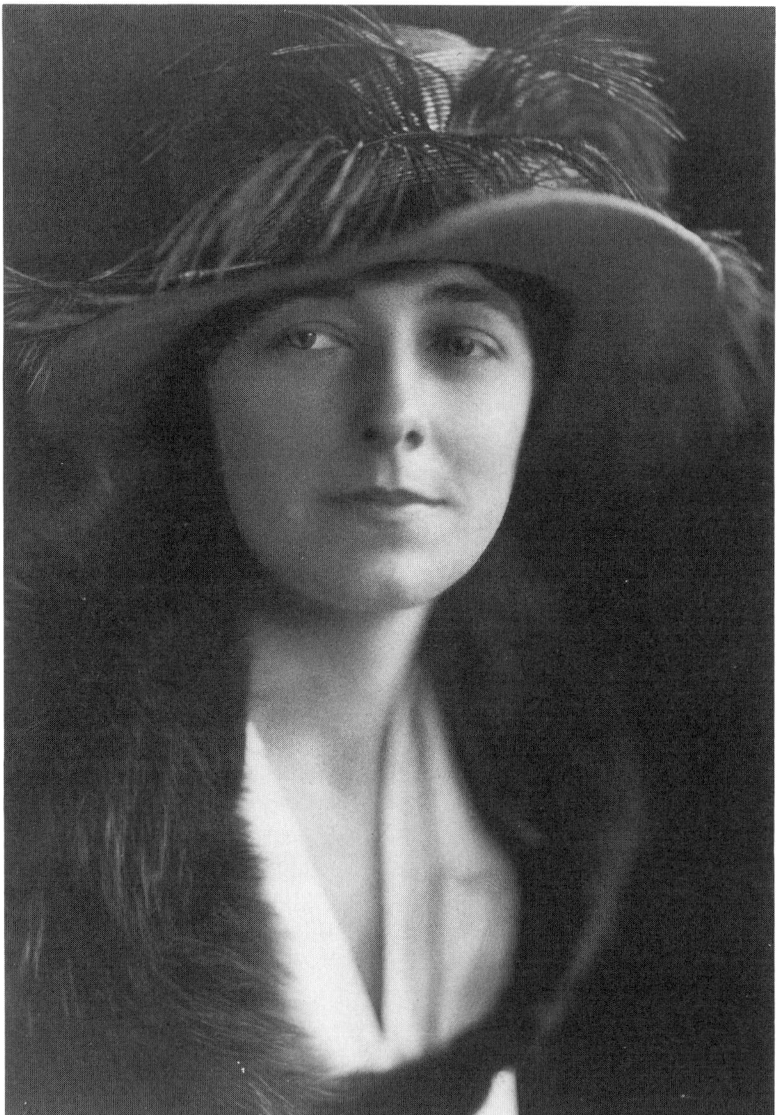

Marie Mikell Lebby (Mrs. Thomas C. Boushall), Public Health Nursing Supervisor, Charleston, South Carolina Chapter of the American Red Cross. (Courtesy of Mrs. Granville Valentine)

The Red Cross was equally pleased with Lebby "who gained for the service many friends among the doctors who, up to that time, were not quite sure what we were trying to give the city." While delighted with Lebby's public relation skills, the Red Cross must have found her intermittent availability discouraging. By September 1920, the Red Cross Board decided they had "demonstrated" public health nursing for Charleston long enough and planned to propose at the January City Council Meeting that the city health department "undertake the responsibility of Public Health Nursing in the city." Despite the health department's interest and a supportive "mass meeting," the city failed to appropriate the necessary funds.[25]

By spring of 1921, Charleston's Red Cross was in crisis. Their treasury was down to $10,519, their chairman had resigned, Lebby was planning to marry a Richmond banker, they had only one nurse left on staff, and they could get no support from Jane Van De Vrede at the Atlanta Divisional Office. That April, determined to terminate their demonstration, Marie Lebby asked the LBS Board to consider taking over the Red Cross Nursing Service. She added that, if they did not, she "would form another organization" for that purpose. In a special meeting called by the LBS Board later that month, Georgia Jatho, chair of the Red Cross Nursing Activities Committee, presented their proposal as a great opportunity for the LBS, but one that required acceptance of the methods and standards established by the Red Cross nationally. Concretely, this meant that the LBS each year would have to raise $8,000 to $10,000 for an office, staff, literature, and nursing supervisor consistent with Red Cross standards. Accepting the Red Cross's methods also meant the work "would be entirely in the hands of a nursing supervisor" and the LBS Board would simply receive monthly reports from her. Jatho was confident that if the LBS did not undertake this work, it would be assumed by another organization and this would be "a great misfortune as it meant the death of the LBS." Lebby contended that Charleston was not rich enough to support two nursing organizations, and therefore, "either one must die or both must hobble on."[26]

The LBS Board took this "golden opportunity" and threat seriously. They consulted with several businessmen, had numerous "animated discussions," and presented the matter to the membership. In the end, they declined the Red Cross challenge "to write for our city a new page in history," accepting instead "the possibility of destruction or a very restricted future."[27]

As they proved in other decisions, the LBS Board was unwilling to trade methods acceptable within Charleston's peculiar traditions for the methods and standards of outsiders. Initially, almost half the LBS Board demonstrated some interest in the Red Cross plan; it was LBS Superintendent Catherine Ravenel's warnings that "all would change" that coalesced opposition. Most distressing was the need to "give up every detail" into the hands of a nursing supervisor. According to Ravenel, all reports would go to the supervisor, who would form all committees, and the board's only responsibility would be to "supply the money." Observing what was happening elsewhere in South Carolina, it must also have been clear to Ravenel that "qualified" supervisors usually came from northern postgraduate public health nursing programs. Accordingly, she cautioned careful consideration, warning that not only would they be giving up the "well organized work which we have striven so hard to establish," but they would also be turning over the LBS's future to the judgment and vision of a "stranger." Sharing Ravenel's sentiments that "a stranger coming here to supervise would find conditions and people very different from elsewhere," the membership unanimously voted to simply place the Red Cross proposal in the minutes as an "informational item." With hardly enough money in the treasury to get through the year, the LBS chose, in the words of Marie Lebby, "to close their eyes to the possibilities and drift on."[28]

Unsuccessful in their negotiations with the LBS, the Charleston Red Cross came to realize that the failure of local organizations to take up this work seemed related to "some objection to the Red Cross supervision." In response, the board sought a "purely local organization" to carry on the service free of Red Cross standards and policies. By January 1922, the task of "safeguarding the health of the community" had been taken up by the newly created Charleston Public Health Nursing Association. The local Red Cross chapter voted to show their support by providing $1,500, selling the new organization the "property" used by the Nursing Activities Committee at half price, and turning over all current nursing records. Watching with "keen interest" and much relief the continuance of their nursing service elsewhere, the Red Cross focused its attention on discovering whether it was viable in any peacetime capacity.[29]

In December 1924 the work and staff of the Charleston Public Health Nursing Association was, in turn, taken over by the recently reorganized Charleston County Health Department. That same year the Metropolitan Life Insurance Company (MLI) opened an independent nursing service in Charleston, having just terminated its contract with the LBS because of complaints from policyholders who "did not like the colored nurses." The record does not explain why the LBS allowed the termination of this beneficial relationship rather than hire a white nurse to care for these grieved patients. Whatever the explanation, discontinuing their contract meant the ladies of Charleston had chosen a very different future for their organization.[30]

By 1925 Ravenel characterized the work of the LBS as "much restricted." Their calls now came from old patients, those the Health Department nurses could not reach, and "those who shrink from asking for city help." Yet, despite this inevitable outcome, simply supplementing the work of the other nursing organizations was more acceptable than having the LBS's mission taken over by outsiders. In the aggregate, the outcome for Charlestonians was a rather confusing collection of small nursing organizations—each driven by its own fragmented perception of community need. Operating mostly in isolation, their interactions remained casual at best. For those seeking nursing care, centralizing all public health nursing services within the LBS might have provided a more rational approach to their needs. For the LBS, however, fragmented and diminished services proved more acceptable than compliance with the dictates of outsiders such as the Red Cross or the MLI.[31] The ladies of Charleston held to the principle that appropriate methods of caring and spheres of usefulness were intimate matters defined at home within locally acceptable boundaries—not by a national agenda guarded by homogenized standards and directed by strangers.

Charleston's story echoed across the country as cities and local voluntary health organizations experimented with the Red Cross's national agenda for health. It confirmed the failure of the Red Cross's scheme for a national nursing service on many fronts. This vast plan to give the Red Cross a peacetime mission and extend the work of the public health nurse across the country to small-town America was valued only by a few reformers like Wald. Standards that sent strangers to small towns where they only "trust the people we know" quickly caused difficulties. Nurses, once again dispatched to do the impossible, were courageous and enthusiastic, but inescapably found themselves unemployed.[32] Most significant, however, was the local chapter members' unwillingness to finance health services that ranked low in perceived importance to their local citizenry.

Karen Buhler-Wilkerson, PhD, FAAN
Associate Professor of Community Health Nursing
School of Nursing
University of Pennsylvania

420 Guardian Drive
Philadelphia, Pa. 19104-6096
Phone: (215) 898-4725

Acknowledgments

This study was supported by the National Center for Nursing Research, National Institutes of Health. I wish to thank the staff of the South Carolina Historical Society, the Carolina Low Country Chapter of the American Red Cross, the archives of the Metropolitan Life Insurance Company, the National Archives Civil Research Branch, the Waring Historical Library of the Medical University of South Carolina, and Marie Lebby Boushall and her daughter, Mrs. Granville Valentine, for their invaluable assistance.

Notes

1. The collection of the American Red Cross, National Headquarters is at the National Archives, Washington, D.C. Lavinia Dock et al., *History of American Red Cross Nursing* (New York: Macmillan, 1949), 1213–15, 1220–21, and Portia B. Kernodle, *The Red Cross Nurse in Action, 1882–1948* (New York: Harper and Brothers, 1949), 71–72.

2. Dock, 1214, 1220–22, and Kernodle, 256–86. For these statistics, see "Public Health Nursing, Changes in Service, July 1, 1919 to June 30, 1930," folder no. 140.18, Public Health Nursing, American Red Cross, National Archives (hereafter cited as PHN, ARC, NA).

3. For an excellent discussion of the "peculiar South," see Drew Gilpin Faust, "The Peculiar South Revisited: White Society, Culture, and Politics in the Antebellum Period, 1800–1860," in *Interpreting Southern History: Historiographical Essays in Honor of Sanford W. Higginbotham*, ed. John Boles and Evelyn T. Noyes (Baton Rouge: Louisiana State University Press, 1987), 78–119.

4. Dock, 1212–15, and Kernodle, 72.

5. For an extensive review of the evolution of Red Cross standards and programs, see Dock, 1211–92, and Kernodle, 71–89. For a more extensive overview of public health nurses efforts toward the creation of standards, see M. Louise Fitzpatrick, *The National Organization for Public Health Nursing, 1912–1952: Development of a Practice Field* (New York: National League for Nursing, 1975).

6. Dock, 1291–92. In 1916, 47 percent of Red Cross visits were for bedside care of the sick, while "instructive" visits to children, infant welfare, prenatal and tuberculosis cases, sanitary inspections, and "other" made up the remaining calls. Rural nurses were also caring for a significantly smaller number of patients than their urban counterparts and tended to make more visits to each patient. For a comparison, see Karen Buhler-Wilkerson, *False Dawn: The Rise and Decline of Public*

Health Nursing, 1900–1930 (New York: Garland Publishing, 1989), 153–55. The Red Cross nursing service changed its name several times, reflecting its evolving mission and/or organizational changes. During World War I it became the Bureau of Public Health Nursing and in the 1920s it was renamed the Public Health Nursing Service.

7. Chatauqua was called the "canvass college of America." It was a very popular traveling program of "enlightenment and entertainment" presented two to three times a day for several days or even weeks under a large tent. Programs ranged from travelogues to plays. Kernodle, 238–41.

8. Buhler-Wilkerson, *False Dawn*, 221–28; Dock, 1293–1351; and Kernodle, 256–86. For Red Cross instruction to chapters, see "The Organization and Administration of a Public Health Nursing Service," 1 March 1919, Form A 701, folder no. 151, PHN, ARC, NA.

9. Ibid. "Public Health Nursing, Changes in Service, July 1, 1919 to June 30, 1930," folder no. 140.18, PHN, ARC, NA. Elizabeth Fox, who succeeded Gardner as director, mentioned the "mother" role in her monthly report, 3 June 1929, folder no. 140.18, PHN, ARC, NA. Gardner "temporarily" rescued the Red Cross by becoming director on 1 April 1918, when the previous director resigned over the Red Cross's failure to "push forward" with the service. Fannie Clements to Frank Persons, 26 March 1918, folder no. 140.12, PHN, ARC, NA. See also, Mary Gardner, "Under the Red Cross," *The Public Health Nurse* 20 (November 1928): 597–99 (hereafter cited as *PHN*), and Elizabeth Fox, "The Development of the Red Cross Bureau of Public Health Nursing," *PHN* 12 (February 1920): 175–81.

10. Kernodle, 278–81. "The Organization and Administration of a Public Health Nursing Service," folder no. 151, and "Report of Public Health Nursing Service, July 1, 1920 to June 30, 1921," folder no. 140.18, PHN; ARC, NA. "Report of the Western Office," May 1919, National Organization for Public Health Nursing, roll no. 27, National League for Nursing Records Collection, New York.

11. This commitment is described in Dock, 1267–68; Kernodle, 267–68, 272, 281–82. Concurrently, the nature of the nursing programs was increasingly limited to bedside care as their preventive programs were taken over by official agencies whose growth was supported by the Rockefeller Foundation, the Children's Bureau, and the Sheppard Towner Act. This trend was financially supported by the Metropolitan Life Insurance Company, which contracted with surviving Red Cross chapters for a considerable portion of the bedside care they provided for policyholders living in rural areas and small towns.

12. Kernodle, 275–78, and Buhler-Wilkerson, *False Dawn*, 221–28. For an example of the variety of letters written by the Red Cross in its effort to assure other organizations that it did not "contemplate the invasion of territory where other organizations are engaged in work of this character," see Rupert Blue (Surgeon General) to Mrs. Ira Perkins, Chief, Child Conservation Section, Council of National Defense, Washington, 3 April 1919, Public Health Service, General File, 1897–1923: 3815, box 372, National Archives. Much of the visiting nurse leadership's "chronically sore and morbidly disposed" feeling toward the Red Cross developed over what they called the Red Cross's "ruthless ambition" at the expense of public health nursing during World War I. See for example, Ella Crandell to Mary Beard, 2 February 1919, roll 31, Wald Collection, New York Public Library, New York.

13. Buhler-Wilkerson, *False Dawn*, 225, and Kernodle, 241, 276–78, 285.

14. Kernodle, 263, 281–83. Between 1920 and 1930 there were 2,959 nursing services created by the Red Cross; 2,323 of these were discontinued, 383 (13 percent) turned over to public agencies, 41 (1 percent) turned over to private agencies, and 1,899 (64 percent) closed due to "lack of funds, interest, etc." As of 30 June 1930 only 636 (22 percent) were still in operation. "Public Health Nursing, Changes in Service, July 1, 1919–June 30, 1930," folder no. 140.18 PHN, ARC, NA.

15. Van De Vrede was born in Wisconsin and moved to Georgia in 1908. "Qualified" nurses were graduates of a two-year nursing course in a general hospital with a minimum of fifty beds (must include men), members of an organization affiliated with the American Nurses Association, registered to practice, and graduates of a recognized postgraduate course. In 1919 there were thirteen educational institutions giving this course that ranged from four to nine months. The only course available in the South was in Richmond, which gave a three-month course. The Red Cross provided scholarships that were paid back through a year of service. Exceptions were made, and eventually supervised experience was recognized as adequate preparation; Dock, 1235–56. Since membership in an organization "affiliating" with the American Nurses Association was required and most black nurses in the South were excluded from these organizations, there were few, if any, "qualified" southern black nurses. They could join the National Organization for Public Health Nursing; Darlene Clark Hine, *Black Women in White: Racial Conflict and Cooperation in the Nursing Profession, 1890–1950* (Bloomington: Indiana University Press, 1989), 91–95. See Jane Van De Vrede, director, Bureau of Public Health Nursing, "Southern Division Report of the Bureau of Public Health Nursing; July 1919 to January 1, 1920," folder no. 149.18, PHN, ARC, NA.

16. Ibid.

17. Dock, 1295–99. Records of the Charleston, S.C., Red Cross Public Health Nursing Service are at the Carolina Low Country Chapter office in North Charleston. Red Cross Executive Committee 13 March 1919, Red Cross, Charleston Chapter (hereafter cited as RC, CC). See memo written by Virginia M. Gibbs and sent by Elizabeth Fox to all Division Directors, Public Health Nursing Service, 1 March 1920, folder no. 140.18, PHN, ARC, NA.

18. Ibid. The Ladies Benevolent Society Collection records (hereafter cited as the LBS Papers) are at the South Carolina Historical Society, Charleston, S.C. The LBS claims to be the country's oldest women's organization, since the Female Benevolent Society of Wiscasset, Maine, which was founded in 1805 no longer exists. Margaret Simons Middleton, "The Ladies Benevolent Society of Charleston, S.C.," *The Yearbook of the City of Charleston* (*YCC*) (Charleston, 1941), 216–39. For a more detailed discussion of the LBS's history see, Karen Buhler-Wilkerson, "Caring in Its Proper Place: Race and Benevolence in Charleston, S.C., 1813–1930," *Nursing Research* 41 (January/February 1992): 14–20.

19. Minutes of the Board, 14 February 1919, LBS Papers.

20. Ibid., and Gibbs Memo, 1 March 1920, LBS Papers.

21. At the end of the first eleven months, the staff of three to five nurses had made 9,182 visits at a cost of $7,641. They cared for an average of 342 patients a month, making approximately 8 to 10 visits a day. Annual Report Red Cross

Nursing Activity Committee for 1921 and April and May 1921, Monthly Report of the Red Cross Board, RC, CC. See also American Red Cross Department of Nursing, Bureau of Public Health Nursing monthly reports for 1920, PHN, ARC, NA.

22. Interview with Marie Mikell Lebby (Mrs. Thomas C. Boushall), February 1991 in Richmond, Va. At the time she was one hundred years old. She is still living and pleased to have her story told.

23. Ibid. Lebby's father would not let her accept a Red Cross Scholarship for her studies or spend her salary on things such as expensive clothes, because he was concerned people would think he could not support her. She apparently went off with her family for several weeks that summer to the mountains where she helped with a well baby clinic.

24. The quote is a comment made by Betty Hamilton, a family friend and neighbor, who has known the Lebby family for years; interview with Karen Buhler-Wilkerson, January 1991, Charleston, S.C. Minutes of the Board, January 1921, 14 February 1919, LBS Papers.

25. Lebby's public relations activities were discussed at the 6 January 1921 meeting. Lebby was finally expected to join the Red Cross on a full-time basis November 1920, but found it impossible to assume these duties. She did agree to stay on part-time until they could secure a permanent supervisor, which they would do "as soon as we know where we stand financially." Report of the Nurses Activities Committee, 4 November 1920. The proposal came from the Nurse Committee to the Executive Committee, 29 November 1920. These plans were discussed with Jane Van De Vrede, the head of the Division Office, who reminded the board that they must insist on the city following the standards required by the Red Cross at the 2 December 1920 Board Meeting. The mass meeting is discussed in the 28 January 1921 meeting. See Board Minutes, RC, CC.

26. Between 1913 and 1931, twenty-eight Red Cross Chapters were operating public health nursing programs in South Carolina. By 1936, only two remained; 48 percent had discontinued operations within the first four years of operation. Almost half had been organized in 1920. See Rosa Hayward Clark, "History and Development of Public Health Nursing in S.C." (South Carolina State Board of Health, February 1942), 14–17, 34. The idea for the LBS to take over the Red Cross service originated with Lebby. See Minutes of the Nursing Activities Committee, 4 April 1921, RC, CC. The Red Cross proposal for takeover was first presented to the LBS Board by Marie Lebby. A week later, Georgia Jatho, chair of the Nursing Committee of the Red Cross, met with the LBS Board to further discuss their plan. See Minutes of the Board, 8 April 1921 and 15 April 1921, LBS Papers.

27. See Minutes of the Society, 21 April 1921, 6 May 1921, and 1 June 1921, LBS Papers.

28. Ibid.

29. The Red Cross decision to abandon their standards was reported in the 26 May 1921 minutes, RC, CC. The vote to support the new organization is reported in the 5 January 1922 minutes of the Annual Meeting. The discussion of the future role of the chapter is reported in the 1924 Annual Report, Charleston Chapter Red Cross. See Clarke, 34. The fortune of the Charleston Chapter of the Red Cross

continued to decline. By 1923 their membership had dropped to 1,472 and there was only $3,486 in the treasury, Annual Report, 1924, RC, CC.

30. Leon Banov, *As I Recall: The Story of the Charleston County Health Department* (Columbia, S.C.: R. L. Bryan Co., 1970). When the Charleston County Health Department took over the Charleston Public Health Nursing Association's work, they employed four nurses, a supervisor, and several other workers who had previously been employees of this association. This was reported in the Annual Meeting Records, February 1924, RC, CC. See also Clarke, 24–27. See the Reports for the Department of Health, *YCC*, 1920, 1922, and 1924. A little over a year later, hearing of MLI's objection to the LBS's "colored nurses," the same association wrote that they would refrain from offering their services to MLI until they found it impossible for LBS to comply with MLI's demand that "white nurses be employed." Minutes of the Board, 9 February 1923, LBS Papers. It is unclear if MLI contracted with the Charleston Public Health Nursing Association to care for their policyholders, but in May of 1924 the company opened an independent nursing service. The Metropolitan Life Insurance Company's nursing service was caring for around 200 cases and making 1,854 visits annually while the LBS visited about 230 cases, making 1,394 visits annually. Louise Tattershall, *Public Health Nursing in the United States: January 15, 1931* (New York: National Organization for Public Health Nursing, 1931).

31. Annual Report Book, 1906–1930, see Reports for 1923–1930 for Patient Data, see especially drafts of the Annual Report for 1924, p. 83; "The Ladies Benevolent Society Elects Its Officers for Ensuing Year," Report of the Annual Meeting for 1925; "The Ladies Benevolent Society Meets," Annual Report for 1923, p. 82, LBS Papers. Ravenel, who had presided over the annual meetings for forty-four years, was unable to attend the 1930 meeting. Ravenel died on 6 March 1933 and had conducted business from her bedroom through the Junior Superintendent for some time before her death. Middleton, 239.

32. In Charleston this saying is such a tradition that one of the local TV stations uses "In Charleston, We Trust the People We Know" as their advertisement. For a Canadian version of the complex local situations nurses are sent to save, see Meryn Stuart, "'Half a Loaf Is Better Than No Bread': Public Health Nurses and Physicians in Ontario, 1920–1925," *Nursing Research* 41 (January/February 1992): 21–27.

"Making Do" with the Midwife

Arkansas's Mamie O. Hale in the 1940s

PEGGE L. BELL
College of Nursing
University of Arkansas for Medical Sciences

The United States Children's Bureau in the late 1930s targeted the development of child-welfare services for rural blacks.[1] Of southern states with high rural black populations, Arkansas ranked ninth. Developing services for the black population included establishing casework programs and using special demonstration units administered by local health departments staffed by black personnel. This article will explore the efforts of one such program developed in Arkansas during the 1940s to try to address the disparity between black and white maternal and infant mortality rates. Its particular focus is on the work of Mamie O. Hale, a black nurse-midwife, and her contributions to a statewide training program for granny midwives.

The Plight of Arkansas's Blacks in the 1940s

In 1940 over two thirds of Arkansas's black and white population lived in rural areas; the state ranked as the third most rural state in the country.[2] As with other rural states, Arkansas suffered from a shortage of physicians, nurses, and hospitals. This shortage of health care providers meant that residents of many rural counties had limited or no obstetrical care. These medical shortages severely affected blacks who lived in the most rural areas of the state.

Racial barriers kept many of Arkansas's black men and women from becoming physicians and nurses and caring for their own. Collegiate programs to educate blacks in these fields were limited and distantly located in large cities like New York and Chicago.[3] In 1941 only twenty-nine schools in the country, other than those exclusively for blacks, were open to black students.[4] Without black nurses and doctors, the health care of Arkansas's black population was left to white physicians in a segregated state. In 1940 the shortage of physicians was so acute in Arkansas—only 1

Nursing History Review 1 (1993): 155–69.

physician for approximately 1,382 people—that many public health programs lacked any medical personnel to provide preventive medicine needed by rural as well as urban blacks.[5] Access to prenatal care was further limited for black women since there were only three board-certified obstetricians in Arkansas in 1941. Medical care during childbirth was even more difficult to obtain. Except for twenty-three beds in the University Hospital of Little Rock, there were practically no hospital beds for black women in Arkansas as late as 1947.[6]

The poverty of Arkansas's blacks also hindered their access to available medical care. Many of the black sharecroppers could afford neither medical care nor the transportation necessary to get to public health services. Using the services of the granny midwife was an economic necessity. For most she was the only link to health care. The granny midwife's influence on the health of Arkansas's rural blacks persisted through the 1950s.[7]

With the bombing of Pearl Harbor on 7 December 1941, the United States committed its resources to a global war. The war depleted the number of physicians in most states but particularly in the southern states. By the end of 1941, there were 1,819 licensed physicians in Arkansas, yielding a ratio of 1 physician to 1,113 people—the national ratio was 1 per 750.[8] By July 1942 the number of physicians in Arkansas declined to 1,019. Despite heavy recruitment of Arkansas's physicians prior to 1942 for the war, the *Journal of the American Medical Association* continued to urge physicians to join the war effort, as an additional 20,000 physicians were needed by the end of the year.[9] Later, in 1944, the physician-to-population ratio in Arkansas rose to what was called a "generally acceptable" ratio of 1 to 1,500 by the Arkansas Medical Society.[10] But it again dropped precipitously in 1945 when the membership of the Arkansas Medical Society fell to only 990.[11]

Thus, diversion of physicians away from the state and from the practice of maternal and child health continued to pose problems even after the war. The Arkansas State Board of Health offered refresher courses in pediatrics and obstetrics to any interested physicians, and then offered them scholarships in the form of tuition, travel, and boarding expenses.[12] Even so, few improvements were made in postwar state health departments because of inadequate staff.[13] Despite the board's desire to provide maternity care to black women through local public health departments, the continued shortage of physicians made "making do" with the granny midwife even more important.

The Status of Maternal and Child Health

Although the country as a whole saw improvements in maternal and child health in general, discrepancies between national black and white mortality rates continued. The maternal mortality rate for white women for the period 1931–1935 was 56.4 per 10,000 live births; it fell to 39.7 in 1936–1940.[14] The corresponding rates for black women were 97.1 during 1931–1935 and 84.1 during 1936–1940. The infant mortality rate for white infants was relatively stable, 44 per 1,000 live births in 1939 and 43 in 1940. The rate for black infants was 73 for both years. The smallest reductions in maternal and infant mortality rates occurred in the southern states of Alabama, Arkansas, Mississippi, and Tennessee. Arkansas's maternal mortality rate for 1931–1935 was 68.1, dropping to 60.4 for the period 1936–1940. Infant mortality rates also improved only slightly from 1939 (25) to 1940 (23.5).

Though more than half of all the live births in the United States occurred in hospitals, less than one fourth of the births in Arkansas were performed in hospitals.[15] By 1941 midwives in Arkansas delivered approximately 25 percent of all babies. As a result of the limited availability of and access to physicians and hospitals, the majority of all babies in Arkansas were born without medical attention.

Midwives were such an instrumental part of Arkansas's maternal and infant mortality that efforts to regulate their practice occurred as early as 1925.[16] Control of granny midwives involved health department annual permits. Initially, these permits were given to midwives who had no formal instruction and merely represented the midwife's reporting to the Bureau of Vital Statistics the births she attended. In subsequent years, the requirements for midwife permits became more detailed. In 1940 midwives were required to have a physical examination, blood Wasserman test, and a clean bag; to sign a pledge card; and to complete a permit form provided by the State Health Department.[17]

The state's attempts to educate and regulate the granny midwife's practice remained largely ineffective. According to a report by the Committee on Study of Midwifery, approximately one third of the active midwives in 1941 not only had no permit for the year but had never had one.[18] Of the 142 deaths among black women, the committee said, 107 could have been avoided under "ideal conditions." They listed these ideal conditions as suitable social and economic status of the patients, available hospitalization, intelligent and cooperative patients, and deliveries attended by properly qualified physicians with competent obstetric consultation. Dr. Jameson, chairman of the committee, used these statistics to recommend that Arkansas's physicians should persuade or coerce midwives to better equip themselves to attend deliveries.

In the following years, the status of child health and welfare remained relatively unchanged. Babies less than a year old accounted for one tenth of all deaths in Arkansas in 1943.[19] The majority of these deaths occurred within the first months, and about one fourth occurred during the first day. Prematurity caused nearly half of all neonatal deaths, and more than half of the deaths due to prematurity occurred within the first day of life.[20] Although the trend of infant mortality in Arkansas mirrored that of the United States as a whole—about 40 deaths per 1,000 live births, state health officials strongly doubted that birth registration in Arkansas was complete. Almost 12 percent of the infant deaths were attributed to "ill defined and unknown causes." In many cases no physician or granny midwife attended the birth.

By 1944 the maternal mortality rate had improved for white women in Arkansas (1.7 per 1,000 live births) but not significantly for black women (5.7).[21] The maternal mortality rate for black women was two-and-a-half times as high as it was for white women in the same year and at about the same level as the rate for white women had been ten years before (5.6). Midwives attended approximately three fourths of all black births, a fact that many members of the Arkansas State Medical Society cited as to the excessive loss of life among black women and their babies.

The society considered abolishing midwifery to try to reduce infant mortality.[22] This solution was not feasible, however, since few hospitals outside of Little Rock provided beds for black maternity patients. Physicians would have to attend approximately 7,637 home births, and since many of these rural blacks were poor, physicians attending home births could expect little, if any, pay. Public funds to pay for this care were not available.[23]

An alternative solution called for replacing the granny midwife with the nurse-midwife. However, there were very few nurse-midwives in Arkansas or in the country, no physicians under whom they could work, and no facilities for hospital care of complicated obstetrical cases. The only viable solution was to attempt to regulate and educate the existing midwives.

In 1944 no law or state board of health regulation required midwives to have permits. The Board of Health had relied on the voluntary cooperation of the midwives to comply with its rules and instructions. These rules and instructions encouraged the midwife to (1) call a physician when any difficulty arose, (2) make no initial examination and use no drugs, (3) be clean, (4) use silver nitrate solution in the infant's eyes, and (5) register all births.[24] State Board of Health regulations only covered birth registration and administration of eye drops.

By 1945 the State Board of Health intensified efforts to address the discrepancy in maternal mortality rates between black and white women by forming a committee to study midwifery. The Committee on the Study of Midwifery, in conjunction with the Arkansas State Medical Society, recommended measures that would make adequate care in childbirth available to all at a price they could afford.[25] They called for the establishment of adequate hospitalization facilities for black maternity cases. This meant supplying at least 500 more beds for the 10,000 annual births. The committee also called for provision of medical care to detect and care for abnormal childbirth cases. The other recommendations focused on the granny midwife. The State Board of Health was committed to "weeding out" the worst midwives and supervising the others as closely as possible. The committee suggested that the State Board of Health adopt a definite regulation against practicing midwifery without a permit, with a penalty for failure to comply.

Making Do with the Midwife

The State Board of Health had hired Mamie Hale in 1942 to work in the Crittendon County Health Department, where she began her work with granny midwives.[26] Three years later, Mamie Hale took the position of midwife consultant for the Maternal and Child Health Division of the Arkansas Health Department. Her promotion to this position on 1 July 1945 marked the date the State Board of Health officially resigned itself to "making do" with the midwife situation.

A graduate of the Tuskegee School of Nurse-Midwifery, Hale was hired to assist local public health nurses with their educational programs for midwives.[27] She was to play an instrumental role in the Division of Maternal and Child Health Nursing's program to promote educational programs for midwives, provide supervision of them at time of delivery, improve birth registration, and register all practicing midwives.[28] With funding

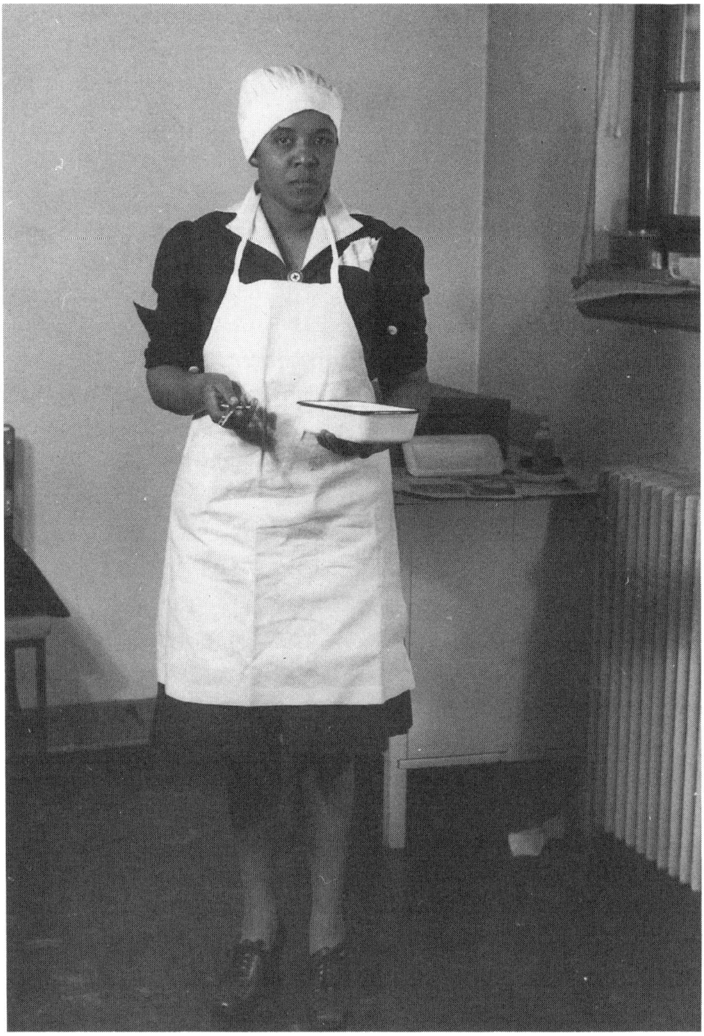

Mamie Hale demonstrating the cleaning of obstetrical instruments for granny midwives attending the state-sponsored training program. (Courtesy of the University of Arkansas for Medical Sciences' Special Collections)

from the Children's Bureau, a statewide training program was started to supplement the midwife classes conducted by local health units. The State Health Department's goal was an annual permit for every practicing midwife. A permit meant that the midwife had attended the training program and successfully passed an examination.

By 1946 "Nurse Hale," as she was called by the granny midwives, was conducting educational programs for midwives in the four health departments of Conway, Faulkner, Lonoke, and St. Francis counties.[29] She presented a series of seven lessons to the local midwives. In addition to classes, Nurse Hale made visits with the midwives to their patients' homes to demonstrate various teaching methods. She also held meetings with parent groups to explain the midwife programs to them. As a result of their training, midwives began to encourage more women to seek early prenatal care. In one county, 366 antepartum patients were identified and added to the program within a three-month period.[30]

Educational programs for the granny midwives proved particularly challenging to Nurse Hale because 75 percent of the midwives could not read or write—only 5 percent could satisfactorily complete a birth certificate.[31] Hale taught the midwives using songs, movies, pictures, and demonstration methods. For example, she instructed midwives to place newspapers in a wood stove until the top and bottom sheets turned slightly brown.[32] The midwives wrapped these papers in cloth and placed them under the mother at the time of delivery. Nurse Hale told the midwives to bake the tape for tying the baby's cord the same amount of time required for baking a medium-sized potato.[33]

Granny midwives were well respected in the community and on the average were between sixty and eighty years of age.[34] Older midwives usually taught the younger midwives, and the majority of these women attributed their position of midwife to a "divine calling."[35] Nurse Hale encouraged this belief by organizing meetings around a religious theme and opening them with hymn singing and prayer. After these preliminaries, Nurse Hale would begin the course of training.

This black nurse-midwife in her mid-thirties commanded respect from black granny midwives as well as white public health nurses and obstetricians. Blacks as well as whites bestowed the title "Nurse Hale" upon her. Support for Nurse Hale was so strong that white public health nurses who traveled with Nurse Hale refused to eat in restaurants where Nurse Hale was denied service.[36]

The Midwife Training Program

The seven-week course was held in churches or schools and depended on the transportation available in the community. An informal first session encouraged the midwives to get acquainted.[37] Nurse Hale's message to the midwives focused on the need to make changes; she described these changes via the metaphor of travel. She talked about the country changing from horse-and-buggy transportation to airplane transportation and encouraged all the midwives to become "airplane" midwives. Occasionally, midwives would call another midwife who adhered to the old ways a "horse-and-buggy" nurse.

The midwives' adherence to the old ways was particularly evident in many of their superstitious beliefs.[38] Some of the superstitions were harmless, but others threatened the health of mother and baby. One common superstition called for placing an axe under the bed of laboring women to cut the labor pains. Other superstitions included biting the baby's fingernails so the baby "wouldn't be a rogue," putting salt on the afterbirth as it was being burned so the mother "wouldn't have no trouble," spitting in the baby's eyes to "keep them from getting sore," and putting soot on the cord to make it "heal up well."

The second session focused on completing a birth certificate.[39] Nurse Hale gave midwives individual assistance in completing these forms in the classroom, as well as in the field, because many were illiterate. Midwives who could not write were encouraged to have family members or neighbors complete the birth certificate.

The third session discussed selection of cases for delivery.[40] Nurse Hale encouraged midwives to consider a woman's willingness to see a physician, the presence of physical handicaps, and her own caseload before taking on additional cases. Further, she encouraged midwives to take only three cases due for delivery in the same week. When a midwife accepted a case, she was to complete a blue card on the mother and have a physician sign the card, which indicated that the physician would see the pregnant woman twice. The physician's physical examination included taking a blood sample for venereal disease.

Nurse Hale urged midwives to make at least three prenatal visits to the patient's home.[41] During these visits, the midwives helped the woman select a place for the delivery and evaluated her diet. The midwife also checked the woman for danger signs such as swelling of hands, ankles and feet, bleeding, severe morning headaches, severe vomiting, and fits or spasms.

The fourth and fifth sessions involved prenatal care.[42] Nurse Hale invited prenatal patients to the fourth session because it focused on nutrition for the expectant mother during labor and the lying-in period. She taught the midwives and prenatal clients to reconstitute dry skim milk and the importance of using milk as a beverage and in cooking during pregnancy.[43]

During the fifth session, Nurse Hale encouraged midwives to seek medical supervision for their cases.[44] Pregnant women were urged to have a physical exam by a doctor, if medical facilities were accessible.[45] Additional instructions focused on diet, rest, exercise, and preparation for delivery. Nurse Hale particularly stressed the importance of using a bag with clean and proper equipment. Each midwife had to have her own bag for the delivery; many used laundry bags.[46]

The sixth session involved a two-hour demonstration of the midwife's role during labor and delivery.[47] Nurse Hale demonstrated the proper setup for labor and delivery and the appropriate care for laboring women. She used a thirty-pound dummy to demonstrate scrubbing, bag inspection, enemas for the mother, and bathing of the mother. She also demonstrated hand-washing techniques. Nurse Hale did not allow the midwives to wear rubber gloves, for she feared they would rely on them instead of proper hand-washing techniques.[48] To prepare for the delivery, Nurse Hale strongly encouraged midwives to prepare the bed for delivery with newspapers, though many believed the floor was the appropriate site for delivery.[49]

Nurse Hale discussed aftercare for the mother and baby in the seventh and final session.[50] She arranged to visit the mothers on their postpartal visit to observe the midwife's care. She interviewed the mothers to make sure the granny midwife adhered to her high standards. Nurse Hale was particularly interested in the cleanliness of the midwife during visits to the home.

Midwives who attended all lectures and met state requirements received permits at graduation ceremonies.[51] They were required to have a medical examination, pledge card, bag equipped according to instructions of the State Health Department, and an application for a midwife permit. The application required the signature of a County Health Officer who could recommend the work of the midwife. Graduation exercises took

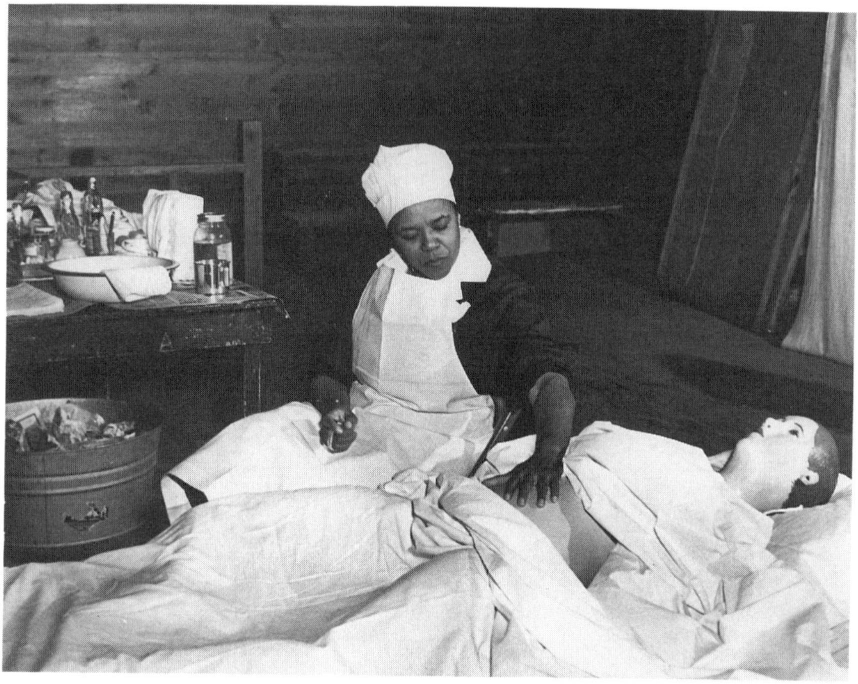

Mamie Hale timing the imaginary contractions of a thirty-pound dummy to demonstrate correct labor and delivery care to granny midwives. (Courtesy of the University of Arkansas for Medical Sciences' Special Collections)

place at a church or school with the minister or principal making welcoming remarks.[52] It was not always possible to having singing or speeches because as many as 80 to 90 midwives graduated in one day.

This one-day graduation ceremony included the local public health nurse reviewing the objectives of the course, a local physician speaking on some phase of maternity care such as "danger signals in pregnancy," and consultants from the State Board of Health giving talks on subjects like nutrition, vital statistics, general maternal and child care, or venereal disease.[53] The ceremonies also included a demonstration of the "modern midwife bag." Dr. Frances Rothert, director of the State Board of Health's Maternal and Child Health Division, addressed the graduates and presented them with permits to practice. Dr. Rothert quoted from Exodus 1:15–17 to impress upon the midwives their responsibilities.[54]

> [15]And the King of Egypt spake to the Hebrew midwives, of which the name of the one was Shiphrah, and the name of the other Puah.
>
> [16]And he said, when ye do the office of a midwife to the Hebrew women, and see them upon the stools; if it be a son, then ye shall kill him; but if it be a daughter, then she shall live.
>
> [17]But the midwives feared God, and did not as the King of Egypt commanded them, but saved the men children alive.

At the close of the ceremony, the midwives would stand, raise their right hands, and solemnly repeat the midwife pledge.[55] The pledge required the midwives to make out a birth certificate on every child, put two drops of silver nitrate in each eye of the baby after delivery, insist that all patients get medical supervision, attend all ongoing midwife classes unless ill or delivering, keep bag clean and equipped at all times, obey all regulations and instructions, and refrain from giving any medicine, performing vaginal examinations, visiting any case when ill, or delivering a woman having a first baby.

Services were also held for retiring midwives. Honorable-retirement certificates were issued to midwives who could no longer attend ongoing midwife classes because of age or ill health.[56] Dr. Rothert thought this a particularly effective method of announcing to the community that the midwife no longer held a permit to practice.[57] Other midwives, as well as members of the community, were invited to these ceremonies to recognize the retiring midwife.

Conclusion

By 1948 new maternal child health clinics and conferences were established in eleven counties in Arkansas.[58] Almost 2,500 women received medical services provided by the maternal and child health service resulting in over 8,500 clinic visits in the same year. The Board of Health encouraged patients to use supervised midwives. For the first time, public health nursing consultants sent in rating sheets on midwives they recommended for permit renewals. During 1948, 569 midwives received annual permits; only 482 of these midwives actively practiced during the year, and they reported 5,026 births.

By 1949, more than 50 percent of the counties with public health nurses were conducting some type of maternity or child health clinic.[59] For the first time since the early years of the war, obstetrical consultation to maternity clinics was available statewide through an agreement with the University of Arkansas on behalf of the Obstetric Department of the School of Medicine.[60] Physicians could enhance obstetrical knowledge compromised by the war efforts at the Postgraduate Refresher Program at the university.[61] The course consisted in making rounds on the wards and in clinics and attending conferences, lectures, and demonstrations.

The improvements in nursing personnel and the statewide establishment of maternity clinics enabled the Board of Health to further monitor and restrict the practice of the granny midwife. In 1943, 1,565 midwives practiced in the state, but six years later the state had "weeded out" the most unfit, leaving 1,024 midwives who reported 7,606 births, almost 17 percent of the babies delivered in the state that year.[62] By 1950 midwife classes were conducted in thirty-two counties, contributing to a marked increase in the number of state-certified midwives.[63] After almost five years of classes, midwives with permits attended 75 percent of all midwife births. The number of black deaths due to pregnancy and childbirth fell from 128 in 1930 to 43 in 1950.[64]

These accomplishments speak highly of the work of Nurse Mamie Hale for she convinced granny midwives to accept the idea that State Health Department classes were important and useful. She found ways to instruct midwives despite their advanced ages, superstitious beliefs, and widespread illiteracy. Midwives who graduated from this training program encouraged their patients to seek medical care during pregnancy. They learned proper conduct for normal delivery and home nursing care of the newborn and mother following delivery. Also, they learned to complete birth certificates, receiving praise for this accomplishment from Dr. Briggs, chairman of the state's Child Welfare Committee in 1951.[65]

The accomplishments of Nurse Hale are even more significant as they occurred amidst a global war and racial prejudice. While Arkansas's physicians were caught up in the war efforts abroad, this nurse-midwife and her granny midwives proved to be effective soldiers at home in the war to improve maternal and infant mortality rates.

Those who knew Mamie Hale personally attribute her contributions to her strong character and belief in black people's ability to address their own problems.[66] Nurse Hale's work with these granny midwives proved she could not only "make do" by improving the midwifery skills of elderly and illiterate women but could help to "make better" the health status of Arkansas's black pregnant women and their children.

Pegge L. Bell, MSN
Assistant Professor
College of Nursing
University of Arkansas for Medical Sciences

3901 South Lookout
Little Rock, Ark. 72205
Work: (501) 686-5374
Home: (501) 661-9698
(501) 664-5731

Acknowledgments

The author would like to give special thanks to the History of Medicine Associates for their partial support of this research.

Notes

1. Vinita Lewis, "Rural Social Services for Negro Children," *The Child* 5 (March 1941): 228–32.

2. Boyce Drummond, "Arkansas 1940–1954," *Historical Report of the Secretary of State*, Arkansas 3 (1978): 175–83.

3. Estelle Riddle and Josephine Nelson, "The Nurse Looks Toward Tomorrow," in *The History of American Nursing*, ed. Susan Reverby (New York: Garland Publishers, 1985), 131–33.

4. Estelle Riddle Osborne, "Status and Contribution of the Negro Nurse," in *The History of American Nursing*, ed. Susan Reverby (New York: Garland Publishers, 1985), 135–40.

5. Frederick D. Mott and Milton I. Roemer, *Rural Health and Medical Care* (New York: McGraw-Hill Book Co., 1948), 29.

6. J. P. Price, "Committee on Study of Midwifery," *Journal of Arkansas Medical Society* 45 (June 1948): 20 (hereafter cited as *JAMS*).

7. Matilda Touhey, "Train Midwives To Aid Work of Health Division," *The Arkansas Gazette* (November 1950).

8. R. B. Robins, "The President's Page," *JAMS* 39 (July 1942): 61.

9. Paul V. McNutt, "The Procurement of Physicians," *The Journal of the American Medical Association* 119 (27 June 1942): 715.

10. W. R. Brooksher, "Distribution of Physicians in Arkansas," *JAMS* 41 (September 1944): 85.

11. Paul Mahoney, "Report of the Secretary," *JAMS* 43 (June 1946): 28.

12. W. R. Brooksher, "Refresher Courses in Pediatrics and Obstetrics," *JAMS* 41 (January 1947): 202.

13. J. P. Price, "Committee on Midwifery," *JAMS* 44 (June 1947): 22.

14. J. Yerushalmy, "The 1940 Record of Maternal and Infant Mortality in the United States," *The Child* 6 (February 1942): 195–206.

15. Ibid., 206.

16. Dr. Frances Rothert to Dr. Dowl K. Eubanks, 27 July 1953, Special Collections, University of Arkansas for Medical Sciences Library, Little Rock, Arkansas (hereafter cited as UAMSL).

17. Dr. W. Myers Smith to Dr. W. B. Grayson, 19 September 1940, Special Collections, UAMSL.

18. J. B. Jameson, "Committee on Study of Midwifery," *JAMS* 39 (June 1942): 23–27.

19. "Premature Birth and Neonatal Death in Arkansas," *Arkansas Health Bulletin* 2 (February 1945): 2–12 (hereafter cited as *AHB*).

20. J. P. Price, W. H. Martin, and T. H. Jones, "Report of the Committee on Study of Midwifery," *Arkansas State Medical Society* (14 April 1946): 1–4.

21. Ibid.

22. Ibid.

23. Jameson, 24.

24. Ibid.

25. Ibid.

26. "Annual Report" (1945), Arkansas State Board of Health, 36–37 (hereafter cited as ASBH).

27. The Tuskegee School of Nurse-Midwifery for Colored Nurses was established in Tuskegee, Alabama, in 1941 with funding from the Rosenwald Fund, Children's Bureau, and State and County Health Departments. Tuskegee Institute and John A. Andrew Memorial Hospital provided the building and cooperated with the undertaking. The school closed in 1945 because of recruitment problems with faculty and students. "Tuskegee School of Midwifery for Colored Nurses Bulletin," 1944, Washington Collections, Tuskegee Institute, Alabama.

28. "Annual Report" (1945), ASBH, 36–37.

29. Dr. Frances Rothert, Director of Maternal-Child Services, Arkansas State Health Department, 1945–1960, interview by author, Hot Springs, Arkansas, 5 September 1991.

30. Claire N. Moody, "State's Midwife Schools Win U.N. Recognition," news clipping of the Arkansas Department of Health, circa 1951, Special Collections, UAMSL.

31. Mamie O. Hale, "Arkansas Teaches her Midwives," *The Child* 2 (October 1946): 66.

32. Interview with Rothert, 1991.

33. Marguerite Burt, Public Health Nurse, Prescott County, 1945–1947, interview by author, Wynne, Arkansas, 2 September 1991.

34. Hale, 66.

35. Interview with Rothert, 1991.

36. Ibid.

37. Hale, 67.

38. Ibid., 66–67; *AHB* (February 1951): 2–3.

39. Hale, 67.

40. Ibid.

41. Ibid.

42. Ibid.

43. "Negro Midwives Trained in State to Cut Death Rate," *AHB* 8 (February 1951), ASBH.

44. Hale, 67.

45. *AHB* (February 1951).

46. Interview with Rothert, 1991.

47. Hale, 68.

48. Interview with Rothert, 1991.

49. Hale, 68.

50. Ibid.

51. "State's Midwife Plan Attracts Wide Acclaim," *Arkansas Gazette* (Sunday, October 1948).

52. Mamie O. Hale, "Arkansas Midwives Have All-day Graduation Exercises," *The Child* 13 (October 1948): 53–54.

53. Ibid.

54. Interview with Rothert, 1991.

55. Hale, "Graduation Exercise," 54.

56. Ibid.

57. Interview with Rothert, 1991.

58. "Annual Report of the Arkansas State Board of Health" (1948), ASBH.

59. "Annual Report of the Arkansas State Board of Health" (1949–1950), ASBH.

60. Brooksher, 202.

61. I. F. Jones, "Maternal Welfare Committee," *JAMS* 47 (March 1951): 190–91.

62. "Annual Report" (1949–1950), ASBH.

63. "Annual Report of the Arkansas State Board of Health" (1950–1951), ASBH.

64. Ibid.

65. B. P. Briggs, "Child Welfare Committee," *JAMS* 47 (March 1951): 191.

66. Interview with Rothert, 1991.

"Exchangees" or Employees? The Exchange Visitor Program and Foreign Nurse Immigration to the United States, 1945–1990

BARBARA L. BRUSH
School of Nursing
University of Pennsylvania

For the past eighty years, the cry "nursing shortage" has been heard repeatedly in the United States. Of different lengths and proportions, each shortage spawned myriad attempts at resolution with divergent outcomes. One often used but rarely discussed strategy is the importation of foreign nurse labor.

In the forty-year span between 1945 and 1985, thousands of men and women moved from their homes in countries like Australia, Great Britain, Ireland, the Philippines, and India to practice nursing in American hospitals. Though this number never represented more than 4 percent of the total domestic nursing work force in the United States, the international trade in nurses is an enduring phenomenon that raises questions about the utilization of nurses—especially during periods of insatiable demand for more nursing care.[1]

Because of the scope and complexity of the phenomenon of foreign nurse immigration and employment, this article elaborates on only one fragment of the mosaic. Focusing specifically on the International Council of Nurses' postwar Exchange Visitor Program (EVP) and its peculiarities, I argue that the Exchange Program fostered two antithetical programs. On the one hand, it promoted the movement of nurses between countries as an avenue for "cultural exchange"; on the other hand, it became a means for nurses from war-torn countries to seek economic refuge as workers in American hospitals. I will show that while the EVP's overlying motives were abstract, extolling a credo of international understanding and world peace efforts through cultural exchange, its underlying effect was quite different. The program became a recruiting mechanism for short-staffed hospitals that augmented depleted nursing staffs with inexpensive foreign workers. Thus, the basic philosophy of the EVP turned out to be quite

Nursing History Review 1 (1993): 171–80.

different from the central motives of the participating nurses as well as the health care institutions. The "exchange" meant different things to the various players involved, setting a precedent for our continued confusion and anxiety about the role and use of foreign nurses in American nursing and hospitals. Ultimately the contradiction between motivation and philosophy created a conflict that pitted efforts to balance supply and demand of nurses in hospitals against public safety and professional welfare.

Exchange Visitor Program

After World War II, many nurses from foreign countries were introduced to American nursing through the 1948 Exchange Visitor Program. Established by the International Council of Nurses (ICN) after the 1947 ICN Congress in Atlantic City, the program, sponsored by the American Nurses' Association (ANA), had two major objectives. First, the EVP offered educational and practical experience to foreign trained nurses under the assumption that they would gain useful knowledge and skills to bring back to their native countries. Second, the EVP promoted "international understanding, good will and the enrichment of world health service."[2] Essentially, foreign nurses were seen as diplomatic emissaries or, as Jeanne Broadhurst labeled them in her 1962 study *Nurses from Abroad: Values in International Exchange of Persons*, "ambassadors of good will."[3]

> What better persons can communicate our achievements to other countries than the nurse with her high code of ethics? What better ambassador can we expect to have? The nurse belongs to an honorable, dignified profession. It is she, who on her return home will mingle both with the average and the influential people of her country. She will tell them about the way of life in the United States.[4]

Broadhurst's study is perhaps the only detailed account of the Exchange Visitor Program and its participants. Funded through the combined efforts of the Rockefeller and American Nurses' foundations, the study investigated the program's effectiveness amidst rising concerns that visitors coming to U.S. hospitals were "arriving in such large numbers that it raised numerous pressing problems."[5] Broadhurst interviewed and recorded the experiences of sixty graduate nurses from fifteen countries who arrived between 1956 and 1961. Though she did not identify the nurses by name or country of origin, most of the nurses in the first decade of the EVP were from Scandinavian or British Isle countries. Between 1948 and 1951, Danish nurses comprised 54 percent of exchangees, followed by nurses from Sweden (11 percent), Great Britain (9 percent), and Norway (6 percent).[6] Nevertheless, Broadhurst's study provides the historian with a valuable glimpse of the foreign nurse's experience from her arrival in the United States to her termination and return home.

Interested nurses from ICN member countries applied to the ANA's International Unit for admission to the Exchange Visitor Program. There were few prerequisites other than previous nurse training, a signed language certificate from the nurse's national nursing association attesting to English language competency, and, most important, the nurse's ability to pay passage to the United States.[7] "The Exchange Program," stated Broadhurst, "is open to anyone who elects to come as a staff nurse if she has the financial means, regardless of her quality as a nurse."[8] Thus, self-subsidization of the trip prevailed over the nurse's level and standard of practice.

Once accepted to the program, the nurse was placed in three or four six-month rotations in participating hospitals for the eighteen-month program.[9] The estimated one hundred affiliate hospitals in twenty-four states were expected to and agreed to provide in-service education and other instructional programs for the foreign nurses in combination with their practical bedside experiences.[10] Further, hospitals provided each foreign exchangee with a small stipend for living expenses in addition to room and board. Stipend amounts varied considerably from institution to institution, averaging anywhere from $35 to $88 every two weeks; this figure compares to American hospital staff nurses earnings of approximately $175 per month or around $2,100 per year.[11] Stipends were also used as measures of competency or as compensation for the lack of required educational programs. One nurse shared with Broadhurst,

> I chose this hospital knowing well that there was no educational program, but I knew, too, that I would receive a higher stipend. In my previous assignment there was no educational program either. I received a low salary and I worked forty hours per week, too. At least in this hospital, I get a financial advantage.[12]

Although foreign nurses visiting the United States on a two-year exchange visa were treated and expected to act as workers, hospitals behaved as though their visitor status justified lower wages. Further, despite the EVP's de-emphasis of nursing capabilities and skills, nurse's stipends and status were often contingent upon them. For example, a foreign nurse deemed poor in language skills or clinically inept was paid a reduced stipend or relegated to a lower paid nurse's aid position until she was "brought up to the standards required of the nursing profession for the safety and welfare of patients."[13] Nursing directors complained bitterly to Broadhurst that inadequate basic training and language difficulties created problems. Broadhurst retorted, "a willingness to accept only those who are highly proficient would be tantamount to asserting, that, being short of nurses, the United States wishes only to receive help and not give it."[14]

Rather than acknowledging the incongruity of the philosophy of the exchange program and hospital practices, hospital and nursing administrators measured and justified the amounts of monetary reimbursement and degree of responsibility given to foreign nurses by "patient safety" standards. Using this criteria, many foreign exchangees faced widespread exploitation. Often treated as low-paid hired hands rather than international trainees, several nurses expressed their discontent to Broadhurst. One nurse stated, "All we do is work forty hours per week like American nurses. We have no lectures, no in-service education, no programs, and receive only a stipend; we are, it seems, used for labor shortage."[15]

The Postwar Hospital and Nursing Needs

The social, cultural, and political forces of the postwar period created and shaped the ways in which the patterns and practices of foreign nurses evolved. Greater emphasis was placed on acute care and the use of hospital versus home care in the years prior to and immediately after 1945. Scientific and technological advances and improvements in the standard of living significantly reduced communicable disease morbidity and mortality.[16] The discovery and use of antibiotics and other pharmaceuticals contributed to altered patterns of sickness, improved outcomes of surgical interventions, and alternate treatment of various forms of chronic illness. Technological improvements for saving and preserving lives were dramatic; extension of that technology to hospital settings received support from hospital professionals, administrators, policy-makers, and the public alike.[17]

By 1945 hospitals became the major employers of nurses and were central to the successful interplay between the postwar emphasis on science and technology and people's expectation of access to care and cure.[18] Concomitantly, the 1946 Hospital Survey and Construction Act (Hill-Burton) enabled the rapid expansion of new hospitals and health centers, so that by 1951 there were nearly one million beds in nearly seven thousand general, mental, tuberculosis, and chronic hospitals.[19]

The combined effect of postwar hospital expansion in both numbers and magnitude, changes in types and amounts of health care, shifts in consumer ideologies about health, greater individual and national economic standings, and postwar recovery strained the U.S. health care system in general and nurses in particular.[20] Demand for more nursing services gave rise to a widespread and critical nursing shortage, despite evidence that nursing numbers actually increased proportionate to numbers of hospital beds.[21]

Hospitals suffering from perceived nursing shortages recruited foreign nurses regularly from the ranks of the Exchange Visitor Program, and they also recruited nurses who were not participants in the EVP.[22] Moreover, recruits were often hired at lower wages than their domestic counterparts. After ten years of sponsorship, the American Nurses' Association began to worry that the misuse of foreign exchangees potentiated unsafe care while adversely affecting the professional and economic status of U.S. nursing.[23]

Perhaps the association's stance was influenced by its active efforts to improve the economic welfare of nurses. Certainly the ANA's criticisms reflected the growing dissatisfaction of U.S. nurses with their own incomes during the widespread nursing shortage. The ANA worked to rectify the working and living conditions of American nurses. The ANA also supported state nurses' associations as bargaining units and tried to eliminate racial and sexual segregation in education and hiring practices. The arbitrary use of foreign nurses by hospitals threatened these national professional organization agendas as well as "international professional concepts of good nursing education and practice."[24]

Raising Supply to Meet Demand

Similar factors probably operated to encourage the combined use of foreign and black nurse labor despite the hospital-based practice of foreign nurses and traditional home-based care by blacks. The postwar period marked the beginning of black nurse integration into the ANA as the National Association of Colored Graduate Nurses voluntarily dissolved its functions into the larger body of the ANA in 1951. The gradual acceptance of blacks into primarily private duty and public health practice occurred at the same time as the utilization of foreign nurses in hospitals during this period of "shortage."[25] The willingness to incorporate black nurses and foreign nurses into a predominantly white female work force was largely the result of an increased demand for nurses and a limited white domestic supply.

Further evidence of supply-side strategies used to alleviate the nursing shortage indicates not only a heterogeneous work force but also a formalized caste system in nursing work. New supplies of nursing personnel came from expanded practical nurse and nurse assistant programs during the 1950s. Numbers of schools of practical nursing increased from a mere 50 in 1947 to over 400 eight years later; the numbers of practical nurses nearly doubled, from 137,000 to 250,000 between 1950 and 1964.[26] The influx of different levels of caregivers spread the work of nursing among more pairs of hands; workers could be trained more rapidly and more inexpensively. The primarily white foreign nurse population, deemed "professionals" but paid less to do the same work as domestic professional registered nurses, did not fit within either the racially or hierarchically segmented nursing work force.

Immigration Law and Foreign Nurse Migration

In 1952, during the height of the McCarthy years, the Immigration and Nationality Act created a xenophobic quota system favoring immigration of individuals from Western hemisphere countries over those in the "Asia-Pacific Triangle."[27] Europeans were given greater access to migration than were individuals from China, India, and the Philippines, for example. As was true of the general pattern of immigration, foreign nurses recruited and admitted during these years were largely from the British Isles countries of Great Britain, Ireland, and Canada.[28] Hence, at first the generally white females from predominantly English-speaking countries did not threaten the Anglo-Saxon hegemony of American nursing. Despite their accents, foreign nurses probably blended into hospital settings relatively easily.

Immigration policy in the late 1960s and early 1970s, a legacy of the Kennedy administration, radically departed from earlier immigration regulations. Under the terms of the 1965 Immigration Act, the national quota system was gradually phased out and preference for immigration shifted from country of origin to family reunification and needed occupational skills.[29] This latter criterion had important implications for nursing, which was again facing a large-scale "nursing shortage." Because countries in the

"Asia-Pacific Triangle" were no longer selectively denied access to immigration, larger numbers of immigrants from a wider range of nations were admitted to the United States. As a result, European immigration declined from 41 percent of the total immigration to 18 percent between 1965 and 1976; Asian immigration, on the other hand, soared from 7.8 percent of total immigration in 1963 to 38 percent by 1976.[30] Again, patterns of nurse immigration mirrored general migration patterns.

By 1970 Filipino nurses comprised the largest number of migrating foreign nurses, making up 43 percent of the total, followed by Canadian (24 percent), British (15 percent), and Korean (4 percent) nurses.[31] While many of these nurses still came to the United States via the EVP, most were recruited directly by hospitals specifically as workers.

Conclusion

Over the past forty years since the inception of the Exchange Visitor Program, considerable change developed in the phenomenon of foreign nurse migration. Changing immigration policies, political ideologies, and social structures have played significant roles in altering the demographic profile of foreign nurses as well as changing sentiments surrounding their utilization in the American health care system. The Exchange Visitor Program was a harbinger of the experience in the next few decades of the international trade of nurses. It was a project of private altruism, cultural promotion, and national propaganda. Its frontline agenda to produce "international understanding and good will" enabled the program to continue and flourish for almost thirty years despite documented institutional misuse of foreign nurse exchangees, inadequately supervised programs, and other "deviations from the original intent" of the EVP.[32] Postwar anxieties over the exploitation of foreign nurses, the manpower "brain drain" from sending countries, threatened wage depression of U.S. nursing salaries, unsafe clinical practice, and the potential substitution of foreign visitors in American nurses' jobs all plagued the Exchange Visitor Program.[33]

Currently, the U.S. General Accounting Office estimates that there are 24,000 foreign nurses working in American hospitals, 75 percent of whom are Filipino nurses working principally in large metropolitan hospitals in the states of New York, California, and Florida.[34] They are the mainstay work force of many inner-city municipally operated institutions. The most dramatic example is the New York City hospital system, where, it is estimated, 20 to 30 percent of employed nurses are foreign nurses on five-year immigration visas.[35] Further, according to the American Hospital Association's most recent survey of nursing personnel (1988), 11.5 percent of hospitals reported shortages of registered nurses and indicated that they use foreign nurse labor.[36]

While there has been an obvious shift from the early internationalism of the Exchange Visitor Program to the contemporary employment of foreign nurses to relieve the perceived short supply of nurses, foreign nurses have been utilized as short-term, temporary workers for nursing shortages in American hospitals throughout the latter half of the twentieth century. Foreign nurses have been present, if not always visible, adjuncts to U.S. hospital nursing staffs for decades. While perhaps the faces and names have changed over time, the recruitment and employment of foreign nurses is emblematic of our persistent preoccupation with inexpensive supply-side strategies to cope with demand-side strains on the U.S. health care system. When demand for nursing care rises, we send for more nurses.

BARBARA L. BRUSH
Doctoral Candidate
School of Nursing
University of Pennsylvania
Research Associate
International Council of Nurses Centennial History Project

8629 Patton Road
Wyndmoor, Pa. 19118
Phone: (215) 836-1285
Fax: (215) 898-6320

Notes

1. Jean S. Arbeiter, "The Facts about Foreign Nurses," *RN* (September 1988): 56–63.

2. Minutes of the Grand Council Meeting, Melbourne, Australia, *Reports of the Standing Committees: Exchange of Privileges Committee* (Agenda Item IX, Annex 4, 1961), International Council of Nurses Archives, Geneva, Switzerland, 58–72 (hereafter cited as ICNA).

3. Martha Jeanne Broadhurst, *Nurses From Abroad: Values in International Exchange of Persons* (New York: The American Nurses' Foundation, Inc., 1962), 9.

4. Martha Jeanne Broadhurst, "Knowing Our Exchange Visitors," *Nursing Outlook* 6 (April 1958): 201.

5. Ibid., 5.

6. Statistics compiled from data, Study Programs and Employment Arranged for Foreign Nurses Who Are At Present in the U.S.A., 15 October 1951, ANA Collection, #N87, box 180, Nursing Archives, Boston University Mugar Library (hereafter cited as BUML).

7. See Martha Jeanne Broadhurst, "Knowing Our Exchange Visitors," *Nursing Outlook* 6 (April 1958): 198–201; "Exchange for Education," *The American Journal of Nursing* 58 (December 1958): 1666–71; Margrethe Kruse, "Exchange of Nurses," *Nursing Times* (12 September 1953): 918–19.

8. Broadhurst, *Nurses From Abroad*, 9.

9. This time period was extended to two years in 1959 in concordance with the U.S. Department of State regulations.

10. Minutes of the Committee on International Affairs, 8 January 1960, ANA Collection, #N87, box 294, BUML. Participating hospitals were not under the jurisdiction of the ANA, rather, they were regulated by the U.S. State Department.

11. Broadhurst, *Nurses From Abroad*, 116; Lily Mary David, "Economic Status of Private Duty and General Staff Nurses," *American Journal of Nursing* 47 (October 1947): 671.

12. Broadhurst, *Nurses From Abroad*, 94.

13. Ibid., 90.

14. Ibid., 89.

15. Ibid., 39.

16. See U.S. Department of Commerce, Bureau of the Census, *Historical Statistics of the United States—Colonial Times to 1970* Part I (Washington, D.C.: U.S. Government Printing Office, 1975), 55. Average life expectancies for white males rose from 62.1 years of age to 66.5 and white females from 66.6 to 72.2 between 1940 and 1950; black men and women experienced prolonged life expectancies as well but at much lower rates overall. Male rates increased from 51.5 to 59.1 and female's from 54 to 62 years of age.

17. For a more detailed discussion of the transformation of hospital care and the effects of science and technology, see Susan Reverby, "The Search for the Hospital Yardstick: Nursing and Rationalization of Hospital Work," in *Health Care in America: Essays in Social History*, ed. Susan Reverby and David Rosner (Philadelphia: Temple University Press, 1987), 206–25; Charles E. Rosenberg, *The Care of Strangers: The Rise of America's Hospital System* (New York: Basic Books, 1987); Dianne E. Long and Janet Golden, *The American General Hospital: Communities and Social Contexts* (Ithaca, N.Y.: Cornell University Press, 1989); Rosemary Stevens, *In Sickness and in Wealth: American Hospitals in the Twentieth Century* (New York: Basic Books, 1989).

18. Donald Yett, "The Supply of Nurses: An Economist's View," *Hospital Progress* 46 (February 1965): 92. Fifty-three percent of active professional nurses were employed in hospitals.

19. "Hospital Beds in the United States," *Public Health Reports* 67 (March 1952): 313; U.S. Department of Commerce, Bureau of the Census, *Historical Statistics of the United States: Colonial Times to 1970* Part I (Washington, D.C.: U.S. Government Printing Office, 1975).

20. Stevens, *In Sickness and in Wealth*.

21. Numbers of active practicing registered nurses increased from 299,067 in 1949 to 532,118 by 1962. U.S. Department of Health, Education and Welfare, *Source Book: Nursing Personnel* (Washington, D.C.: U.S. Government Printing Office, 1973).

22. Meeting of the Committee on Nursing in International Affairs, 9 December 1965, ANA #N87, box 460, BUML. Chairman of the committee, Dorothy J. Sutherland stated, "these people disappear in the United States that immigration can't find . . . we are sure [they] are working as nurses some place."

23. Louise Flanagan, *Braving New Frontiers: ANA's Economic and General Welfare Program* (Washington, D.C.: American Nurses' Association, 1984).

24. ANA Statement on Practices Relating to Nurses From Abroad, 2 March 1960, ANA Collection, #N87, box 180, BUML.

25. Darlene Clark Hine, *Black Women in White: Racial Conflict and Cooperation in the Nursing Profession, 1890–1950* (Bloomington: Indiana University Press, 1989); G. R. Smith, "From Invisibility to Blackness: The Story of the National Black Nurses Association," *Nursing Outlook* 23 (April 1975): 225–29. Black nurses who were employed in hospitals during this period were still primarily segregated in black hospitals and training schools and did not enter "mainstream" hospital staff nursing until the 1960s.

26. Lucille Petry Leone, "Trends and Problems in Practical Nurse Education," *The American Journal of Nursing* 56 (January 1956): 51–53; National Commission on Community Health Services, National Task Forces Project, *Health Manpower: Action to Meet Community Needs* (Washington, D.C.: Public Affairs Press, 1967), 52.

27. I. R. H. Rockett, "American Immigration Policy and Ethnic Selection: An Historical Overview," *The Journal of Ethnic Studies* 10 (April 1983): 1–23.

28. A. Mejia, H. Pizurski, and E. Royston, *Physician and Nurse Migration: Analysis and Policy Implications* (Geneva: World Health Organization, 1979).

29. Rockett, 15.

30. Ibid., 17.

31. United States Department of Health, Education, and Welfare, *Survey of Foreign Nurse Graduates*, DHEW Publication No. 76–13 (Bethesda: U.S. Government Printing Office, 1976): 25.

32. ANA Statement on Practices Relating to Nurses From Abroad, 1960, ANA Collection, #N87, box 180, BUML.

33. Board of Directors Meeting, *Report of the Exchange of Nurses Committee*, 6 June 1949, ICNA, 26–28; Francis Elder, "Are Our Hospitals Exploiting Foreign Nurses?" *RN* 17 (September 1954): 38–42, 68; "Protecting Our Exchange Visitors and Nursing Practice," *The American Journal of Nursing* (December 1953): 698.

34. United States General Accounting Office, *Information on Foreign Nurses Working in the United States under Temporary Work Visas* (Washington, D.C.: Government Printing Office, 1989).

35. Booz, Allen and Hamilton, Inc., *Characteristics and Labor Market Impact of Persons Admitted Under the H-1 Program: Final Report* (Washington, D.C.: U.S. Government Printing Office, 1988).

36. "Foreign Nurses Play Critical Role During Shortage," *AHA News* (April 1990): 18, 22.

A Profession in Caricature

Changing Attitudes Toward Nursing in the *American Medical News*, 1960–1989

JUDITH A. CHANEY
School of Nursing
Southern Illinois University at Edwardsville

PATRICK FOLK
Department of History
McKendree College

"Increasingly we live in a symbolic world, a world which is 'make believe,' but a world which has very real consequences."[1] Modern mass communications have created a society in which much of our perception of reality is composed of a complex mixture of impressions, images, symbols, and stereotypes manufactured and delivered by the media. The mass media is probably the most important agent of socialization in our culture today, critically influencing how we see our world, our fellow human beings, and even ourselves. We live in a social universe created by radio, television, movies, magazines, and newspapers. "By selecting out of the culture certain existing tendencies, patterns of behavior, attitudes, and values and by repeating them over and over again" the modern media is able to "not merely *reflect* the society but *shape* it by reinforcing those characteristics they select for attention."[2] Thus, mass communications also impact dramatically on our value systems, since they "help indicate the elements which make for power, success, and happiness in society and provide models for behavior."[3]

The popular image and status of any group in society is constantly being defined and redefined by the mass media. The three most important sources for status ranking in the United States are probably race, gender, and occupation. Membership in the first two of these categories is biologically determined, but the last is, at least partially, a matter of voluntary individual choice. While any group must be vitally concerned about its public image, occupational groups are especially vulnerable to popular perceptions since new members are attracted, or repelled, by that image. A negative occupational status ranking may attract only recruits with low self-

Nursing History Review 1 (1993): 181–202.

esteem, eventually depressing the self-image of the entire group. This will retard the occupation's prestige, power, and financial standing, and lead to increasing job dissatisfaction in the ranks.[4]

Clearly, nursing has long suffered from low public image. Philip and Beatrice Kalisch noted a 1979 federal report ranking the occupational prestige of 122 professions. Physicians came in first, with social workers, clergy, school teachers, physical therapists, librarians, and dental hygienists all listed in the top 90 professions. Nurses ranked ninety-first, "just ahead of embalmers."[5] Although the public at large may know nurses only through movies, television, radio, and the printed page, surely those who work most closely with the profession have formed a more realistic image. What perception of nurses is held by those at the top of that professional prestige ladder, the physicians?

Any examination of doctors' images of nurses must begin with a recognition that nursing is almost entirely a female occupation, while the medical profession remains predominantly male. According to Suzanne Gordon, women are still in the majority of those in the caring professions, comprising 97 percent of the nation's nursing professionals. While most of the 2.1 million nurses are women, only 16 percent of the 585,597 doctors in the United States are female.[6]

This fact raises a serious question. Is the view of nursing held by the medical profession, and that of the public in general, based solely on gender? Janet Muff certainly thinks so: "The image of a 'nurse' is that of a female. . . . There are certainly men in nursing . . . but the image and identity problems of *nursing* are female."[7] Anne Hudson Jones also argues that "the nurse is a metaphor for all women. The tensions within the profession of nursing today and the conflicting images of nurses reflect historical and contemporary conflicts about women's role."[8] In their preface to *The Changing Image of the Nurse*, Kalisch and Kalisch cited a recent Gallup poll in which 99 percent of those questioned agreed that women made better nurses than men. No other occupation (not even truck driving) received such a high gender-role stereotype rating.[9]

Because doctors have close personal and professional contact with nurses, their perceptions may include non-sex-role elements. One major problem in assessing medical views of nursing arises, however, from the attempt to separate those elements of the image grounded in gender perceptions and those arising from other sources. This would be difficult to accomplish even if attitudes and images remained constant over time. But the obvious fact that the role of women and of the nursing profession have both undergone dramatic changes in the last few decades exacerbates the problem. Have physicians' views of nurses changed during this period? If so, have those changes resulted primarily from challenges to male supremacy in society at large, or from shifts in power relationships between the nursing and medical professions?

Such questions cannot easily be answered by studying traditional medical sources. Attitudes toward others, especially those with whom we work and on whom we depend, are often consciously or unconsciously camouflaged. This is especially true if displaying such attitudes might bring retribution. Even those who seem to hold little power can make the workplace a living hell if aroused. In Suzanne Gordon's *Prisoners of Men's Dreams*, one female doctor recounted what her teachers warned her: "All I was ever taught about nurses in medical school is . . . you'd better get along with the nurses because if you don't they can *hurt* you."[10]

Not only nurses have developed a capability to inflict damage on antagonists. Since 1960, public expressions of hostility toward women increasingly carry the potential of triggering social, economic, political, or even legal sanctions. Attitudes that cannot be openly voiced are often communicated in humor: "And in an era of great tension, humor seems more important . . . than ever before."[11] A longitudinal study of medical humor about nurses covering the period of the past few decades could reveal much about how doctors really regard nursing.

In this article we examine the cartoon because it is "communication to the quick," a freer form of humorous expression than the written word. "In an era when media are increasingly fast-paced and visual, the cartoon seems to capture the best—and perhaps the worst—of modern communication." It is symbolic and pertains to the emotions rather than the intellect. The cartoon "deals in images and stereotypes which . . . may be out-of-awareness; it persuades without taking responsibility, and its arguments are difficult to articulate or to refute on a rational, logical basis."[12] The cartoon represents a perfect idiom for modern life, where our world is increasingly a symbolic creation of our mass media. Within this process, "anything can happen—anything the cartoonist can conceive or the viewer imagine. The creation of this make-believe world has deep roots in human perception, memory, fantasy, and communication."[13] By their very nature, cartoons convey perceptions by portraying stereotyped representations of their subjects.

Although cartoonists ideally try "to avoid the prejudicial and hackneyed to the extent possible, the demands of the medium make it almost impossible to shun stereotypes completely."[14] These stereotypical representations, however, have become a vital vehicle for social commentary that can often find no other outlet. "Because the cartoon makes us laugh, it may not seem serious. But by most standards—social, psychological, economic, political, or artistic—the cartoon is a unique force in modern society." European scholars, who have long studied the cartoon, believe that the cartoon, a living medium, at once mirrors the inner workings of society and in turn molds that society's perceptions.[15] These perceptions are often negative rather than positive. "The cartoon deals in racial, ethnic, and sexual stereotypes . . . it conserves and perpetuates some of the worst elements of popular culture." Since "the cartoon is humorous . . . in commentary or serious discussion, its 'sugar-coated' contents may be swallowed—no matter how lethal."[16]

The only major medical publication that is aimed at all doctors and that has included cartoons since its inception is the *American Medical News*. This newspaper has been continually published as an official organ by the American Medical Association (AMA) since 1958. Originally titled the *AMA News*, the paper adopted its present title in 1969. The *News* uses a brief, nontechnical format that can be read quickly. Its purpose is to keep physicians informed about new research and treatment methods and to keep them abreast of political trends affecting the profession. Reports from national specialty meetings and human interest stories are also included. A newspaper for the practicing physician, its size has increased dramatically, reflecting the information explosion that has taken place in health care.

In the beginning the *News* was a biweekly publication. By July 1960 it was the most widely distributed medical publication in the United States. An AMA survey found that 89.6 percent of America's physicians, or some 220,000, were reading the *News* regularly.[17] In 1965, it became a weekly publication. In its tenth anniversary issue, an article entitled "Medical Publications . . . Big Business and Booming" boasted that the *News* had the most vigorous growth of all medical publications, reporting 365,000 subscribers, despite the fact that sixty-three medical periodicals had been born in the last decade. The paper's editors promised to keep news reports and articles as simple and brief as possible, and to "continue to serve a great profession by providing accurate, reliable reporting by investigating and reporting on issues of concern, and by acting as a means whereby physicians can express their opinions, through letters to the editor as well as in news stories reporting their activities."[18]

By 1981, *American Medical News* was only one of many publications of the AMA, which claimed to be the largest medical and scientific publisher in the world. With a growing list of publications in French, Flemish, German, and Chinese, the AMA in the 1980s was reaching out for liaisons with medical groups worldwide. The *News* remained its official voice and still boasted a readership of well over 300,000 weekly, placing it above the nine AMA specialty journals whose combined subscribers totaled 215,000 per month. The *News* and other publications were trumpeted as "another part of the AMA's role as the leading professional medical organization for all American physicians, and for its additional role as a world leader in advancing the art and science of medicine."[19]

From its inception, the paper's editors made clear their intention to make the *News* a major factor in creating a more organized and articulate body of medical opinion. "Our goal is to make the *AMA News* medicine's greatest conduit of communication. And through our editorials, we hope to help stimulate, challenge, and strengthen the moral and intellectual foundations of the democratic way of American medicine."[20]

Because of the broad spectrum of doctors in its reading audience, and their long-term loyalty, the *American Medical News* undoubtedly reflects social attitudes held by a wide range of practicing physicians far more accurately than any specialty journal. Indeed, as the official organ of the AMA, the *News* consciously seeks to advance the interests of the medical profession as a whole, and it can, therefore, be assumed to reflect attitudes typical of its professional clientele. The inclusion of cartoons in the *News* since its inception indicates that its editors believe their readers find them humorous. One expert on cartoons explained that the audience must first be considered when placing a gag cartoon.[21] The cartoonist must sometimes convince an editor that the audience will appreciate his work. "The editor is the gatekeeper who stands between the cartoonist and the audience. . . . The editor is likely to know and enforce the concerns of the sponsor. The editor gauges what will find favor—or disfavor—with the public."[22] Thus, although most cartoonists complain about editors, these same editors help to shape the cartoonist's thinking.[23] And the editor's thinking is, as noted, shaped by his bosses: "When the sponsor pays there is, of course, usually a reason. The sponsor hopes to sell a product, build a readership . . . persuade, educate, or propagandize."[24] A longstanding tendency by a periodical to select and publish materials reflecting any particular viewpoint indicates an editorial assumption that readers share (or at least do not disfavor) that attitude. Reader loyalty over significant time periods clearly reinforces and validates that assumption.

A complete collection of the *News* since 1960 exists in the Library and Archives of the American Optometric Association in St. Louis. Over a period of two years, we evaluated every cartoon from May 1960 to August 1989; data collection then stopped and full analysis began. Originally, we selected only those cartoons depicting nurses. It seemed, however, that cartoons portraying female patients were as common as those about nurses. This suggested the possibility of using this second group of women as a control to help sort out gender-based attitudes from other potential determinant factors.

During the three decades covered by this study, the *News* published 3,045 cartoons. Of this total, 416 (14 percent) included nurse or female patient caricatures. Two hundred and fifty-eight cartoons depicted nurses, while 267 showed female patients; 109 of the 416 cartoons collected included members of both groups and were, therefore, counted in each total. In order to make our discussions and descriptions more understandable and readily comparable, all cartoon totals will also be expressed as a *percentage of the total base sample* of 416 cartoons collected that contained nurses or female patients (unless otherwise specified).

After our data collection was complete, we reviewed the material many times, letting the categories emerge out of the data—a qualitative technique that we felt to be important to the validity of the study. The first rudimentary viewings led to breaking the data into positive and negative depictions. Seven categories began to surface from the cartoons about nurses. These categories were based on the shared perception that certain attitudes were portrayed consistently through the decades. Each researcher independently viewed and categorized every nurse cartoon. This process was repeated three times, at three-month intervals, with all previous categorizations hidden from view. The fact that we both independently arrived at the same results, with virtually no changes, reassured us that the categories clearly defined the data and that they were valid and reliable.

These seven categories included three negative, one neutral, and three positive groupings. The smallest negative category portrayed the nurse as a sex object. Only 11 cartoons (2.6 percent of the 416 collected) fit into this category. Nine have been published since 1979 (see Cartoon 1).

A second group included cartoons depicting nurses as simple employees, performing menial or unimportant tasks not associated with the nursing profession. This category included only 22 cartoons (5.3 percent), and only one has appeared since 1984.

The final negative category showed nurses as incapable of professionalism. This inability was ascribed to such traditional "female" characteristics as excessive emotionalism and inability to think rationally. This category included 42 cartoons (10 percent), the largest negative group and second largest concentration of nurse depictions in the study (see Cartoons 2 and 3).

One category portrayed nurses in a neutral manner. Cartoons in this group used nurses purely as set decoration or as indicators of a medical setting. Twenty-seven cartoons (6.5 percent of the sample) were judged to belong in this group (see Cartoon 4).

Three categories emerged in which the image of nursing seemed positive. One group depicted the nurse as a professional engaged in important medical activities, although usually under a physician's direction. Thirty-five cartoons (8.4 percent) were found to fit this category (see Cartoon 5).

The largest category of nurse cartoons depicted a collegial relationship between the nursing and medical professions. The nurse was seen as a collaborator engaged in a joint effort. These cartoons often pictured good-natured jousting, with the nurse usually delivering the punch line. Of those collected, 112 cartoons (27 percent) were placed in this category (see Cartoons 6 and 7).

The smallest grouping showed nurses superior to doctors. These cartoons depicted the physician as absentminded or ineffectual and suggested the nurse could replace him. Such depictions were clearly unpopular with the medical profession, since only 9 (2.2 percent) of them appeared in three decades, with only 2 since 1969 (see Cartoons 8 and 9).

The earliest conclusion of this study quickly became obvious from even a cursory review of our data: the cartoon nurse was female and the physician was male. In thirty years of *American Medical News* cartoons, we found one male nurse and two female doctors. The male nurse occupied the same cartoon as one of the female physicians, and the humor was derived from a male patient's befuddlement at these reversed sex roles. The other female physician was clearly a pediatrician (dealing with small children has always been acceptable for females) and the joke is that a tiny male patient is refusing to undress for her. His mother is obviously too flustered to help.

Since nursing was seen by *News* cartoonists as a gender-determined profession, apparent attitudes toward nurses in particular might merely reflect perceptions of women in general. That is why we also collected cartoons about female patients. We expected to map changing attitudes toward women patients and to compare them with attitudes toward nurses. This would demonstrate the extent to which perceptions of nursing were gender-based. We were shocked to discover that the cartoon view of female patients *never* changed. In thirty years, the *News* published 267 cartoons showing female patients. *Not one of those cartoons was positive*. Female patients were depicted as overweight, illogical, overemotional, ignorant, hypochondriacal, pampered, self-indulgent, and generally mindless. One cartoon included in this group did not actually portray a female patient, but merely showed the male doctors of a gynecological society drinking a toast to "the ladies!" These cartoons also portrayed insensitivity on the part of doctors toward female patients (see Cartoons 10 and 11; also see Cartoon 5).

To be sure that the unrelenting hostility directed toward female patients was not due to their role as patients, rather than their gender, a random sample of cartoons featuring male patients was collected. Though they appeared far less frequently, male patients were generally also perceived negatively. But serious differences became obvious. Male patients were sometimes portrayed neutrally, as helpless patients rather than the butt of a joke. It was also male patients, not doctors, who primarily saw nurses as sex objects. The male patient, unless helplessly sick, was normally his own advocate. Finally, male patients were occasionally viewed with some compassion. One angry patient pointed out to his doctor that he had already received three hours of complete rest in the waiting room and it had not helped one bit.

While the unswerving hostility toward female patients was clearly gender-linked, it would take a full-scale study of attitudes toward females as patients to analyze the possible ramifications of that negativity. Such a study was clearly not within the scope of this research, nevertheless, the uniformly negative nature of depictions of female patients allowed us to use them as a rough barometer of hostility toward women. Any significant increase in a *frequency* of cartoons featuring women patients could reflect increased gender-based tensions.

Cartoons featuring female patients totaled 267, or 64 percent, of the total sample of 416 cartoons collected in the study. Figure A shows the incidence of these cartoons as percentages of the total sample organized into five-year cohorts. Thirty-two percent (half of all female patient cartoons) appeared from 1965 to 1974. Hostile cartoons skyrocketed from a mere 5.5 percent in the early 1960s to 14.5 percent in the latter part of the decade. In the early 1970s, they jumped to 17.5 percent. In the late 1970s and early 1980s, the incidence dropped back to single figures, only to escalate to 10.5 percent in the 1985 to 1989 period. Cartoons depicting nurses also peaked from 1965 to 1974. As Figure B shows, nursing cartoons doubled

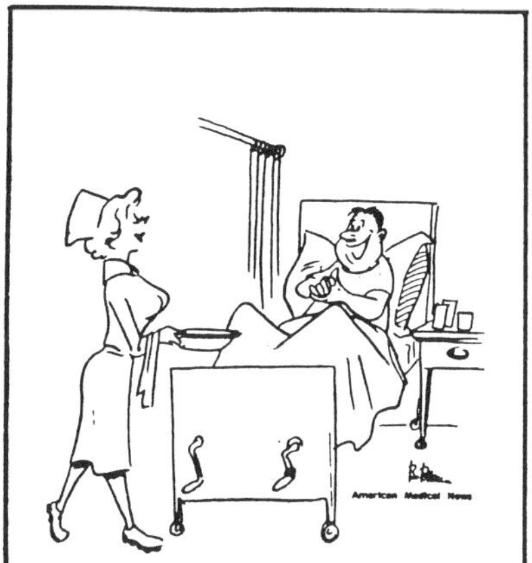

"Time for our bath? Boy, oh boy!"

Cartoon 1. Nurse as sex object. Includes male patient. (*AMN*, 14 July 1969, p. 2)

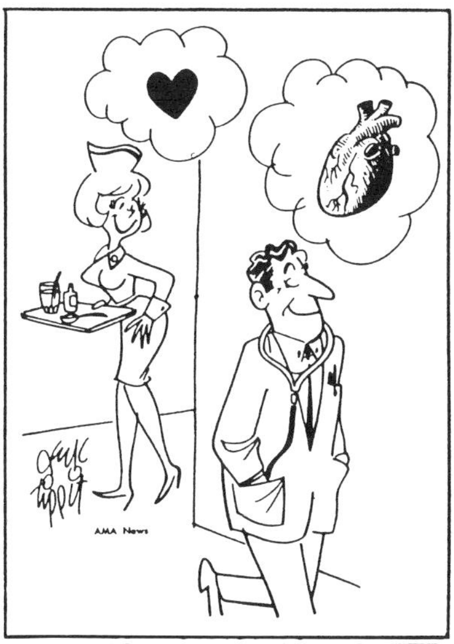

Cartoon 2. Nurse incapable of professional conduct. (*AMAN*, 27 May 1963, p. 11)

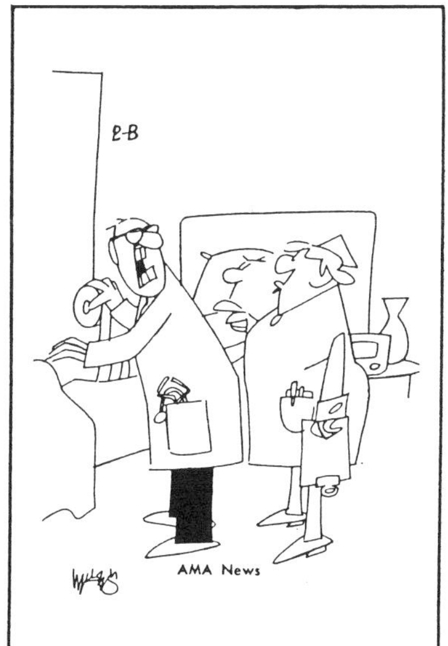

"I don't care **how** *Dr. Kildare does it!"*

Cartoon 3. Nurse incapable of professionalism. (*AMAN*, 20 August 1962, p. 12)

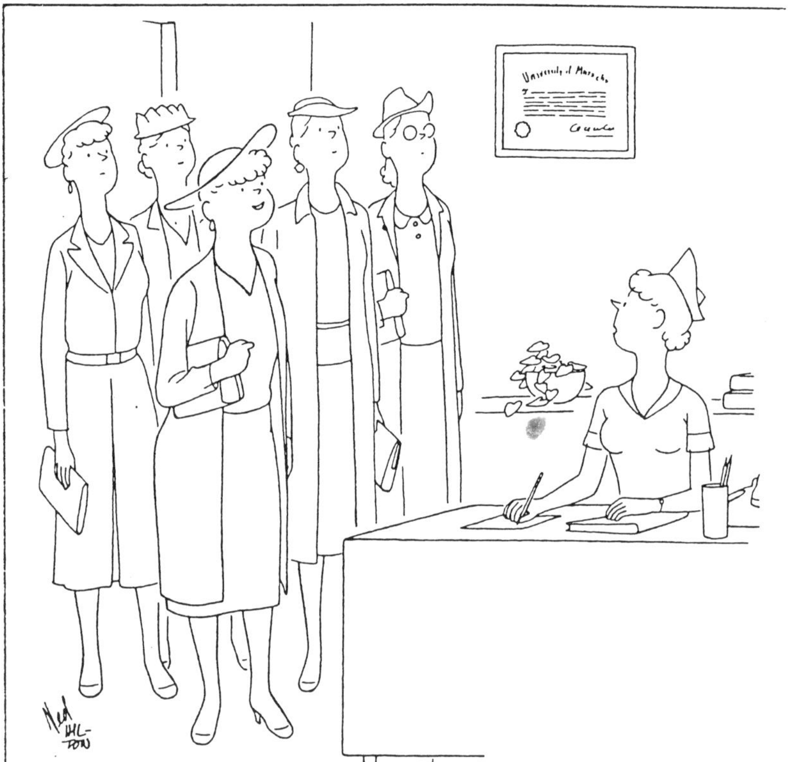

AMA News

"If only one of us goes in and describes everybody's symptoms, won't it count as just one office call?"

Cartoon 4. Nurse portrayed in medical setting; female patients shown as mindless; nurse neutral toward cartoon's hostility to patients. (*AMAN*, 6 August 1962, p. 8)

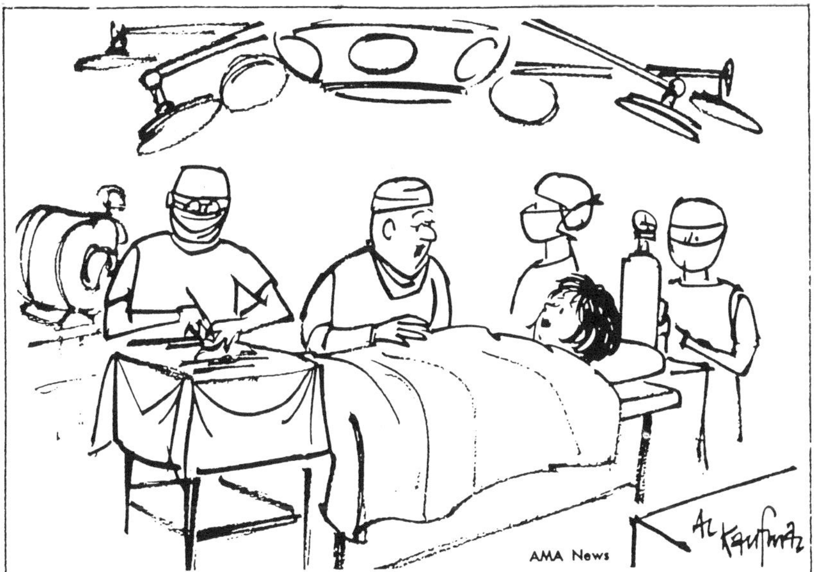

"I don't have a brochure of scars to show you. You'll just have to take potluck."

Cartoon 5. Nurses portrayed as professionals assisting in operation; patient portrayed as mindless; nurses neutral toward patient. (*AMAN*, 24 October 1966, p. 9)

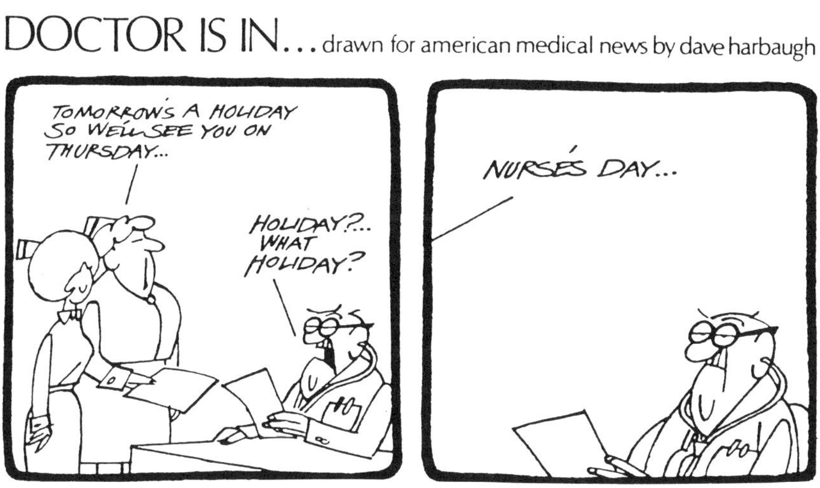

Cartoon 6. Collegial nurse-doctor relationship. (*AMN*, 16 March 1970, p. 5)

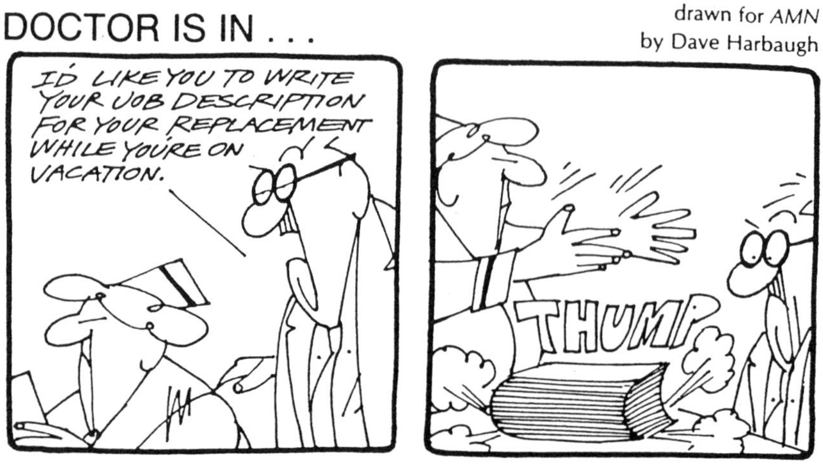
DOCTOR IS IN . . .
drawn for AMN
by Dave Harbaugh
I'D LIKE YOU TO WRITE YOUR JOB DESCRIPTION FOR YOUR REPLACEMENT WHILE YOU'RE ON VACATION.
THUMP

Cartoon 7. Collegial nurse-doctor relationship. (*AMN*, 9 October 1987, p. 32)

from the early to late 1960s, dropped off slightly in the early 1970s, and then fell back to the levels of the early 1960s.

The similarity of these curves indicates that cartoonists focused their attention on women during this period. Indeed, 49 percent of the 416 cartoons collected for this study were published from 1965 to 1974. These 416 cartoons represent 14 percent of all cartoons published by the *American Medical News* from 1960 to 1989, but nearly half of them are concentrated in one decade.

This focusing of attention should not be too surprising to students of recent history. As the basic assumptions of their traditional worldview came under increasingly effective assault in the late 1960s and early 1970s, men often reacted with bitterness and hostility. These feelings were clearly mirrored in the cartoons published in the *News*. Increasing attention was directed toward women, and the frequency of hostile cartoons aimed at female patients mushroomed. Half of all the cartoons about women patients appeared from 1965 to 1974, and they peaked in the early seventies. During the peak of their frequency in 1970 to 1974, nearly 77 percent of all cartoons taken in the sample for those five years included barbs aimed at female patients.

This high tide of feelings against women as patients certainly owes something to their rising militancy during that period. The Women's Health Care Movement was making increasingly insistent demands during the early 1970s for more power in determining their own treatment. The

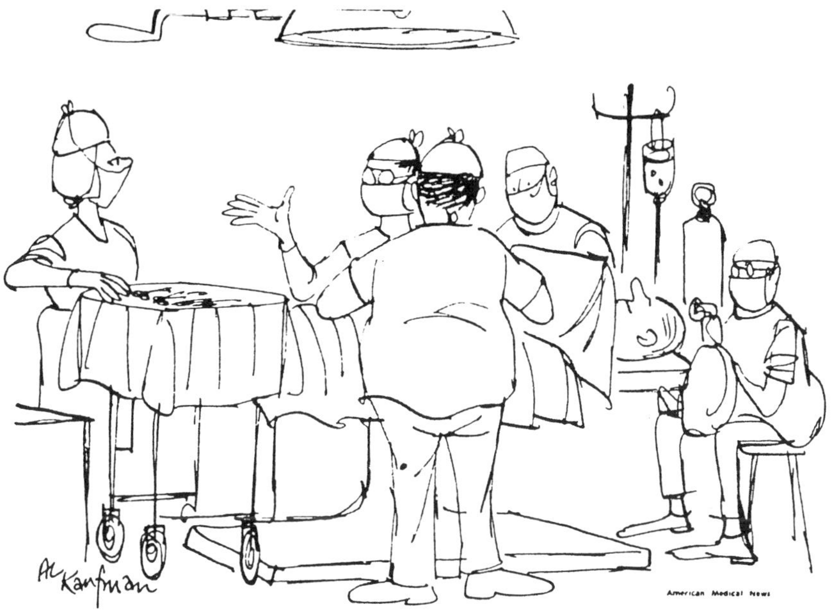

"You're not concentrating, doctor. You just asked for your 'number 3' iron."

Cartoon 8. Nurse's professionalism as superior to doctor's. (*AMN*, 22 October 1973, p. 5)

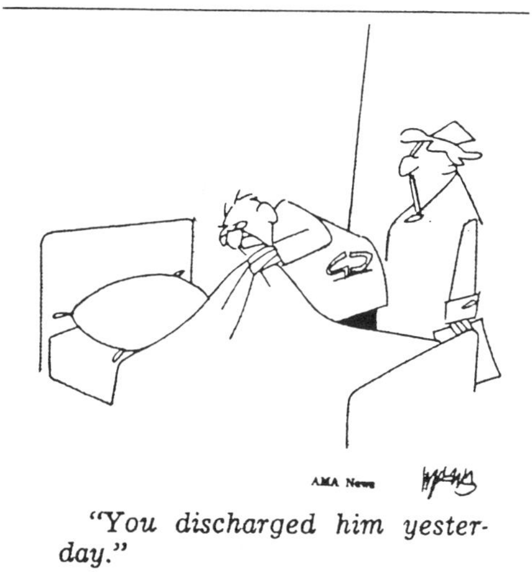

"You discharged him yesterday."

Cartoon 9. Nurse superior to absentminded doctor. (*AMAN*, 22 January 1962, p. 10)

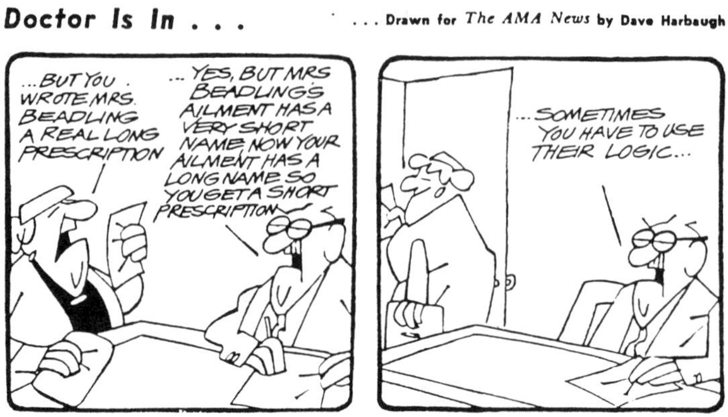

Cartoon 10. Female patient as illogical. (*AMAN*, 14 March 1966, p. 14)

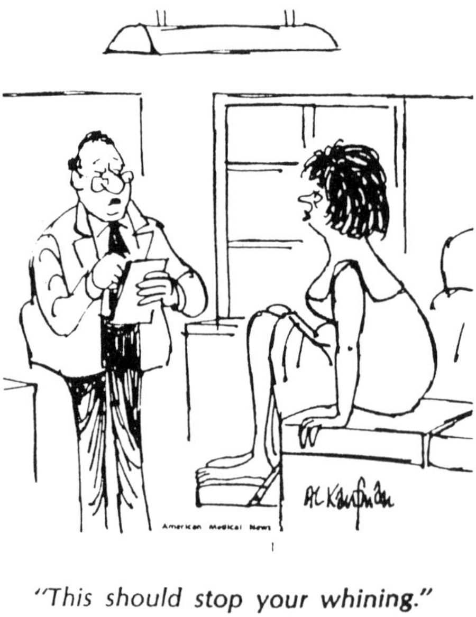

Cartoon 11. Female patients assumed to be hypochondriacs. (*AMN*, 14 December 1973, p. 2)

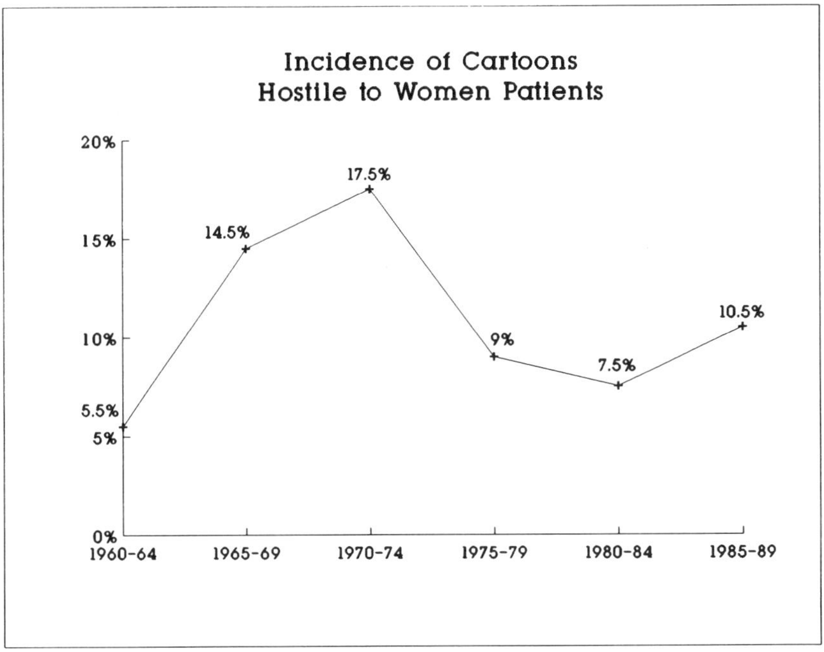

Figure A.

movement was largely ignored by the *News* editorial columns until 7 October 1974, when they devoted five pages to explaining "what these women want," to a readership described as suffering from "simple confusion."[25] But, one *News* cartoon doctor had seen the movement coming in 1970. His simple prescription—physical violence—can be seen in Cartoon 12.

Even if we grant some probability of incremental instances of hostility toward female patients specifically because of male physician fear of the women's health care movement, it does not change the unremittant nature of that hostility. The women's health care movement was one direct impact of feminism on the medical profession. There were many others. The cumulative effect of these hammer blows against one of the most powerful and sacrosanct of male preserves was a predictable backlash of frantic outrage directed against women. This is shown in our sample by the dramatic increase in the frequency of cartoons portraying female patients. Joyce Hammond's study, "Gender Inversion Cartoons and Feminism," likewise found a widespread increase of cartoons directed against women during the same period of the late 1960s and early 1970s.[26]

If perceptions of nursing were solely gender-based we would expect them to follow a same general pattern, with negative categories rising and positive categories moving lower during the 1965 to 1974 period. But the data refused to follow that pattern. The three combined negative categories indeed continued to escalate from 1964 to 1969, rising from 3 to 8 percent. All three negative categories peaked in the late 1960s, with more than twice as many cartoons as during any other cohort. Forty-four percent of all the cartoons showing negative attitudes toward nursing appeared from 1965 to 1969. But by the early 1970s, the negative categories dropped to around 2 percent where they hovered until the late 1980s. Only 3 cartoons since 1985 have depicted nurses negatively.

The three positive nursing categories also fail to fit the gender pattern. Positive cartoons rose lazily from 1960 to a high of 9 percent in 1970 to 1974, then settled back to a level around 6 percent. The fact that positive views of the nursing profession peaked during the same time as did hostile depictions of female patients clearly indicates that cartoon attitudes toward nurses are *not* based solely on gender perceptions.

The evidence shows that while nursing is still viewed as a feminine profession, it seems to have been divorced from the hostility generated toward women in general. The image of nursing emerging from the study of these cartoons shows that significant positive shifts in attitudes toward the nursing profession occurred in the past three decades. We believe this shift results from the dramatic changes in the organization, education, and

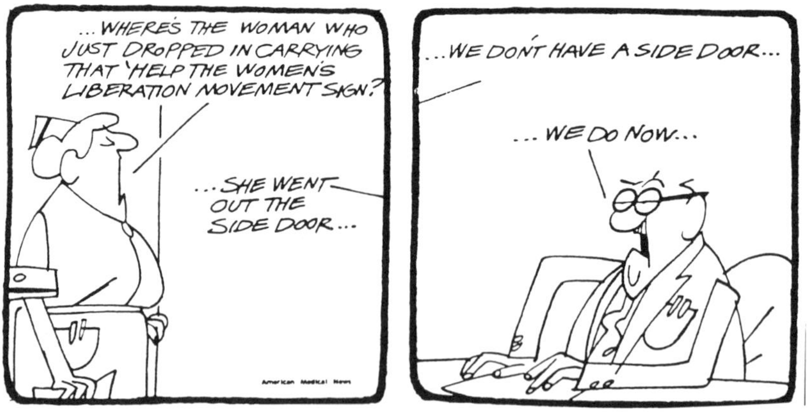
...WHERE'S THE WOMAN WHO JUST DROPPED IN CARRYING THAT 'HELP THE WOMEN'S LIBERATION MOVEMENT SIGN?
...SHE WENT OUT THE SIDE DOOR...
...WE DON'T HAVE A SIDE DOOR...
...WE DO NOW...

Cartoon 12. Liberated female patient bashed; nurse depicted neutrally; nurse neutral toward female patient. (*AMN*, 28 September 1970, p. 5)

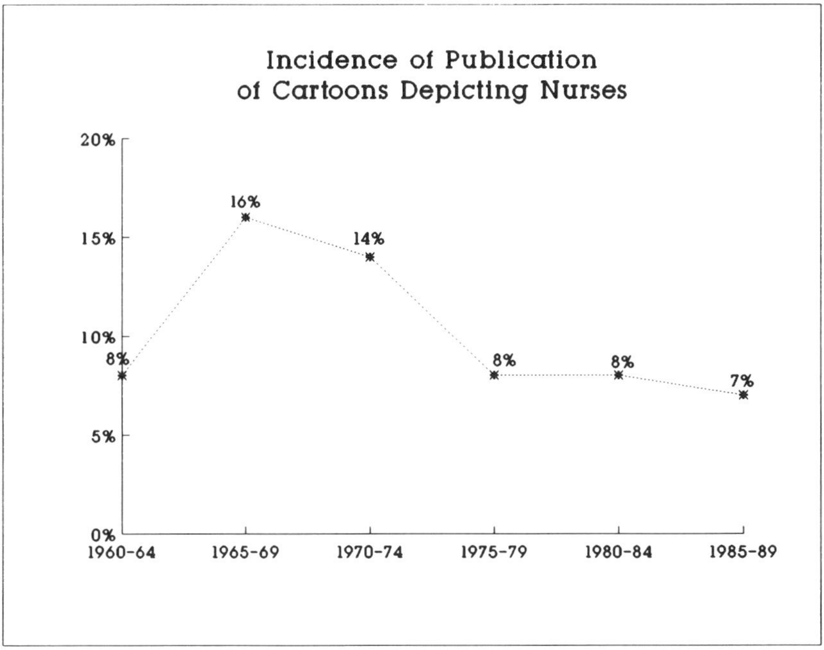

Figure B.

preparation of nurses, which occurred during the period covered by this study.

Increasing calls for more comprehensive education of nurses began to be heard in the early 1960s. The attention of the medical profession was drawn toward the nursing profession and the frequency of cartoons about nurses doubled (see Figure B). But the reaction of the doctors, as mirrored by cartoons in the *News*, was ambivalent. Many saw the movement as catastrophic since it threatened to end the "physician's handmaiden" idea of nursing. Negative cartoons rose from 3 percent to 8 percent of the sample in the late 1960s. The years from 1965 to 1969 are the *only* period during these three decades when negative cartoons about nursing appeared more frequently than positive depictions, but the picture was not uniformly bleak. Positive cartoons rose from 5 percent to 7 percent during the same period.

By the early 1970s, the movement was clearly irreversible. Even politicians, the last to sign on in any new movement, recognized the strength of the nursing profession with legislative decrees. The medical profession was largely convinced of the value of the "new nurse," as negative perceptions

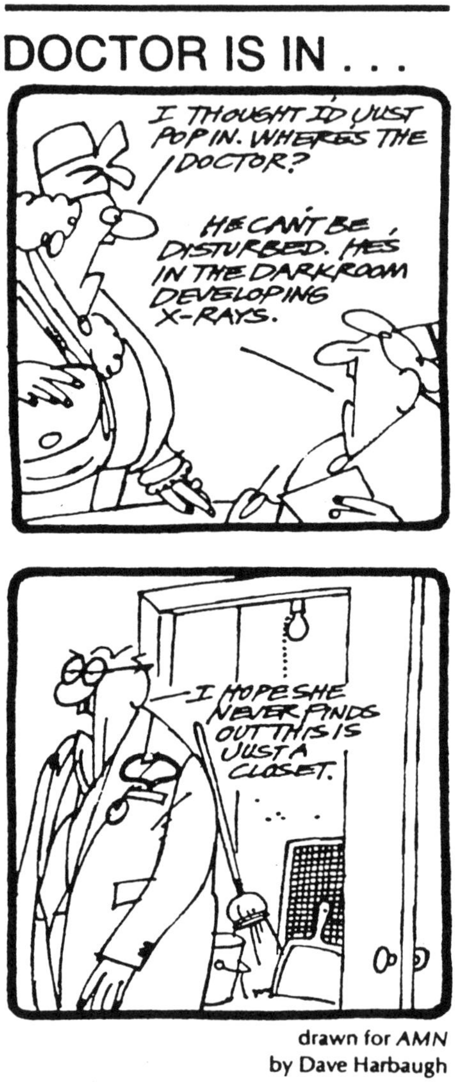

Cartoon 13. Nurse has collegial professional relationship; female patient fooled; nurse joins in charade. (*AMN*, 14 February 1986, p. 6)

melted away and positive cartoons reached their zenith. After 1974, interest in nurses returned to a normal frequency level of about 8 percent of our sample.

The nature of this more positive view of the nursing profession emerges from a study of both positive nurse cartoons and some of those depicting women patients. The incidence of cartoons depicting a collegial relationship between the nursing and medical professions rose from 2.5 percent of the sample in 1960 to 1964 to 6.5 percent ten years later. Collegial cartoons provide the bulk of those published annually since 1975, with more depictions than all other categories combined.

But gains often include hidden losses. The cartoon nurse who awakened the physician from his golf reveries or reminded him that the bed was empty because he discharged the patient is gone. Only 2 cartoons since 1969 dared suggest that nurses might be good enough to replace physicians. Perhaps some jokes strike too close to find humor in them.

Another chilling perception emerged from analysis of the 109 cartoons that depicted both nurses and female patients. The perceived attitudes of the nurses toward the patient fell into three categories. Nurses were depicted as sharing the cartoon's hostile attitude, as neutral toward the female patient, or as showing compassion toward a sister in need. The empathetic nurse appears in only 1 percent of the sample, and only 1 cartoon since 1974 has depicted a nurse showing compassion for a female patient. One method depicted in many cartoons whereby nurses achieve a collegial relationship with physicians is the sharing of professional disdain for female patients. Cartoons showing nurse hostility toward such women peaked in 1970 to 1974, when positive views of nurses also reached their apogee (see Figure A and Cartoon 13).

The category of cartoons that tops all others combined depicts nurse neutrality to the hostility shown toward female patients. These neutral cartoons may indicate ambivalent or undecided attitudes toward the nursing profession. Those cartoon groups featuring a neutral nurse with, and without, a female patient both peaked in 1970 to 1974. Perhaps part of the medical profession was unsure about the new trends in nursing, and especially about how nurses might feel toward their sisters who happened to be patients. The rise in both neutral categories in the recent years might reinforce the argument about ambivalence (see Cartoon 5).

However, the cartoons could also reflect an assumption by medical physicians that nurses share, but do not always voice, similar hostile feelings toward female patients. The nurse may be seen as a silent accomplice in playing out these hostile scenarios. When hostility to female patients first began to peak in 1965 to 1969, nurses only appeared in 17 of the 60 hostile cartoons. By 1970 to 1974, 73 hostile cartoons included 36 nurse depictions. Clearly one price of the acceptance of nursing as a collegial profession divorced from gender-based attitudes was a perception that nurses could no longer remain invisible when gender issues arose. They had become silent partners in the hostility shown toward women patients.

One last point must be raised based on our survey of these cartoons. Philip and Beatrice Kalisch found in their study of the profession's changing image that, since the mid-1960s, a preoccupation with nurses' sex lives has governed all other thematic elements in the mass media: "Nurses are depicted as sensual, romantic, frivolous, irresponsible, and promiscuous."[27] On the surface, our findings seem to refute that viewpoint entirely. Only 11 cartoons, none of them published since 1979, viewed the nurse as a sex object. Although their study of popular mass media uncovered a nursing image literally dripping with superheated sexuality, our cartoon nurse's world was asexual, perhaps even antisexual. The stereotypical nurse in this world was overweight, clearly postmenopausal, and showed not the slightest propensity for sexual propinquity. She was almost as unappetizing and uninterested as her frumpy sister, the female patient. Even the doctor was portrayed as having all the masculine sex appeal of a balding, presbyopic bore. This desexed cartoon world was only occasionally visited by any character with the least animal magnetism. The sex object nurses were extremely attractive, but only fat, loutish male patients ever made any advances (Cartoon 1). The nurse in Cartoon 2 looks like a stereotyped "dumb blonde" looking for "true love," but her would-be lover sees her only as a heart valve, not a heart throb. The operating room nurses in Cartoon 5 are so covered by gowns and masks as to be just barely recognizable.

The only "sexy" cartoon characters who appeared regularly were a dizzy young blonde nurse (see Cartoon 6) and a Don Juanish new doctor who appeared in the "Doctor Is In" series created for the *News* by artist Dave Harbaugh. Both appeared for a short time in the early seventies, then both disappeared. It can only be assumed that the readers objected to this intrusion of overt sexuality into a normally sexless cartoon world.

Perhaps the difference between the "hot" Kalisch media world and the "cold" *News* cartoon image stems from the moral superiority of the *AMA News*; or perhaps the medical world may simply be immune to trends in the public mass media. Each of these possibilities seems unlikely. Perhaps the cartoon medical world of the *American Medical News* is so totally devoid of sex because physicians prefer that sex be one complication left out of the simplified stereotypical universe of the professional media cartoon.

Our major findings on the perceptions of nursing illustrated by the cartoons in the *American Medical News* from 1960 to 1989 are summarized as follows:

1. Nursing is clearly perceived as a dependent, gender-determined, female profession. There was only one depiction of a male nurse and no depiction of an independent nurse practitioner in thirty years of cartoons.
2. Women patients were viewed with unrelenting disgust and hostility, with no positive depiction in thirty years.
3. Cartoons depicting females peaked in the decade from 1965 to 1974; nearly half of our sample came from this period. We ascribe this interest to the feminist challenge to established patterns of male dominance.
4. Hostility to nurses peaked in 1965 to 1969 as new trends in nursing education and organization challenged traditional roles. This hostility died quickly to be replaced by a growing acceptance of the nurse as a professional.
5. We ascribe the increasingly positive view of nursing as evidence of an acceptance of nurses as professionals. This acceptance means that, despite the fact that it is viewed as clearly feminine, the nursing profession has become divorced from the hostility often generated against women in general and female patients in particular.

Judith A. Chaney, RN, MS
Instructor
Southern Illinois University at Edwardsville
Edwardsville, Ill. 62026-1066
Phone: (618) 692-3956
Fax: (618) 692-3854

38 Red Oak Drive
Highland, Ill. 62249
Phone: (618) 654-7107

Patrick Folk
Deneen Memorial Professor of American History
McKendree College

Lebanon, Ill. 62254
Phone: (618) 537-2583

Notes

1. Randall P. Harrison, *The Cartoon: Communication to the Quick*, The Sage Commtext Series, vol. 7 (Beverly Hills, Calif.: Sage Publications, Inc., 1989), 10.

2. Philip A. Kalisch and Beatrice J. Kalisch, *The Changing Image of the Nurse* (Menlo Park, Calif.: Addison-Wesley Publishing Company, 1987), 4. Emphasis in original.

3. Ibid.

4. Ibid., 2–7.

5. Ibid., ix.

6. Suzanne Gordon, *Prisoners of Men's Dreams: Striking Out for a New Feminine Future* (Boston: Little, Brown and Company, 1991), 125, 143, 149.

7. Janet Muff, "Of Images and Ideals: A Look at Socialization and Sexism in Nursing," in *Images of Nurses: Perspectives from History, Art, and Literature*, ed. Anne Hudson Jones (Philadelphia: University of Pennsylvania Press, 1988), 219, note 1. Emphasis in original.

8. Jones, xxi.

9. Kalisch and Kalisch, ix.

10. Gordon, 122. Emphasis in original.

11. Harrison, 28.

12. Ibid., 11, 115, 10.

13. Ibid., 55.

14. John Adkins Richardson, *The Complete Book of Cartooning* (New York: Prentice Hall Press, 1986), 43.

15. Harrison, 9.

16. Ibid., 115.

17. *AMA News* (25 July 1960): 4.

18. Ibid. (23 September 1968): 12–13, 5–6.

19. *American Medical News* (16 October 1981): 4.

20. *AMA News* (22 September 1958); quoted in *AMA News* (23 September 1968).

21. Richardson, 124.

22. Harrison, 41.

23. Ibid., 42.

24. Ibid., 34.

25. *American Medical News* (7 October 1974): 14–18.

26. Joyce D. Hammond, "Gender Inversion Cartoons and Feminism," *Journal of Popular Culture* 24, no. 4 (Spring 1991): 145.

27. Kalisch and Kalisch, 161.

The Origins of Geriatric Nursing

The Chronically Ill Elderly in Almshouses and Nursing Homes, 1900–1950

Ellen Schell
Department of Physiological Nursing
University of California, San Francisco

> Of all the classes and kinds of destitute and vicious who were once promiscuously consigned to the poorhouse [almshouse], these, the aged and infirm, remain as the irreducible minimum, the irremovable residue, of the poorhouse population.
> —Caroline Bartlett Crane to the Nurses' Associated Alumnae, 1907[1]

Nurses' concern for the elderly poor of the almshouse foreshadowed the birth of geriatric nursing, a specialty conceived in the womb of the almshouse, a marginalized, stigmatized institution.[2] The almshouse, a dreaded place of last resort, became a target of the reform effort of one of nursing's luminaries, Lavinia L. Dock. Though the attempt to establish almshouse nursing failed, nurses' concern for the aged and chronically ill who inhabited these places continued. The institutions that arose to carry on the charge of the almshouse—nursing homes—inherited the stigma attached to the almshouse and struggled with many of the same problems. Nurses who examined conditions within these marginalized institutions were among the first to address the unique needs of the chronically ill elderly.

The Early American Almshouse

Almshouses existed in America from colonial times and served as institutions for the care of the poor and destitute. Initially, almshouses provided shelter for the poor of all ages and conditions, sick and well together; prostitutes; children; the elderly; the insane; and vagrants.

From their inception in this country, almshouses were stigmatized as sorry, inhospitable places that sheltered the lowest ranking members of society. Historian Charles Rosenberg discussed at length the experience of Ezra Stiles Ely, a Presbyterian minister who preached in the New York City almshouse hospital from 1810 to 1813. Rosenberg used Ely's diary to paint a vivid picture of life in the almshouse, also providing a fascinating analysis of the piece.

Nursing History Review 1 (1993): 203–16.

Given Ely's reaction to what he saw, it is remarkable that he persisted so long at his mission. Ely's catalogue of his feelings of revulsion and scorn included his horror at nearly being touched by one inmate. The putrid, filthy wards were filled with the "depraved and miserable of our race," and "blasted, withered, dying, females [prostitutes]."[3] He described their destitute lives amid the dead and dying, the dreadful smells, and hostile atmosphere.

Ely judged the majority of inmates as victims of their own sin and depravity, suffering from conditions brought about as a "consequence of making a god of animal appetite."[4] Ely's condemnation of the almshouse inmates reflected the opinions of the society in which he lived and the perceived division between the worthy and the unworthy poor. The worthy poor were honest, hard-working laborers, whose misfortune of illness left them unable to earn a living. This group was deemed deserving of compassionate, decent treatment. But the unworthy poor warranted their fate within the almshouse's demeaning walls; they justly suffered the consequence of indolence, intemperance, and immorality. According to Rosenberg, one of the prime motivations in the development of the American hospital was to spare the worthy poor from the indignity of the almshouse.[5] The philanthropists who established the first hospitals took great care to distinguish their institutions from almshouses, admitting only the deserving poor to their institutions. Some hospitals even required a letter of recommendation for admission as a patient.[6]

The Twentieth-Century Almshouse

At the dawn of the twentieth century, almshouse conditions had changed little from the sorry state described by Ely in 1810. They remained unsanitary, cheerless places of last resort.[7] Disease spread easily and the sick were poorly attended to. Inmates lacked adequate food and proper clothing.

Census data revealed a demographic shift in the almshouse population. From the beginning, almshouses had sheltered substantial numbers of elderly. In the first decade of the twentieth century, the proportion increased to reach a majority; by 1920, 66.6 percent of the almshouse population was over sixty.[8]

Specialized institutions for care of the poor and sick drew away a portion of the original almshouse residents. Tubercular patients were sent to sanitaria, children to orphanages, and the mentally ill to insane asylums. Who remained in the almshouses? "Homeless, friendless poor old men and women."[9]

As an institution, almshouses developed a characteristically American pattern of diversity. Many were run by county governments and were therefore controlled by local elected officials whose main goals were to keep undesirables off the streets at the lowest possible public expense. These facilities varied widely from place to place in size, characteristics of inmate populations, and patterns of care or relief provided.

In some communities, civic authorities contracted with private individuals to house and care for the poor. These profit-making, private almshouses relied on public funds for income, foreshadowing the proprietary nursing homes of today.[10]

Care of the Elderly in Other Settings

Private charitable old-age homes represented another important model of care for the elderly.[11] These homes were founded by church, service, and ethnic groups in the second half of the nineteenth century. Typically small and culturally homogeneous, these institutions provided custodial rather than medical care for the residents. In some regions, charitable homes housed substantial proportions of the aged living in institutions. For example, in Massachusetts, residents of these facilities constituted fully 43 percent of the total population of institutionalized elderly.

These fascinating and important institutions, about which little is known, merit further study. In their focus on the social and psychological needs of the elderly, these early homes present an intriguing model for the restructuring of long-term care today.[12] While some nursing occurred within their bounds, most of these homes catered to the well elderly. In this respect they differed substantially from the almshouses where such a high proportion of the elderly residents were sick. Chronic conditions such as rheumatism, stroke, and senility made the almshouse population especially dependent and vulnerable. The crying needs of these elderly almshouse residents attracted the attention of reformers and nurses like Lavinia Dock.

Lavinia Dock and Social Reform

Dock's interest in the almshouse poor reflected her socialist agenda. For some twenty years she lived and worked with Lillian Wald at the Henry Street Settlement where she confirmed her intuitive "sympathy with oppressed classes."[13] Her encounters with workers involved with the labor movement strengthened her socialist leanings. She sought ways to improve the life of oppressed people for she firmly believed in progress and the betterment of human beings.

Views of the plight of the poor held a century before and represented by men like Ely contrasted sharply with Dock's view. She made no distinction between the worthy and unworthy poor. Rather, consistent with her socialist views, Dock saw the poor as victims of economic and social injustice. These views formed the backdrop of her argument for the advantages of almshouse training for the pupil nurse:

> Where else could she better learn . . . tolerance and pity for ignorance and misfortune and the sympathy which prompts the ameliorating of the sad conditions of human life as much as lies in one's power?[14]

Dock, as well as other nursing leaders of this period, had a clear vision of nursing's social mission and an unflagging belief in the profession's ability to bring social change. As she stated in a speech to the Nurses' Associated Alumnae Convention in 1907, "human society can be voluntarily and consciously built into nobler and fairer forms than those of the past."[15] Lystra Gretter, one of the respondents at the convention, voiced nursing's role in this crusade: "Until every man, woman and child has the benefit of trained, skilled nursing, the noble aim of our profession will not have been fulfilled."[16]

Borrowing an image from Jane Addams, a prominent social reformer, Dock described the society as a household in which women held a special trust. Dock referred to this image when she addressed the 1907 meeting of the Nurses' Associated Alumnae:

> The problems of the modern city are almost entirely housekeeping questions on a vast scale. The cleanliness and healthfulness of the city must be simply extensions of the cleanliness and healthfulness of the home.[17]

For Dock, women's ability to accomplish social reform was inextricably linked with the suffrage issue. The vote would empower women, allowing them to make their reforms stick. Without it, she cautioned, "we shall not know when we may get up in the morning to find that all we had gained has been taken from us."[18]

The Attempt to Establish Almshouse Nursing

As a contributing editor of the *American Journal of Nursing* (*AJN*), Dock used her position to champion almshouse nursing. The first editorial on the subject, in 1906, reported the efforts of Caroline Bartlett Crane, chairman of the Charity Organization Department of the Women's Improvement League of Kalamazoo, Michigan. Crane had addressed the Michigan State Nurses' Association, detailing the appalling conditions of the almshouses in that state. Crane proposed an alliance between the State Nurses' Association and the Michigan State Federation of Women's Clubs to provide nursing care in almshouses. The nurses' association would supply the nurses and the women's clubs the required salary. At that meeting, the nurses agreed to begin the project with a survey of almshouse conditions.

In 1907 Crane brought her ideas to the annual convention meeting of the Nurses' Associated Alumnae of the United States.[19] In her impassioned speech, she detailed the plight of almshouse residents and called for reform. She praised Dorothea Dix's work and noted Dix's role in emptying almshouses of the "destitute insane . . . the blind, dumb, epileptic, idiots and—destitute children!"[20] She added, "of all that motley assemblage of human beings who were once carelessly consigned to oblivion in the county poorhouse, presently none will be left except—the aged and infirm!"[21]

Throughout her speech, Crane repeated this point, emphasizing the needs of the elderly almshouse resident. She pointed out that the majority of sickness in the almshouse was chronic in nature and promoted the almshouse as a place for training in the care of the chronically ill. "The great variety of chronic cases—the cases in which the hospital training-school is most deficient—will constitute a post-graduate opportunity of great value," she asserted.[22]

At that same meeting, L. J. Lupinski, a nurse, reported on the progress of the Michigan alliance.[23] The group had funded the building of a hospital wing on the Muskegon almshouse and had plans to hire two nurses to staff the hospital.

Lupinski also reported on a failed attempt to place a nurse in an almshouse in another county (unnamed in her report). The women's group in that county offered to fund an almshouse nurse for six months on a demonstration basis. The county supervisors rejected the plan in spite of the provision of seed money for the project. Lupinski speculated the supervisors were wary of a plan that would eventually result in the county assuming additional costs, thereby increasing the county budget and jeopardizing their chances of reelection. While disheartened by the action of the supervisors, Lupinski was even more discouraged by the fruitless search for a nurse willing to apply for the position. Lupinski blamed the lack of applicants on the low salary offered ($50 per month).

Following Lupinski's presentation, Dock make a motion to support development of similar alliances between women's clubs and nurses' associations in all the states. She suggested the groups begin their work by making a survey of all almshouses, detailing the number of people in almshouses requiring nursing care and the types of cases involved.

The plan moved forward in two states, Michigan and Illinois. In 1908 Crane and a group of Michigan taxpayers investigated the Kalamazoo County Almshouse and published a scathing report on conditions there.[24] The report drew much criticism from local politicians who attacked Crane personally.

Dock reported the Michigan story in *AJN* and proclaimed again the special trust of women as the housekeepers of society. She emphasized the need for women to gain political power. She ended her report:

> Conditions such as these go far to show why women—intelligent and able women, not servile ones, should have, not only *positions* in such institutions, but a share of *power*, so that these evils, all of which lie strictly in the sphere of *housekeeping* and *nursing*,—two spheres which have always been lauded as women's own—might not occur. How I wish that our women's eyes everywhere might be opened to realize that only by possessing their rightful share of our municipal and state and national government can they ever hope to claim their right and their duty of carrying the standards of good homes into public institutions. What selfishness to think only of one's *own* home![25]

In Illinois, a committee of volunteers composed of nurses and members of the Federation of Women's Clubs set out to collect information on almshouse conditions and to construct a plan to provide nursing care for the residents. The plan proposed that visiting nurses include almshouses on their rounds and suggested that training schools include an almshouse rotation in the curriculum.[26]

This brief editorial reporting the progress of the Illinois group is the last mention of Crane's almshouse project in *AJN*. What happened to the project is hinted at in Dock's 1912 *History of Nursing*.

> The committees [almshouse committees of state nurses' associations] are ready to ally themselves with women's clubs and some have already accomplished definite things in almshouse reform. Even more than other institutions, however, almshouses are in the grasp of petty and venal politicians. Until women attain full citizenship no thoroughgoing improvement can be made in them.[27]

Political entanglements, low pay, low status, job insecurity, and lack of women's political power appear to have combined to hamper the progress of almshouse nursing. Twenty years passed before the journal published another article on the subject. Those years were filled with dramatic events that transformed the nation. World War I forced an unwilling America into the role of a world power. Great waves of immigration continued to change the character of America's population. The 1920s brought a heady optimism and prosperity that ended with the astonishing stock market crash of 1929. But this tumultuous period brought little change to the American almshouse.

The Depression Era Almshouse

In 1930 Helen W. Munson reported on the care of the sick in almshouses in New York, Virginia, and North Carolina.[28] Her article suggested that almshouse conditions had changed little. Most of the residents were elderly: 62 percent were over sixty-five years old. The report found that 30 percent of the residents were in need of nursing care but that the overwhelming majority were not receiving it. Munson emphasized the necessity for a focus on care of the chronic conditions that composed the majority of health problems in this population and lamented that chronic illness had eluded the concern of medical, nursing, and public health interests.

Her report showed that nursing had made little impact on the almshouse population. Of the twenty-seven almshouses studied, only three had trained nurses on staff. She noted that "neglect, indifference, and poor management through ignorance as to be almost medieval" was apparent in many facilities.[29] She reported the same stumbling blocks described by Dock:

> Control of almshouses is entirely local and the conditions within an individual almshouse reflect the degree of social enlightenment reached by the community in which it happens to be. This, of course, is variable. Although yearly inspection of almshouses is made by agents of state boards of charities, for the most part these boards have not power to enforce any recommendations which they may make. Hence conditions stay about as they are from year to year.[30]

Munson's article suggested that women's organizations continued to be concerned with almshouse conditions. Some of her information is drawn from a report on almshouses in four states compiled by the Woman's Department of the National Civic Federation and State Charity Boards. She does not mention the state nurse associations. The strong alliance between nursing and the women's groups envisioned by Dock and

Crane had not come to fruition. Whether some state nurses' associations continued an organized interest in the almshouse population is unclear.

The Death of the Almshouse

While county politics had hampered the establishment of almshouse nursing, the waning of the almshouse itself dried up interest in the experiment. Beginning in the late 1930s, the almshouse began to a slow death. From an estimated high of 135,000 in the early 1930s, the almshouse population dropped to 72,000 in 1950.[31]

Developments in social policy hastened this demise. Though reformers had not managed to improve almshouse conditions much, they had raised public concern. Policymakers responded with efforts to close the facilities down. The Social Security Act of 1935 reflected this agenda in its stipulations barring residents of public institutions from receiving Social Security benefits. Almshouse residents were specifically excluded in Title I of the act.[32] This policy was intended to support home care as an alternative to the almshouse by providing funds to people for remaining in or returning to the community. The act was intended to make the almshouse unnecessary and hasten its demise.

One Institution Replaces Another

Despite its goal of deinstitutionalization, the Social Security Act inadvertently fostered the transfer of the chronically ill elderly to private and voluntary nursing homes. While the bill was intended to promote a return to home and independence, many elderly needed the support and care offered through an institution. Commercial nursing homes moved in to fill part of the gap left by the almshouses, capitalizing on people's ability to pay for their services with Social Security funds.[33]

Some of the senile elderly were shifted to institutions for the mentally ill. This trend had begun prior to Social Security when, in the early part of the century, several states enacted laws requiring the state to be responsible for the mentally ill. Local authorities in charge of almshouses, eager to shift the burden of care to the state, reclassified senile elderly residents as mentally ill, thereby forcing state mental hospitals to admit them. Through this process, large numbers of the aged senile were transferred from almshouses to mental institutions, further depleting the almshouse population.[34]

As the number of almshouses declined, the number of nursing homes mushroomed. An article in 1947 pointed to two other factors that contributed to the increase in nursing homes.[35] First, the numbers of chronically ill elderly needing institutional care grew rapidly, reflecting the aging of the general population. Second, changes in the structure of the American family increased the demand for nursing home care. Adult children moved away from aging parents to follow jobs in the service or wartime industries. Women, traditional caregivers of elderly parents and in-laws, sought employment outside the home in increasing numbers. Their new jobs left women less time for caregiving. Smaller homes meant less living space available to house elderly relatives needing care.

The problems found in almshouses were transferred to private nursing homes. Like almshouses, nursing homes in the 1940s were unregulated, and many provided poor care. Many were small proprietary facilities run by unscrupulous operators. Although they were called "nursing homes," few of these facilities employed professional nurses to administer or supervise care. Nurses saw the problems in these facilities and wrote about the need for improvement and regulation. Examples of these writings are drawn from two leading nursing journals: *AJN* and *Public Health Nursing* (*PHN*).

In 1947 Maude Carson, chief of Public Health Nursing in Illinois, discussed the first attempt in that state to set up a voluntary licensing system for nursing homes.[36] The Department of Public Health used public health nurses to carry out inspections of facilities. Carson described the deficiencies found in many of the homes inspected and the need for education of operators on topics so basic as sanitation, nutrition, and pasteurization of milk.

In their effort to improve standards in nursing homes, nurses focused on the special problems of the chronically ill elderly. One article entitled "A Community Plans for Its Aged and Chronically Ill" described the role of the public health nurse in a program of nursing home inspection in Milwaukee.[37] The program included consultation, supervision, and instruction of nursing home operators by public health nurses. The article also detailed the activities of a nurse-directed voluntary agency for the chronically ill. Agency personnel visited and evaluated private nursing homes and made these evaluations available to the public. Throughout the article, the author emphasized the importance of encouraging facilities to adopt a rehabilitative focus in the care of the aged chronically ill.

Shining Examples

In the 1940s, nursing journals painted a generally bleak picture of nursing homes; writers focused on efforts to regulate and improve care. But a few articles described some facilities that were shining exceptions. For example, in a 1941 article for *AJN*, Edith Marsh discussed the progress of the Cuyahoga County Nursing Home, an innovative, publicly-funded facility in Ohio.[38] Marsh, a graduate of Lakeside Hospital in Cleveland, had a long and multifaceted career as a pediatric nurse, a nurse anesthetist, and a midwife with the Frontier Nursing Service. She became the Cuyahoga County Nursing Home's first superintendent. Of course, as administrator of the program, Marsh was hardly an unbiased reporter, but her description of her facility for *AJN* demonstrates her commitment to promulgate new ideas in the care of the elderly.*

The home was opened in 1939 in response to "all the mistakes gleaned through experience in the placement of relief clients in privately owned nursing homes in Cleveland."[39] The enlightened Board of Commissioners formed nursing and medical advisory bodies to hire personnel and develop policy. The Nursing Advisory Committee included Marion Howell, the dean of nursing at Western Reserve University; Edna Newman, superintendent of nurses at St. Luke's Hospital; M. Anna Gillis, superintendent of nurses at Mt. Sinai Hospital; and Elizabeth Folckemer, director of the Visiting Nurse Association.

Exceptionally well staffed for its time, the home had 179 beds and had hired nineteen graduate nurses as well as attendants to provide bedside care. It also served as a training site for students completing attendant training.

The program of care maintained a rehabilitative focus, employing physical and occupational therapists. The staff reported considerable success; 200 patients out of 480 admitted over eighteen months were returned to their homes in the community, and some of these returned to work.

Some important innovations, now considered standard good nursing care, were part of the program at the Cuyahoga home. The staff gave attention to such problems as maintaining activity, preventing pressure sores, and managing incontinence. Moreover, Marsh entirely eliminated the use of physical restraint at the home, saw the value of activity for the agitated patient, and wrote about the dangers of overusing sedatives and

*See Strumpf and Tomes, this issue.—ED.

hypnotics.[40] The home placed considerable emphasis on entertainment, recreation, and useful occupations; residents acted as receptionists and switchboard operators. Marsh also gave careful attention to the food service and employed a graduate home economist to supervise diet preparation.

> We feel that a poor cook is an expensive investment, so from the beginning we have had a most excellent chef. As our well-seasoned, well-cooked meals are relished, there is very little food that finds its way into the garbage can because it is not palatable.[41]

The articles about the Cuyahoga home describe a remarkable, forward-thinking program and are testimony to what could be accomplished when talented nursing leadership was involved.

Another article in the 1940s reported innovations in institutional care. It discussed a program of orientation, education, and in-service for nurses at a Jewish home for the aged in New York that was concerned with staff development in an institutional setting.[42] The program covered nursing care of common conditions of the elderly such as cardiac and respiratory disorders. It placed a strong emphasis on the psychosocial aspects of care and called for individualized care sensitive to the "characteristics accompanying the aging process."[43] Groups from the Division of Nursing Education at Teachers College were invited to participate in the program with the hope "that in their future contacts with student nurses, they will present the whole concept of geriatric nursing more attractively."[44]

These articles in leading nursing journals suggest some innovative projects were evolving—testimony to an emerging consciousness about the special needs of the geriatric patient and the attempt to shape a nursing response. It is probable that more such projects existed. Innovative nurses are not always writers, and their work results in much unpublished documentation that is difficult for historians to retrieve.[45] Projects such as Marsh's were forerunners of the best in modern institutional geriatric care.

Conclusion

The 1950s brought significant changes in the care of the institutionalized elderly. Policymakers moved forward in addressing the social needs and health concerns of the rapidly increasing aged segment of the population. Gerontology became a recognized discipline as its first professional and scientific organizations founded in the late 1940s became firmly established. The special nursing care needs of the elderly were sufficiently well recognized to merit the publication of the first geriatric nursing textbook in 1950.[46]

Important developments in gerontological nursing continue today, including heightened interest in care of the elderly in community and acute hospital settings. But the nursing home of today, like the almshouse and nursing home of the first part of the century, remains at the center of long-term health care for the elderly. The difficulties that beset Dock and others in their attempt to improve care for the institutionalized elderly continue to plague us today. Nursing has failed to seize the opportunity to take control of the institutional care of the aged. It may be time to push for excellence in gerontological nursing, to recruit the best and the brightest into nursing home care, and to recapture the enthusiasm for reform and excellence in care held by nurses like Lavinia Dock and Edith Marsh.

Ellen Schell, RN, MS
Doctoral Candidate
Department of Physiological Nursing
University of California, San Francisco

877 Rhode Island Street
San Francisco, Calif. 94107
Phone: (415) 647-8149

Acknowledgments

The author wishes to acknowledge Janna Dieckmann for her insights on care of the elderly in almshouses.

Notes

1. Caroline Bartlett Crane, "Almshouse Nursing: The Human Need; the Professional Opportunity," *American Journal of Nursing* 7 (September 1907): 874–75 (hereafter cited as *AJN*).

2. The nursing specialty of care of the elderly is now termed "gerontological nursing." In this article, however, I will use the term "geriatric nursing," which was the term used prior to 1950, and, indeed, is the title of the first textbook on the subject (Kathleen Newton, *Geriatric Nursing* [St. Louis, Mo.: Mosby, 1950]).

3. Charles E. Rosenberg, *The Care of Strangers* (New York: Basic Books, 1987), 15.

4. Ibid., 17.

5. Ibid., 19.

6. Ibid.

7. Lavinia L. Dock, "The Crusade for Almshouse Nursing," *AJN* 8 (April 1908): 520–23.

8. Gerald N. Grob, "Explaining Old Age History: The Need for Empiricism," in *Old Age in a Bureaucratic Society*, ed. David Van Tassel and Peter N. Stearns (New York: Greenwood, 1986), 34–35.

9. Crane, 874.

10. Richard J. Margolis, *Risking Old Age in America* (Boulder, Colo.: Westview Press, 1990), 149.

11. Muriel R. Gillick, "Long-Term Care Options for the Frail Elderly," *Journal of the American Geriatrics Society* 37 (December 1989): 1198–1203.

12. Ibid.

13. Lavinia L. Dock, "Lavinia L. Dock: Self-Portrait," in *Pages From Nursing History* (New York: American Journal of Nursing Company, 1984), 55.

14. Editorial, "A Neglected Field of Nursing: The County Almshouse," *AJN* 4 (May 1906): 494.

15. Lavinia L. Dock, "Some Urgent Social Claims," *AJN* 7 (September 1907): 895–901.

16. Report of the Tenth Annual Convention, Nurses Associated Alumnae of the United States, *AJN* 7 (September 1907): 886.

17. Dock, "Some Urgent Social Claims," 900.

18. Ibid., 901.

19. Crane, 872–81.

20. Ibid., 873.

21. Ibid., 874.

22. Ibid., 880.

23. L. J. Lupinski, "The Professional Opportunity," *AJN* 7 (September 1907): 882–85.

24. Dock, "The Crusade for Almshouse Nursing," 520–23.

25. Ibid., 523.

26. Editorial, "Almshouse Nursing," *AJN* 10 (April 1910): 540–41.

27. Lavinia L. Dock, *A History of Nursing Vol. III* (New York: Putnams, 1912), 228.

28. Helen W. Munson, "The Care of the Sick in Almshouses," *AJN* 30 (October 1930): 1226–30.

29. Ibid., 1228.

30. Ibid., 1230.

31. *Encyclopedia Britannica*, 15th ed., s.v. "almshouse."

32. W. Andrew Achenbaum, *Shades of Gray: Old Age, American Values, and Federal Policies since 1920* (Boston: Little, Brown and Co., 1983), 40.

33. Gillick, 1201.

34. Grob, 41–42.

35. Maude B. Carson, "Improving Standards in Nursing Homes," *Public Health Nursing* 39 (June 1947): 312–14 (hereafter cited as *PHN*).

36. Ibid.

37. S. Gertrude Mulaney and Theda L. Waterman, "A Community Plans for Its Aged and Chronically Ill," *PHN* 42 (October 1950): 568–73.

38. Edith L. Marsh, "The Care of the Chronically Ill at the Cuyahoga County Nursing Home," *AJN* (February 1941): 161–66.

39. Ibid., 161.

40. Edith L. Marsh, "Stabilization Instead of Restraint in the Care of Elderly Patients," *AJN* 44 (November 1944): 1849–50.

41. Marsh, "The Care of the Chronically Ill," 164.

42. Blanche D. Gubersky and Vera M. Burke, "A Modern Home for the Aged," *PHN* 41 (November 1949): 582–86.

43. Ibid., 582.

44. Ibid., 584.

45. Janna Dieckmann, personal communication, 12 March 1992.

46. Kathleen Newton, *Geriatric Nursing* (St. Louis, Mo.: Mosby, 1950).

From Almshouse to City Nursing Home

Philadelphia's Riverview Home for the Aged, 1945–1965

JANNA L. DIECKMANN
School of Nursing
University of Pennsylvania

The almshouse was the established method of institutional relief for economically dependent elderly people from early in the nineteenth century until recent decades. Tacit acceptance of almshouse methods was, however, frequently countered by appeals for their abolishment.[1] When Social Security payments became available to the aged in 1940, noninstitutional relief was advocated. Almshouse care came to be seen as not only undesirable but also unnecessary. Yet reducing the almshouse population proved difficult. Increasing numbers of the aged and the emerging chronic illness "problem" of the 1940s provoked a reassessment of institutional relief, ultimately transforming many almshouses into homes for the aged.[2]

Who was to care for the aged sick? While each city and county reached slightly different accommodations based on local circumstances, Philadelphia's story reveals themes found elsewhere: the political shape of health problems, and the difficulty in designing—and paying for—health services to meet the needs of the poor and chronically ill. In 1951 Philadelphia's Riverview Home for the Aged was reborn from the Home for the Indigent almshouse. Struggling to fulfill the needs of the long-term sick, Riverview's reform leadership sought to establish a public nursing home. How Philadelphia failed to transform its almshouse before 1965 suggests the limitations on municipal institutional care for the aged in the two decades between World War II and the 1965 legislation approving Medicare and Medicaid.

The Almshouse Past

The Home for the Indigent opened in the late 1910s as part of the redistribution of responsibilities previously carried by Blockley Hospital and Almshouse.[3] It relieved overcrowding from the hospital, now renamed Philadelphia General, and accommodated the hospital's new mission of

Nursing History Review 1 (1993): 217–28.

scientific medicine and acute care. The home took over certain unwelcome patient categories from the hospital, including the aged, blind, and chronically sick, as well as vagrants, epileptics, alcoholics, and the mentally ill. Between 1920 and 1950, the Home for the Indigent housed 900 to 1,500 inmates at the remote, northeastern edge of Philadelphia.[4]

Before 1950 male inmates of the home outnumbered women three to one, and 80 percent of inmates were over age fifty.[5] Confined to a social welfare mission, the home's goals included the provision of shelter and food, but rarely caregiving. In 1947 the *Bulletin*, Philadelphia's afternoon newspaper, complained: "The senile, feeble-minded, crippled and incontinent, alike are herded into barn-like rooms with hard benches and slated rockers to spend their days, and into huge barracks at night to sleep."[6] Home inmates had no privacy and few comforts; they had little more to do than play cards and smoke, for the men, and sew, for the women. The demeaning aspects of inmate lives even extended to efforts to aid them, as when inmates were bribed with lollipops to attend chapel.[7]

Prisoners from the neighboring House of Correction comprised the home's work force and substantially controlled daily life. Paid staff supervised the prisoner work force and provided minimal direct patient assistance. Paid staff to patient ratios varied from one to twenty-five during the day, to one for one hundred inmates at night. Medical care was sparse, with physicians called in for emergencies. The few nurses handed out medications during day shift only. Able-bodied inmates assisted the more dependent, out of kindness and because of the lack of a real staff. The home was popularly stigmatized as a poorhouse; the presence and complex needs of sick, frail, and disabled persons were overlooked.

Criticism of Home Practices

Criticism of the pre-1950 home focused on visible concerns, such as the structural problems, the absence of physical maintenance and sanitation, and the bleak institutional atmosphere, rather than complex problems such as the absence of inmate classification. For example, neither tuberculosis patients nor the "senile and mentally incompetent" were specially treated.[8] Who was responsible for them? Was it the home's management, families who abandoned their aged members, inadequate city appropriations, or Philadelphia's taxpayers?[9] Finding the home's conditions worse than those in the neighboring prison, Philadelphia Grand Jury examiners reported that "old age and poverty [seemed] more sins and crimes than assault and battery, robbery, manslaughter or almost any felony."[10]

Deterring would-be residents from such homes seemed an accepted goal of poorhouse management; persons should have foresight as working adults to set aside funds for later years. Nationally, the care and treatment of long-term, chronically ill aged was poorly understood and organized, complicated by the perception that chronic illness was inherent and irreversible in the aging process. New ideas of physical rehabilitation, flowing from the military medicine of World War II, only slowly had an impact on institutional practices.

Real conditions at the pre-1950 home were invisible to both the city's elite and its everyday people; Riverview's remote location limited the public's awareness, knowledge, and involvement. Sensational news, such as human bodies found on the grounds after inmate drinking parties, or the mysterious enteritis deaths of thirty inmates, or the collapse of basement dormitory ceilings just days after inmates were relocated, drew limited public attention.[11] In 1939 a wide-ranging State Welfare Department investigation attributed problems to the lack of personnel, particularly of registered nurses who "understand the idiosyncrasies of aged persons."[12]

But political graft at the home was so pervasive, from the home's sloppy construction to the theft of food and money, that before 1950 no reform could be sustained. Philadelphia was a model of how corrupt a city could become when one political machine retained control too long. This corruption, producing neglect of both public institutions and social needs, seemed generally accepted by Philadelphia's residents.[13] Scandal at the Home for the Indigent seemed to be accepted in light of its essential function to shelter the outcast.

The Reform Movement at Riverview

The transformation of the Home for the Indigent into Riverview Home for the Aged was part of citywide changes following the 1951 election of Joe Clark, the first Democratic mayor since the 1890s. The Democratic reform movement adopted a mid-twentieth-century philosophy of "good government" as institutional and economic action rather than moral appeal. Deep changes in the city charter and city government, as well as growing intolerance of corruption, sparked a reconstruction of previously neglected city services. Municipal government embraced a special responsibility "for the care, the guidance, and the rehabilitation of certain classes of its citizens."[14] Community responsibility for the long-term sick shifted from "mere institutionalization" to "recognition of [inmate's individual] needs as a living, growing personality."[15]

Although Riverview was a relatively minor beneficiary of the reform movement, substantial improvements in quality of care occurred during the middle to late 1950s. The changing needs of the aged Riverview population and attenuation of reform efforts in the early 1960s, however, ended immediate hopes to establish a public nursing home. The reform movement initiatives do reveal areas in which municipal reorganization and innovation were possible. These changes, reflecting the new view of government and the individual, addressed four major areas: (1) classification of patients, (2) repairs to and construction of the Riverview buildings, (3) financing, and (4) medicalization, or espousal of a medical model of care.

Classification

Classification restructured Riverview itself, creating an explicit mission of care for the aged and infirmed. Specialization in the care of aged, chronically ill patients would enable Riverview to develop population-specific services, a first step in gaining control of the institution and elaborating the nursing role. Social workers were employed to manage classification initiatives, explicitly limiting Riverview's use as a "dumping ground" by other institutions.[16] Sick persons requiring extensive medical or psychiatric care were refused admission, regardless of their age.[17] Hospital transfers were screened, and some were directed to the growing network of nursing homes.

Construction

The second feature that transformed the almshouse into Riverview was a $2.5 million program of construction and major repairs that implemented the classification mission and raised quality of life. The home was originally built with substandard materials on unstable land, and sewage seepage had been a long-standing problem. During World War II, shortages of employees and construction materials compounded long-term failure to make repairs. An increased proportion of sick and frail elderly residents rendered the frame construction of many buildings unsuitable: by the 1960s second floors in these buildings were abandoned because of the absence of elevators and danger of fire.

Underlying the capital improvement plans, and reflecting the reform motive, was a goal to "restore to the elderly residents the respect for themselves and others that they may have lost . . . [and to] retain their human dignity . . . [through] a decent home and good care."[18] New building designs accommodated the physical limitations of the new residents with the use of ramps and handrails. Large windows, a designer's touch of color, and an interest in patient privacy separated the new facilities from the old. When the units opened, the Arlene Francis national television show broadcast live from a circus tent on the grounds of Riverview, celebrating it as an ideal nursing home.[19]

As did most Philadelphia homes for the aged during the 1950s, Riverview remodeled and staffed an infirmary for its most frail residents: plans were made in 1956 to replace two small sick wards.[20] A forty-year-old building was remodeled in 1961 as a central infirmary of two large dormitory wards, each with sixty patients. The infirmary was originally intended for Riverview residents requiring a high level of care; however, political pressure forced accommodation of direct admissions.[21] Many people with acute illnesses were treated there to avoid the fourteen-mile journey in a police wagon to Philadelphia General Hospital.

Financing

Improved financing was the third enabling factor. Family financial responsibility was newly enforced, yielding a modest institutional income. After 1950 old age assistance payments could be used for persons in public homes. Most important, for the first time in Riverview's history the reform city council provided it with near-adequate appropriations. This income was primarily used for construction and represented a visible, enduring, popular distribution of funds to remedy "the shame of Philadelphia." But city spending for everyday items, such as food and clothing, could not keep pace with rising inflation.

Medicalization

The fourth major change at Riverview Home for the Aged was the adoption of a medical model of care. Riverview increasingly focused on the care of the medically indigent, articulating and producing a new class and a new mission. The credibility and acceptance of this change in institutional mission was supported by (1) a recognition of chronic illness as a sickness category; (2) an increasing medicalization in all phases of society; and (3) an increasing confidence in the medical model as a viable method, as opposed to the traditional moral model of charity subsistence care.

Professionalization was key to medicalization. Appointment of a new Riverview administrator reflected professional rather than political criteria. The medical program at Riverview was redesigned to promote the care and rehabilitation of the residents, many of whom had chronic illnesses. Sick calls at the infirmary were now held in the morning and afternoon; people referred for diagnosis and follow-up care were sent to Philadelphia General Hospital. Psychiatric personnel evaluated and classified the entire resident population of the institution. Some "disturbed" residents were treated with medications, some were given therapy, and some were referred to Philadelphia General Hospital and the state psychiatric system. Registered and practical nurses and nurses' aides were hired for the infirmary and dispensary, although not for residential areas. Registered nurse roles were limited to either supervision or teaching, with some clinical involvement. Physical and occupational therapy programs were initiated and relevant equipment provided, "designed to keep the residents constructively occupied, healthy and happy."[22] Facilities for segregating and treating tuberculosis and infectious disease patients were finally arranged. Dentists, podiatrists, and optometrists generally visited on a volunteer basis. Even with these limited initiatives, identification and prompt treatment of illness was more likely than before.

Limitations of Reform at Riverview

In the early 1960s, the Philadelphia reform movement collapsed, possibly because it had focused more on particular projects than on broader social goals, and possibly because of its inability to sustain reforms that separated politics from government.[23] The reform movement "eroded," plagued by funding problems and a sense that this American city could not rebuild. In the opinion of one local historian, "reform in Philadelphia provided emergency surgery, especially downtown, and it also provided a temporary transfusion. What this town needed [and never received] was a change of its genetic code."[24] At Riverview the reform goal of establishing a nursing home remained incomplete. Adequate medical and rehabilitation services were never offered to all Riverview's residents. Long-term municipal attitudes kept the Riverview "an unpleasant place where the City likes no one, including itself, to peer too closely."[25]

Changing Functions of Related Institutions

City council and ward leaders continued to use Riverview for their own political ends—as a source of patronage jobs and as a haven for the neediest of their aging constituents. Politicalization of individual admissions also circumvented classification initiatives at Riverview. And the home was obliged to accept transfers from the city's public hospital system and prisons, and from the state psychiatric system. These institutions continued to flood Riverview with patients needing care outside its stated mission and resources. While Philadelphia General Hospital received the unwanted—invalids, alcoholics, and chronic patients—from the city's nonpublic hospitals, Riverview received what Philadelphia General Hospital would not keep. Riverview Home remained the last hope for many.

In the 1950s Riverview was forced to admit nearly three hundred "non-violent, senile aged" transferred from state psychiatric hospitals. The state system had been "burdened with chronic cases" and with increasing custodial referrals for mentally impaired elderly.[26] Faced with severe institutional overcrowding and an increase in younger mental patients having potential for cure, state mental hospitals demanded to be relieved of chronic, senile, aged patients. In addition to reducing patient numbers through the transfer, the state saved money by shifting the cost of care to the city.

Riverview was unable to stem municipal court commitments and transfers of city prisoners, which remained at an average of thirty percent of all admissions until 1962.[27] Some former prisoners had long records of sex offenses and violent crimes; one was charged with murder of an aged Riverview resident. Many were physically or psychologically frail, needing sheltered care but rarely the complex care Riverview sought to provide. Riverview transfer relieved the prisons of those deemed inappropriate for corrections—the homeless, vagrant, and alcoholic—who were picked up randomly during police sweeps of Skid Row. Also, care at Riverview was thirty-percent cheaper than care at any city prison.[28]

These three transfer programs—from acute care, psychiatric, and corrections systems—supported the "primary mission" of other public institutions. As a result, Riverview sheltered people in various states of health, requiring many different degrees of care, "simply because there's no other place they can go."[29] The limitations of Riverview were symptomatic of the larger, systemwide failures to care for all of Philadelphia's aged, but particularly the poor, sick aged at every level of need.

Changing Needs of Philadelphia's Aged

While many county homes elsewhere were converted into nursing homes and chronic care hospitals, Philadelphia's political leadership permitted no change in Riverview's use as "the last hope"—Riverview served the rest of the system too well. As long as Riverview could not control its admissions, it could not control the shape of the institution and its programs. The type of care needed by those admitted to Riverview became progressively more complex. Needy Philadelphians were ever older and more dependent. Residents requiring medical and nursing services, rather than residential care, rose from 36 percent of the total to 75 percent in 1965.[30] As the numbers of the well and ambulatory aged at Riverview decreased, the slow process and limited goals of medicalization proved inadequate to the increasing nursing care needs of residents.[31] More and more of Riverview's patients needed the structured care of a nursing home rather than a home for the aged with a modest infirmary.

The increased numbers of sick Riverview residents never received adequate care. Caregivers were always too few for the number of patients. Riverview staff also received unsuitable and wasteful assignments; registered nurses could be found scrubbing walls and cleaning lavatories. Physicians and nurses were reluctant to approve patient transfers out of the infirmary, where nursing care was assured, back into other buildings with few services.[32] Rehabilitation failed as well; blind men, who could walk, were in wheelchairs for years for lack of training and assistance. Other patients were depressed and disinterested in their surroundings and had not spoken in years. Neither a nurse nor a physician was available at Riverview on the night shift in either the infirmary or the dispensary.[33] A dietitian's position was unfilled for years, until a meat-cutter was promoted into it. Personnel recruitment remained difficult as the home was so isolated. Half the nursing positions were generally unfilled.[34]

In 1967 the nursing staff added to the growing public outcry regarding Riverview with public charges of poor patient care. Their concerns unanswered, seven of ten registered nurses resigned, triggering a state investigation. With the added impact of the new Medicaid regulations setting standards of care for reimbursement, Riverview was reorganized with a 30 to 40 percent reduction in patients. Nursing and personal care staff increased almost 20 percent, yielding a staff-to-patient ratio of 1 to 2.4 in 1974, compared to one staff for 6.2 patients in 1965.[35] Although never an outstanding institution, Riverview was finally a nursing home.

Conclusions

Nursing's lack of involvement in almshouses was challenged in 1908 by Lavinia Dock and a network of advocates.[36] If nursing could reform the hospital, would not nursing's methods change the almshouse? Nursing's absence from the almshouse is as much a story of the profession as is its advancement in the hospital. Nursing has been ambivalent about chronic care and reluctant to make a stand in institutions other than hospitals.

Most professionals, as well as politicians and the public, chose to ignore the poor and chronically ill. Many Philadelphians found a certain satisfaction in the reforms at Riverview, particularly those who believed Riverview to be the direct descendant of the original almshouse. It looked better, and it provided adequate food and reasonable shelter. Those who looked for a good quality nursing home remained dissatisfied as Riverview failed to reach this goal. In Philadelphia, as in many other cities, long-term care for the chronic sick remained unresolved.

Who should Riverview serve, a patronage network, or the dependent sick? The dilemma between achieving an institutional mission for care of the poor aged and maintaining a traditional role as a safety valve for other city institutions persisted. While Philadelphia's experience was distinct from other cities, all shared a concern and fundamental obligation to care for the aged, dependent sick. Philadelphia's reform of Riverview outlined the aspirations as well as the limitations of municipal long-term care in the years leading up to Medicare and Medicaid.

JANNA L. DIECKMANN
Doctoral Candidate
School of Nursing
University of Pennsylvania

76 East Logan Street
Philadelphia, Pa. 19144
Phone: (215) 848-5541

Acknowledgments

I would like to acknowledge support from an NRSA Pre-Doctoral Fellowship from the National Center for Nursing Research; The American Nurses' Foundation, "Agnes Olson, R.N., Scholar" grant; and a dissertation fellowship from the

Program for Assessment and Revitalization of the Social Sciences, University of Pennsylvania.

Notes

1. Estelle M. Stewart, *The Cost of American Almshouses*, Bulletin of the U.S Bureau of Labor Statistics, no. 386 (Washington, D.C.: Government Printing Office, 1925), 52.

2. Jacob Fisher, "Trends in Institutional Care of the Aged," *Social Security Bulletin* 16 (October 1953): 9; Raymond M. Hilliard, "The Development of County Homes for Care of the Chronically Ill," *Public Welfare* 3 (December 1945): 266.

3. The Philadelphia Almshouse was established in 1731; it moved to Blockley Township in 1834. Efforts to separate the almshouse and hospital functions began by 1873 and were implemented between 1910 and 1920, forming Philadelphia General Hospital (with a Blockley and a Northern/Contagious Division) and the Home for the Indigent (later Riverview Home for the Aged).

4. *Annual Report 1950*, City of Philadelphia, Bureau of Charities and Corrections, box A-561, City Archives of Philadelphia, Pennsylvania (hereafter cited as CAPP).

5. Ibid.

6. "Home for Indigent Needs $100,000: Amount Must Be Spent for Repairs, Charities Bureau Head Says," *Bulletin*, 4 January 1947, Temple University, Urban Archives, Bulletin Collection, "Riverview Home—Miscellaneous (RH-Ms), 1951 and Prior" (hereafter cited as TUUA, BC).

7. L. S. Willis, "Petty Rackets and Big Hearts Found By Disguised Scribe at Indigent Home," *Evening Ledger*, 3 April 1940, TUUA, BC, "RH-Ms, 1951 and Prior."

8. "Facilities at Three Institutions: Asks More Funds for Improvements," *Philadelphia Inquirer*, 29 July 1950, TUUA, BC, "RH-Ms, 1951 and Prior."

9. "Jailed Drug Addicts Neglected, Grand Jury's Report Charges," *Bulletin*, 29 December 1950, and "City's Care of Poor 'Shocks' Grand Jury," *Bulletin*, 2 July 1947, both TUUA, BC, "RH-Ms, 1951 and Prior"; "Grand Jury Presentment for December 1950 and June 1950 Terms," box A-4363, CAPP.

10. Grand Jury Presentment for December 1946 Term, box A-4363, CAPP.

11. "Hint Rum-Running in City Poorhouse: Coroner to Probe 'Shocking' Conditions Linked to Two Deaths in Marshes," *Evening Ledger*, 16 October 1939 (for example), and "Dysentery Kills Thirty-Three in Poorhouse," *Evening Ledger*, 15 October 1937, both TUUA, BC, "RH-Ms, 1951 and Prior"; and "Test Buildings At Indigent Home: Woodruff Orders Careful Examination as Result of Ceiling Collapse, No One Was Hurt," *Evening Bulletin*, 13 March 1933, TUUA, BC, "RH—Buildings."

12. "Will Weed Out Inmates: Feeble-Minded To Be Shifted, Officials Say," *Philadelphia Inquirer*, 21 October 1939; TUUA, BC, "RH-Ms, 1959 and Prior."

13. Jim Nicholson, "Crusading Mayor Joe Clark Dies at 88," *Philadelphia Daily*

News, 15 January 1990, p. 13; Kirk R. Petshek, *The Challenge of Urban Reform: Policies and Programs in Philadelphia* (Philadelphia: Temple University Press, 1973), 15.

14. Dennis Clark, *Proceedings from Philadelphia's Political Reform Movement, 1946–1961*, Historical Society of Pennsylvania, 27 February 1988 (Philadelphia: The Historical Society of Pennsylvania, n.d.), 39.

15. *Towards Human Dignity: The Story of the New Philadelphia Department of Public Welfare and the People It Serves, 1952–1955* (Philadelphia: Department of Public Welfare and Office of the City Representative, circa 1955).

16. *Annual Report 1953*, City of Philadelphia, Department of Public Welfare, box A-561, CAPP, p. 61 (hereafter cited as DPW, CAPP).

17. *Annual Report, 1955*, DPW, box A-561, CAPP, p. 20.

18. Mary Ellen Gale, "Large Modern Cottages To Be Built At Riverview at Cost of $2 Million," *Evening Bulletin*, 9 February 1964, TUUA, BC, "RH—Buildings."

19. *Annual Report, 1956*, DPW, box A-561, CAPP, p. 16.

20. "Asked for $300,000 for Infirmary at Riverview," *Evening Bulletin*, 27 March 1956, TUUA, BC, "RH-Ms, 1952–1956."

21. Pennsylvania Economy League, *Caring for Philadelphia's Needy Aged* (Philadelphia: Pennsylvania Economy League, 1968), I-4.

22. *Design for Human Dignity: The Story of Philadelphia's Department of Public Welfare* (Office of the City Representative, 1959?), p. 18, box A-561, CAPP.

23. James Reichley, *Art of Government: Reform and Organization Politics in Philadelphia* (New York: The Fund for the Republic, 1959; reprint, Dubuque, Iowa: Brown Reprints, 1972): 114. Edward Schwartz, *Proceedings from Philadelphia's Political Reform Movement, 1946–1961*, Historical Society of Pennsylvania, 27 February 1988 (Philadelphia: The Historical Society of Pennsylvania, n.d.), 66.

24. Dennis Clark, 45.

25. Editorial, "Home for the Indigent," 10 October 1939, TUUA, BC, "RH—Editorials."

26. *Annual Report, 1953*, DPW, box A-561, CAPP.

27. *Annual Reports, 1951–1960, 1962–1964*, DPW, box A-561, CAPP, p. 20.

28. *Background Material* (February 1956), DPW, box A-561, CAPP; George R. Staab, "Visitor Finds Riverview Clean, Cheerful; Philadelphia Officials Irked at Jury's Criticism," 2 January 1955, TUUA, BC, "RH-Ms, 1952–1956."

29. David M. Cleary and Gary Brooten, "Key to a Controversy: What Does the City Want at Riverview?" *Sunday Bulletin*, 23 July 1967, TUUA, BC, "RH-Ms, 1963–1973."

30. Pennsylvania Economy League, *Philadelphia's Needy Aged*, I-7.

31. Raymond J. Groller, "Riverview Fact Sheet," circa 1960, TUUA, BC, "RH—1959–1962."

32. "Report to the Trustees of Riverview," January/February 1964, box-5839, CAPP, p. 3.

33. David M. McCleary, "Good Things Happen at Riverview Thanks to Medicare and Dr. Papa," *Sunday Bulletin*, 9 June 1968, TUUA, BC, "RH-Ms, 1963–1973." Kos Semonski, "Take Riverview Patients 'Out of Life of Hell,' Foglietta Urges," *Bulletin*, 23 June 1967, TUUA, BC, "RH-Ms, 1963–1973."

34. "City's Home for Aged Plans New Drive to Recruit Nurses," *Bulletin*, 27 March 1967, TUUA, BC, "RH—Nurses."

35. *Annual Report, 1965*, DPW, box A-561, CAPP; City of Philadelphia, Department of Public Welfare, *Annual Report, 1973–1974* (Philadelphia: Department of Public Welfare, 1974).

36. Lavinia L. Dock, "The Crusade for Almshouse Nursing," *American Journal of Nursing* 8 (February 1908): 361–63.

The Legacy of Domesticity
Nursing in Early Nineteenth-Century America

PATRICIA O'BRIEN D'ANTONIO

The heart of nursing is, and has been, the care of the sick. Through most of history, the responsibility for nursing has rested with women: with mothers, daughters, sisters, and neighbors who cared for their sick children, spouses, parents, and friends in the home. Here lies the domestic roots of modern nursing practice. Prior to the establishment of formal training schools, and well before the drive toward professional status through the registration movement, nursing revolved around the image and the activities of mothers caring for the sick in their own homes. In the domestic world of the early nineteenth century, the time and place where this story begins, the nursing of family and friends took place at home because most sickness, birthing, and dying centered in the home. Further, in a historical world where women's domestic duties were tied tightly to notions about women's innate capabilities and their loving responsibilities, such nursing was an almost unquestioned part of their lives. The care of a sick family member, in the words of one chronicler of the early nineteenth-century domestic world, was to be "commended" to a "woman's benevolent ministries."[1]

Yet, even as the image of nursing has been framed by the historic duty of women to care for the sick at the domestic bedside, how that duty found its form in the actual work of nursing changed in the first half of the nineteenth century. It changed as ideas about expert knowledge, correct social order, viable occupational options, and the centrality of therapeutic alliances in the caring process changed. I argue in this article that, long before Florence Nightingale brought her vision of nursing reform to the late nineteenth-century hospital bedside, earlier nineteenth-century physicians and nursing women, at the bedsides of their patients in the home, had

Nursing History Review 1 (1993): 229–46.

already reworked certain fundamental assumptions about nursing's work and nurses' relationships with physicians. I am going to argue that this reform was driven by the tension between physicians and nurses as each sought to assert the centrality of their alliance with the sick patient. The legacy of this domestic reform not only influenced the later structuring of the first nurses training schools in Philadelphia, as one particular case study, but also continues to resonate in today's debate about what kinds of nurses should do what kinds of work.

* * *

This story begins in the 1830s, a time when the best in medical as well as nursing care centered in the home. Much has already been written about the chaos of early nineteenth-century medical practice—most particularly the rise of competing medical sects; the frightening and unpredictable quality of infectious diseases, which, like most diseases, had yet to be understood as specific entities; and the growing dissatisfaction and disillusionment with the traditionally heroic measures of bleeding and purging. But it is important to remember that, through it all, physicians, nurses, and patients continued to share beliefs on certain fundamental issues. Most important, all shared what historian Charles Rosenberg has described as the central metaphor dominating early nineteenth-century assumptions about health and illness: in health the body existed in dynamic equilibrium with both itself and its environment; in illness the body lapsed into disequilibrium. And all shared, to some degree, assumptions about the efficacy of those therapeutics (stimulants, purgatives, emetics, and bleedings) that produced the visible, physiological effects (the energy, evacuations, vomiting, and relaxation) associated with the careful regulation and regaining of that delicate equilibrium.[2]

Indeed, because of such deeply shared assumptions, domestic dosing (individuals prescribing their own remedies) remained the norm. Stimulants, emetics, purgatives, and, occasionally, even opium and laudanum were within easy reach of any member of the family who wished to prepare his or her body for the upcoming seasonal change or who was plagued by minor and irritating ills.[3] Physicians of all persuasions knew, accepted, and even promoted these practics, although within limits. Philadelphia physicians compiled careful lists of therapeutics necessary for the early nineteenth-century domestic medicine cabinet, but frequently omitted botanicals, as one physician wrote, "from a conviction that nothing is so injurious as affording the means of quackery to nurses and ignorant mothers."[4]

Such "quackery" in early nineteenth-century Philadelphia was most noticeably, but not solely, associated with the Thomsonian practitioners. The Thomsonians shared the fundamental belief in the idea of equilibrium. They believed that the cause of all disease was cold and that the only cure was the restoration of the body's natural heat. They took issue, however, with traditional therapeutics, preferring botanical preparations and steaming. The Thomsonians had lists for the domestic medicine cabinet, containing various combinations of lobelia (an emetic long used by native Americans) and stimulating peppers. They gave considerably more responsibility to the families for the actual treatment of diseases, but they also had their limits. One practitioner, despairing over the interference of opinionated nurses, flatly declared that "Thomsonian practitioners, to have justice done to either the system of practice, or the patient, require Thomsonian nurses."[5]

One breed of nurses that traditional physicians and Thomsonian practitioners both could denounce as "quacks" were the midwives. They agreed that a long catalog of problems associated with both mother and child—ills ranging from bloody noses through childbed fever and infant convulsions—could be laid squarely at the hands of the untrained and uneducated midwife.[6] They joined to ridicule her delivery techniques, her treatment of the infant, and her language. One Thomsonian practitioner in Philadelphia, Dr. J. W. Comfort, agreed with the famous allopathic practitioner William Buchan who protested the midwives' practice of purging the infant; Comfort chided the midwives' colloquial use of the word "economy" for the medical term "meconium." Not one to miss an opportunity, however, Comfort went on to add that, while it was gratifying to see allopathic physicians "exposing the malpractice of nurses giving physic to 'purge off the meconium,'" his readers should recollect "that it was the *medical profession* that first instituted this abominable practice."[7]

Here Comfort rather casually underlined a significant connection between the midwives and the regular medical practitioners: the midwives' therapeutic traditions drew heavily from both the prescriptions of standard medical practice and their own experience. In their use of emetics and purgatives during labor, their practice of dosing of infants with castor oil and goose grease after birth, and their plan for a stimulating diet for the postpartum mother, they bound themselves both to the beliefs and to the therapeutic practices of their regular medical contemporaries. Indeed, the most strident complaint medical practitioners could lodge about midwives' actual practice was that it was outdated and, hence, potentially dangerous, not that it was conceptually wrong.[8]

The ultimate efficacy of this system of belief and practice must be understood, as Rosenberg points out, in relation to its social setting and emotional context. Patients, midwives, and physicians participated in an almost ritualized patterning of relationships in the home. The shared cognitive understanding of sickness, and its treatment provided a framework for a relationship in which practical therapeutics could be at once emotionally reassuring to the patient and socially legitimating to the practitioner. But using a therapeutic agent, that is, actively manipulating elements of a physiological equilibrium toward healing, depended on a "shared faith"—a "conspiracy to believe" between patient and practitioner—for its effect.[9] It depended on what we might today call the therapeutic relationship. For physicians in the early nineteenth century, the crucial problem with the midwives, as with other nurses, involved the threat they posed to the sanctity and the reciprocity of the physician-patient relationship.

Midwives were notorious for their opinionated and independent behavior at the bedside. They would refuse to assist physicians of all persuasions if they disapproved of their proposed course of treatment. One midwife, for example, told a Thomsonian accoucheur that she would leave if he persisted in his valor bath. Another refused to administer an injection of lobelia as "she did not approve of it." Regular physicians fared little better. They saw their orders countermanded, their medicines discarded, and their patients' sickrooms inadequately prepared for both delicate therapeutic interventions and the necessary convalescence. Worse still, midwives' descriptions of afterbirth in terms that implied a fair degree of judgment and experience—describing the flow of the lochia as "just about right," "too much that way," or "not as much as ought to be,"—were perceived as entirely inadequate for proper medical assessment.[10]

The crux of the problem, however, lay within the midwife's relationship with her patient. As Joseph Warrington, a Quaker physician at the Philadelphia Dispensary, ruefully pointed out, "the opinions of the nurse are not infrequently demanded by the nervous and timid lady." Warrington initially had what he thought the simplest solution—refer the lady back instead to her physician for answers.[11] Few midwives paid attention. They freely answered questions from their patients and not infrequently offered their own comments on the course of therapeutics. "Dr. ———," said one midwife after watching her patient swallow a particularly noxious dose, "would not have given you such a medicine." Another, observing preparations for a Thomsonian vapor bath, commented to her patient that she herself would suffer death before steaming.[12]

Warrington turned to another, more complicated solution to ensure the physician's authority: to train working-class women of good moral character as adjuncts to the physician. These nurses would still be available to care for other women in childbirth, but, unlike the midwives, they would be trained by a physician, responsible to him rather than to the parturient woman, and, in important ways, they would be an extension of his more "scientific" services. In 1839 Warrington founded the Nurse Society of Philadelphia. The society trained worthy, working-class women in such areas as the management of the lying-in chamber, convalescent diet, and care of the new mother and infant. The society sent the women into the home to assist the physician during childbirth and the mother during the postpartum period. Despite close control over the practice of these nurses, Warrington still felt obliged to carefully delineate proper spheres of authority. His training of nurses was designed, he wrote, "less with a view to create the business of nursing into an *independent* calling, than to impress those who engage in it with the importance of understanding their relations with a class of men who devote years to the acquisition of the *science* and then exercise themselves for years besides."

Relatively few working-class women agreed with Warrington's prescriptive, hierarchical ordering of roles between themselves and the physician. The physician's wish for such nurses always exceeded the number willing to work for the Nurse Society. For the nurse the promise of such a dependent role would be either a well-paid invitation into the lying-in chambers of the city's social elite, or the altruistic satisfaction of knowing that another poor, birthing woman was saved from the humiliation and the danger of Philadelphia's lying-in hospitals. One can speculate that these nursing women, knowing they could "profess" their skills on their own within their own communities, found Warrington's price too high.[13]

Physicians, though, had a clear and persistent sense of what was at stake: the challenge posed by the midwives' confidence in their own therapeutics and their own relationships with their patients undermined the fragile emotional bond between physician and patient. The physicians believed they had to have the patient's complete confidence to begin any treatment or effect any cure. For one physician, Anthony Thomson, treatment became possible only after the patient had been "impressed with the belief that [the physician] is not only duly qualified for the investigation and cure of diseases, but that he is deeply interested in the case" as well. Indeed, the proper role for family, friends, and attendants involved promoting, "in every instance, the efforts of the physician to secure the confidence of his patient."[14]

Midwives were the most obvious but by no means the only threat to this fragile confidence. Nurses in general made difficult the necessary therapeutic alliance—but here we begin broaching the thorny issue of defining just who is "the nurse." Some women, with reputations in the community as good nurses, came into families as hired help when one member took ill. These nurses, as did midwives, came to families armed with their own experience and therapeutics—cold keys for nosebleeds, sulphur for measles, and leeches for fevers.[15] More often a servant would be pressed into duty. In fact, one very erudite patient expressed her preference for the care of servants over that of her willing family. "In so far as the help is mechanical," she wrote, "the relation is sustained with the least amount of effort."[16]

More often, however, members of the family were called on to nurse. More specifically, mothers, daughters, and sisters nursed their families and, depending on these women's financial and social resources, they were aided by their friends, hired nurses, or servants.[17] It was these middle-class nurses with family ties who posed the strongest threat to the fragile relationship between the physician and his patient. Opinionated, educated, connected to the patient through emotional ties, and equal to the physician in shared middle-class background—formidable in her prescribed role as guardian of the home and preserver of its health—she presented a threatening challenge to the sanctity of the physician-patient relationship. What was the physician to do? When he would prescribe a light diet, the family would produce a rich broth. When he would allow visitors, relations would enter, survey the scene, and disconcertingly shake their heads. "I wish," said one to the patient, "you had been under dear Dr. ———; he did so much good in a case exactly the same as yours. Yes! he is the Physician I shall always recommend."[18]

The problem, of course, was hardly new. Physicians had to deal with the family from the first time they entered the home. Threats had been a useful strategy. "Nurses take care!," one late eighteenth-century English physician wrote in a book to families about nursing, reprinted in Philadelphia in 1804. "If you indulge relations at the expense of your patient's life, how will you satisfy your conscience afterwards?" Conduct within the healing relationship was fairly straightforward. "It behooves the patient," this physician continued, "to regard his [physician's] rules, the nurse to see them punctually observed, and both, to be cautious about how they deviate from them; as fatal consequences may sometimes arise."[19]

Rules described at the turn of the century had subtly changed as the Civil War approached. Obedience to the physician's orders remained the norm, confidence in his therapeutics the ideal. But the authoritarian high-handedness of the physician had yielded somewhat in acknowledgment of the growing public dissatisfaction with traditional heroic medical therapeutics and, particularly, in acknowledgment of the growing power of middle-class nursing women within the physician-patient relationship.[20]

Popular ideas about domesticity and the role of women changed in the first half of the nineteenth century as urbanization, industrialization, and immigration reshaped both the economy and the social landscape. In Philadelphia, for example, the population rose fourfold between 1830 and 1860 as a result of the devastating Irish potato famine, political upheaval in Germany, and economic depression of the countryside causing farmhand migration. Industrialization, spurred by the new technologies and the river mills in Philadelphia and other growing towns, moved much of women's traditionally domestic work out of the home and into factories. Cloth, for example, was no longer spun and woven at home; the mills along Philadelphia's Schuylkill River did a much more efficient job producing a range of fabrics for sale that no one woman could create on her own. But fabric was not the only thing being bought and sold in Philadelphia. With industrialization, work itself became a commodity to be bought and sold in the market like any other object of exchange. Economically, the early decades of the nineteenth century brought with it the emergence of a new urban middle class, those able to buy work for the factory or for the home, and its counterpoint, the urban working class, those selling work for wages.

The most compelling change in the domestic world of early nineteenth-century women, though, came as a response to industrialization's new and dramatic separation of the home and workplace. The first half of the nineteenth century redefined the purpose of the home and women's role within it. The home had lost its place in economic production—domestic tasks moved into mills, and husbands and fathers left each morning to practice their professions or trades in offices or factories—to be recast in the rhetoric of the time as a social haven from the harsh work world and as an emotional nest for the rearing of children. Women's prescribed roles changed concurrently. Time that had been spent on economic tasks was now spent on more social and emotional responsibilities. The domestic rhetoric created a "cult of true womanhood," as it has been called by historians. A "lady's" proper role, now that she could buy from factories the cloth she previously had to spin and weave, became that of guardian of her family's morals, manners, and health; she became the symbol of her family's economic prosperity. At least in the popular literature, if not always in fact, the authority and the responsibility for the ideal middle-class home had shifted from men to women by the end of the 1860s.[21]

Middle-class nursing women took this authority and responsibility to heart, turning to the resources available to them. They listened to speakers, usually other middle-class women traveling the urban lecture circuit, who outlined the then current facts of basic anatomy and physiology, nutrition and hygiene, sexuality, and family planning. They read a growing genre of domestic medicine and nursing manuals that, by 1861 when the first American edition was published, included Florence Nightingale's own *Notes on Nursing*. Also, they looked to their traditional resource, the hired nurse, or what historian Susan Reverby has named the "professed nurse."[22]

Because of Reverby's research, historians know something about some of these "professed nurses." They tended to be white, native-born in rural areas, and daughters of farmers or skilled workers. They tended to enter the market at ages older than other women workers, usually pushed there by the poverty and destitution that so often accompanied the widowhood, divorce, or abandonment of working-class nineteenth-century women. And, as noted earlier, they entered the market, which, of course, was the middle-class home, armed with the practical experience gained at the bedsides of their own families and often with their own particular therapeutics.[23]

The domestic bedside of the mid-nineteenth-century patient was crowded and tense. Physicians, middle-class nursing women, midwives, and professed nurses gathered there, sharing beliefs about the causes of the illness but competing for the faith of the patient in the efficacy of their idiosyncratic therapeutics. In Philadelphia, Joseph Warrington's earlier attempt to align some working-class nurses with physicians in a hierarchical relationship had failed, but the need to assert the centrality of the relationship with the patient remained. Physicians, absorbing the domestic rhetoric of their time, saw their patients as "children"—capricious, demanding, truculent, and vulnerable. Vulnerable, in every instance, particularly "to the advice of ignorant nurses and misguided friends."[24]

In this carefully worded characterization lies the thrust of the mid-nineteenth-century movement to reform the work and the role of nursing women and their relationships with physicians: professed nurses were "ignorant" and middle-class women who nursed, "misguided"; working-class women who nursed threatened the physician-patient relationship through their "prejudices" while middle-class women did so through their misleading "affection."[25] To gain middle-class allies in the fight for control of the therapeutic relationship, physicians played to increasingly meaningful class distinctions among nursing women. They sought to align the perceived chaos of relationships at the patient's bedside hierarchically—with the physician supervising the middle-class woman, who, in turn, would supervise the hired nurse.

This reform proposed a realignment that resonated with the middle-class woman's domestic experience. Popular ideas about domesticity gave the woman control of the home, but they did not ask that she actually perform the physical labor required in a home. Rather, a "lady" would hire and manage the working-class "help,"—persons, both men and women, now trading their labor for money in an industrializing economy. In fact, the middle-class woman was already managing the servant, cook, washerwoman, and the gardener in her home. She was now being asked to manage the nurse.

Of course, to intelligently manage and supervise one's help, a woman had to know enough about their work to recognize when tasks were or were not being performed properly. Not surprisingly, then, "education" became the operative word in the proposed reformation of alliances between physicians and middle-class nursing women. Regrettably, as one physician pointed out, "few ladies, even those who are wives and mothers, have any acquaintance with the arrangement of the sick room, and the management of an invalid; they are consequently, too often forced to be guided by, and to rely for instruction of, the nurse, instead of being able to superintend her conduct, to ascertain that she performs her duties, and to correct her feelings."[26]

The plan to correct the "misguided" and the "ignorant" developed along several interrelated lines. First, mothers who nursed had to be drawn away from their alliance with other women—nurses working for pay—and into a new relationship with the physician as his eyes and ears and as his superintendent in the sickroom. Interestingly, though, she was not his hands. The physical work of caring for the patient—bathing, turning, cooking, feeding, administering treatments—remained in the hands of the hireling. That work requiring judgment and intellect—watching for changes in the course of the disease, attending to the labile disposition and temper of the patient, deciding the wisdom of pursuing one course over another if alternatives were available—would be the work of "ladies."

The alliance of ladies with nurses could hold across class lines only insofar as it was felt that hired nurses offered the ladies something of value:

tried and true methods of affording relief and cure. The nurses' experience, however, next came under attack. "Experience," one physician wryly noted, "is a quality to be much and justly prized in a nurse, were the term not too frequently misapplied, and confidence placed in the nurse merely because she is advanced in years and has seen much, without any inquiry as to her capacity for observing and making proper use of what she has seen." Regrettably, he continued, "it is well known, that, in the lower ranks of society, no habit is so little cultivated as the habit of attention. Thousands pass from cradle to grave without seeing correctly a single object which passes before them, and if we reflect how essential this faculty of mind is for the improvement of intellect, the importance of not trusting the domestic management of the sick wholly to hired nurses surely requires no comment."[27]

Education, on the other hand, was an attribute much prized in a nurse. Where the old and the ignorant could appeal only to experience, the educated nurse could appeal to her carefully cultivated spheres of knowledge and judgment and then apply them to the care of her patient. Working, as did the physician, within the framework of both knowledge of the laws of disease and its convalescence, and within the boundaries of her intimate knowledge of both the patient and the family, the nurse could even justify her "pausing in the plan laid down for her guidance, until the physician is sent for." Indeed, "her reasons for the deviation will be listened to by the physician; and, without lowering his dignity, a useful hint from an intelligent nurse may be adopted and acted upon, much to the advantage of the patient."[28] The problem, however, was that too few educated women knew how to "properly" care for the sick.

Where Joseph Warrington had sought to train working-class women in the 1830s, his colleague, Ann Preston, dean of the Female Medical College of Pennsylvania, and one of the founders of the Woman's Hospital of Philadelphia, set her sights on the middle-class women of the 1860s. Her idea of "proper" education involved teaching such women the scientific rules of ventilation, sanitation, and convalescent diet; she instructed through public lectures, through her book, *Nursing the Sick and the Training of Nurses*, and through a formal school, established in 1861 and the first in Philadelphia, for "the practical training of nurses" at the Woman's Hospital.[29] Her idea of "proper" education, however, like those of her medical brothers, had nothing to do with the actual diagnosis and treatment of diseases—that remained within the physician's realm. Therapeutics remained peripheral to nursing—the nurse's responsibilities would be limited to making the doses as palatable as possible. Preston, like her women physician colleagues in Boston and New York, did take special interest in the nursing education of middle-class women. However, her training of nurses emphasized a hierarchical therapeutic alliance with the women of the family in support of the primary relationship of the patient to the physician over any other possible configuration along gender lines—as did that of her medical brothers, the physicians.[30]

However hierarchically defined, Preston did advocate a new configuration of relationships based on class: all nurses should be middle class. Whether in the hospital or in the home, all nurses needed to be "high toned and well trained," as well as "enlightened and refined." Indeed, at public lectures in Philadelphia on the nursing care of the sick sponsored by the newly incorporated Woman's Hospital, women nursing at home and those nursing at the hospital sat side by side in the lecture room. Apart from sporadic ward supervision by Woman's Hospital physicians and a differing fee structure—lay women paid two dollars for a course of ten lectures, nurses in training paid seventy-five cents—there was little to differentiate the instruction of mothers from that of their few middle-class sisters in the hospital.[31]

While Preston had little trouble attracting middle-class women to the Woman's Hospital public lectures on nursing, she had tremendous difficulty attracting such women to the hospital training school and to hospital work. She did try; in 1855 she and Hannah Wright published a pamphlet urging single, middle-class women to consider nursing an acceptable life's work. Her book, published in 1863, was as much instructional as it was a strategy to excite those single women who read it with the value of nursing as a lady's vocation. But the numbers of women accepted for training rarely exceeded one or two during the 1860s, as "the fine combination of qualities, that union of judgement, kindliness, tact, and efficiency which makes the accomplished nurse is not always to be found in applicants."[32] There were applicants, but not the right, middle-class type. Preston had stumbled on the inherent problem in her generation's efforts at nursing reform. The reworking of relationships among physicians, middle-class nursing mothers, and working-class professed nurses at the bedside of the patient in the home was based on the assumption that the actual work of caring could be hierarchically structured on the basis of class, or its code word, education. This hierarchical ordering of middle-class nursing women with the physicians as their educated superintendents in the domestic sickroom did create a meaningful managerial role for these women. However, this ordering implicitly devalued the physical aspects of nursing care. This was now the domain of the hired help, the working-class woman. While a middle-class nursing mother had to know how to ventilate a room, how to prepare a nutritious diet, and how to keep her loved one comfortable in bed, the actual airing, cooking, turning, and bathing remained the purview of the hired help. Middle-class women would supervise such work; they would not do it. In 1864 Preston herself articulated the inherent contradiction in creating class-based alliances in nursing. While emphasizing publicly that "the nurse alone, who intelligently cooperates with the healing powers of nature is, in certain stages of the illness, more important and effective than the physician," she could not avoid hoping, privately and pragmatically, that an increase in the number of applicants to her training school might allow the hospital to "do away with the necessity of chamber-maids," as the necessary nursing duties included so many, more menial tasks.[33]

* * *

It would be later in the nineteenth century when the reforms associated with Florence Nightingale and the trained nurse would reframe such "menial tasks" into a higher form of service to the sick and to the suffering in hospitals—and thus touch, at least for a time, the aspirations of the "right kind" of middle-class woman. In Philadelphia, to continue this case study, Ann Preston saw the number of appropriate applicants to her training school rise slowly but steadily through the 1870s as the romantic image of nursing strangers in hospitals, an image fed by the popular literature, meshed with some women's need for respectable, paid work. For the early 1870s graduates of the Woman's Hospital Training School, seeking to reconcile their need and desire for paid work with their society's rhetoric about appropriate roles for women, it was the Nightingale image, not the substance of her reform, that provided the essential respectability. Nightingale forged the link with the world of the home. Nurses' work became a "calling," not a job; their family all the sick, not just parents, brothers, and sisters. The difference between them and women nursing their families at home would reside not in the duties performed but in the location of such work. The Nightingale image allowed women who needed to work to keep body and soul together.[34]

The reformed vision of nursing's work and nursing's relationship to the physicians worked out a generation earlier by middle-class nursing women in the home more directly influenced the way in which the Ladies

Visiting Committee went about setting up their own training school for nurses at the better known Hospital of the University of Pennsylvania (HUP) in the early 1880s. Frustrated by the less than respectable showing of the hospital's domestic departments, the male managers and physicians at HUP turned to their wives, sisters, and mothers in 1874 for advice and sorely needed help. The newly formed Board of Lady Visitors took to their mandate with an enthusiasm borne of some middle- and upper-class women's need for meaningful and socially acceptable volunteer work. A "lady" may have had a primary moral obligation to her own home and family, but once these obligations were fulfilled, she could and did extend the scope of domesticity to schools, orphanages, and, of course, hospitals.

The Board of Lady Visitors left little of the HUP's domestic world untouched. They supervised the kitchen and tasted the food; they inspected the ventilation system and checked for odors; they visited the patients and provided them with clothes. Even the laundry did not escape their careful review. They described washing conditions as "immoral" and suggested stationary tubs and heated hot water to save the nurses time and energy. But the board took on more than they either could or wanted to handle. Unable and unwilling to perform all the routine chores needed to recreate efficient domesticity at the institutional bedside, these women looked for someone to do the physical work of nursing. This "someone" would have to share these women's middle-class sense of domestic duty and responsibility, but not necessarily their social status. The Board of Lady Visitors saw this "someone" as a trained nurse. As early as 1878 they pushed for a nurses training school. They finally succeeded in 1885. Trained nursing came to HUP, less as a professionalizing strategy and more as a means of producing "the help."[35]

* * *

At this point in the late nineteenth century, traditional histories of professional nursing in the United States usually begin. However, to begin modern nursing history at this time overshadows a more important story played out in an earlier time and in a different historical context. By the end of this earlier story, the framework that structured the development of nursing in the United States had already been established. In the late 1860s and early 1870s nursing still centered in the home, but the ways in which the actual work of nursing would be accomplished had been substantially reformed. Middle-class nursing women had gained a meaningful managerial role in the hierarchical ordering of relations with physicians, one which trained nurses themselves were able to draw on in the next generation. At HUP, in fact, trained nurses did not remain "the help." Some nurses—many of whom would later become leaders in the drive to professionalize modern nursing practice—themselves became managers of the domestic life both on the wards and in the school. In exchange for this domestic authority, the hierarchical ordering of relationships remained sacrosanct. In matters of clinical care of the patient, the physician had "absolute" command.[36]

This reform, like all reforms, had its costs. It came at the expense of middle-class women's traditional alliances with their professed nursing sisters; it came at the expense of the social value placed on physical nursing care. With the actual work of nursing split along class lines, prestige and status followed. This, too, became a theme throughout modern nursing practice. By 1900, as nursing became a more viable and accessible occupational option for working-class women, training schools became flooded with applicants that the nursing elite explicitly called the "wrong kind" of women—working-class women whose care had been devalued a generation earlier.[37] The legacy of this reform—the giving and the taking of the prerogatives of nursing on the basis of class, or its codeword, education—resonates today. It can be heard in today's tension between the head-work and the hand-work in nursing and in the debate about what kinds of nurses should do what kinds of nursing work.

We can also find the legacy of early nineteenth-century reform in today's disciplinary tensions between nurses and physicians. As this study suggests, the patterns of the relationships that have arisen between nurses and physicians involve more than simple boundary disputes over clinical practice, or, as historians have suggested, mere economic self-interest. It also reflects an ongoing, tortuous groping toward new ways to care for the sick when older ways lose their validity and power.

More important, the reform of the early nineteenth century touched on a topic that has always been known and is now being rediscovered: the faith and trust that patients place in their caregivers. The shared belief among caregivers, patient, and family that what is being done is right, good, and necessary is as important to healing as the most sophisticated technology and the most powerful drug. Without the technologies and without the drugs, early nineteenth-century physicians and nursing women experimented with different ways to reassert the centrality of the therapeutic relationship. They did not leave us an unambiguous legacy; it is a part of the past we carry with us when we meet at the bedside of the patient—wherever it may be.

PATRICIA O'BRIEN D'ANTONIO, RN, PhD
231 Avon Road
Merion, Pa. 19072
Phone: (215) 668-1957

Acknowledgments

An early version of this article was presented at the Colloquium in Nursing History, University of California, San Francisco, in September 1988. The author wishes to thank Marilyn Flood and Joan E. Lynaugh for their generous comments.

Notes

1. This quote is in Susan Reverby's *Ordered to Care: The Dilemma of American Nursing, 1850–1945* (New York: Cambridge University Press, 1987), 12. For a sensitive and sophisticated treatment of physician-nurse tensions after 1875, see Joan E. Lynaugh's "Narrow Passageways: Physicians and Nurses in Conflict and Concert Since 1875," in *The Physician as Captain of the Ship: A Critical Reappraisal*, ed. Nancy M. P. King, Larry Churchill, and Alan Cross (Boston: D. Reidel Publishing Company, 1988).

2. Charles Rosenberg, "The Therapeutic Revolution: Medicine, Meaning, and Social Change in Nineteenth Century America," in *The Therapeutic Revolution: Essays in the Social History of American Medicine*, ed. Morris Vogel and Charles Rosenberg (Philadelphia: University of Pennsylvania Press, 1979), 3–25. For overviews of nineteenth-century physicians, practices, and diseases that have particularly informed this work, see Paul Starr's *The Social Transformation of American Medicine* (New York: Basic Books, 1982); William G. Rothstein's *American Physicians in the Nineteenth Century* (Baltimore, Md.: Johns Hopkins University Press, 1972); and Joseph Kett's *The Formation of the American Medical Profession* (New Haven, Conn.: Yale University Press, 1968).

3. Rosenberg, "Therapeutic Revolution," ed. Guenter B. Risse, Ronald L. Numbers, and Judith Walzer Leavitt, *Medicine Without Doctors: Home Health Care in American History* (New York: Science History Publications, 1977).

4. Anthony Todd Thomson, *The Domestic Management of the Sick Room, Necessary in Aid of Medical Treatment, for the Cure of Diseases*, with revisions and additions by R. E. Griffith, MD (Philadelphia: Lea and Blanchard, 1845), 312. Thomson was, in fact, a Fellow of the Royal College of Physicians in London, and his book was originally published in England. Griffith, an American, orchestrated

the publication of the first American edition (1845). He carefully delineated his own revisions and additions; his contribution was primarily to underscore those sections that addressed the necessity for those nursing the sick to support the interventions of the physician.

5. J. W. Comfort, *Thomsonian Practice of Midwifery, and the Treatment of Complaints Peculiar to Women and Children* (Philadelphia: Aaron Comfort, 1845), 84. Comfort also published *The Practice of Medicine on Thomsonian Principles, Adapted as well to the Use of Families as to that of Practitioners* (Philadelphia: Lindsay and Blakiston, 1850). While this paper emphasizes strands of similar attitudes between Thomsonian and allopathic practitioners with regard to nurses and midwives, it is also important to note that important differences existed. In general, Thomsonian practitioners gave families more information about diseases, differential diagnoses, and treatments than their allopathic contemporaries.

6. See, for example: Comfort, *Thomsonian Practice of Midwifery*; and Joseph Warrington, *The Nurses Guide* (Philadelphia: Thomas Cowperthwait, 1839), 23–24.

7. Comfort, *Thomsonian Practice of Midwifery*, 63–64.

8. Descriptions of midwives' practices are in Comfort, *Thomsonian Practice of Midwifery*, and Warrington. For an overview of midwifery practices, particularly later in the nineteenth century, see Judy Barrett Litoff, *American Midwives: 1860 to the Present* (Westport, Conn.: Greenwood Press, 1978).

9. Rosenberg, "Therapeutic Revolution."

10. Comfort, *Thomsonian Practice of Midwifery*, 83. Warrington, 62.

11. Warrington, 14, 27.

12. Thomson, 335. Comfort, *Thomsonian Practice of Midwifery*, 83.

13. Warrington, iv. For an analysis of the influence of Warrington and his nurses school on the development of nursing in Philadelphia, see Patricia O'Brien's, "All a Woman's Life Can Bring: The Domestic Roots of Nursing in Philadelphia," *Nursing Research* 36 (January/February 1987): 12–17.

14. Thomson, 335. Despite the similarity in names, Thomson, it should be noted, was an allopathic, not a Thomsonian practitioner.

15. Thomson, 42, 57, 110. Because this paper locates the patient's bedside in the home, nuns are not included in the summary of who nursed. For an excellent description of the backgrounds and work imperatives of the "born" or "professed" nurses, as well as one of the best analyses of the development of nursing, see Reverby.

16. Harriet Martineau, *Life in the Sick Room: Essays by an Invalid* (London: Edward Moxon, 1845), 34–35.

17. Reverby.

18. Thomson, 335–36.

19. Robert Wallace Johnson, *Friendly Cautions to the Heads of Families and Others Very Necessary to be Observed in Order to Preserve Health, and Long Life* (Philadelphia: James Humphreys, 1804), 137–38, 141. This was the first American edition of a book originally published in England. The American editor added careful footnotes calling attention to those sections that described specific instructions to those supervising nurses of the sick.

20. Compare, for example, Johnson's straightforward commands (1804) with Thomson's (1845) more careful etiquette and rules (108, 335–38).

21. See Stephanie Coontz's *The Social Origins of Private Life: A History of American Families, 1600–1900* (London and New York: Verso Press, 1988); Mary Ryan's *Cradle of the Middle Class: The Family in Oneida County, New York, 1790–1865* (New York: Cambridge University Press, 1981); Gerda Lerner's "The Lady and the Mill Girl: Changes in the Status of Women in the Age of Jackson, 1800–1840," in *A Heritage of Her Own: Toward a New Social History of American Women*, ed. Nancy F. Cott and Elizabeth H. Pleck (New York: Simon and Schuster, 1979), 182–96; and Kathryn Kish Sklar's *Catherine Beecher: A Study in American Domesticity* (New York: W. W. Norton and Co., 1973).

22. For an analysis of women's roles in nineteenth-century health reform, see Regina Morantz's "Making Women Modern," *Journal of Social History* 10 (1977). For one description of the use of domestic medicine manuals, see Ronald L. Numbers, "Do-It-Yourself the Sectarian Way," in *Sickness and Health in America: Readings in the History of Medicine and Public Health*, ed. J. Leavitt and R. Numbers (Madison: University of Wisconsin Press, 1978).

23. Reverby, chap. 1.

24. For a specific reference to patients as "children," see Ann Preston's *Nursing the Sick and the Training of Nurses* (Philadelphia: King and Baird, 1863). For "vulnerability," see Thomson, 105.

25. Ibid., 104.

26. Ibid., 102.

27. Ibid., 103.

28. Ibid., 100.

29. Minutes of the Board of Managers, Woman's Hospital of Philadelphia, March 1861, Women in Medicine Archives, Medical College of Pennsylvania, Philadelphia, Pennsylvania (hereafter cited as WMA, MCP). A straightforward history of Ann Preston and the Woman's Hospital can be found in Guliema Fill Alsop's *A History of the Woman's Medical College, 1850–1950* (Philadelphia: J. B. Lippincott, 1950).

30. Patricia O'Brien, "Nursing the Sick and the Training of Nurses at the Woman's Hospital of Philadelphia," *Collections: The Newsletter of the Archives and Special Collections on Women in Medicine* (1986), 1–2. Virginia Drachman's *Hospital with a Heart: Women Doctors and the Paradox of Separatism at the New England Hospital for Women and Children, 1867–1969* (Ithaca, N.Y.: Cornell University Press, 1984) also suggests that women physicians and nurses in Boston maintained the same hierarchical configuration at the hospital bedside at the expense of an alternative reordering on the basis of gender.

31. Preston, 3, 15. O'Brien, "Nursing the Sick." The few graduates of the Woman's Hospital Training School, however, were influential in the introduction of hospital training schools in the later nineteenth century. Amanda Judson (1871) became the head nurse on the newly formed training ward at Bellevue Hospital in New York. Emily Bayard (1872) became the first superintendent of nurses at the Connecticut Hospital Training School for Nurses in New Haven.

32. Minutes of the Board of Managers, 18 January 1865, WMA, MCP.

33. Minutes of the Board of Managers, September 1864, WMA, MCP.

34. O'Brien, "All a Woman's Life can Bring."

35. Julie Fairman, "Voluntarism, Upper Class Women and Nursing: The

Nurses Training School at the Hospital of the University of Pennsylvania, 1874–1886" (Paper presented at the Third Annual Meeting of the American Association for the History of Nursing, September 1986). I am grateful for Fairman's help in drawing this connection.

36. For the opinions of two prominent nursing leaders on this hierarchical "quid pro quo," see Isabel Hampton, "Educational Standards for Nurses," and Lavinia Dock, "The Relation of Training Schools to Hospitals," *Nursing of the Sick, 1893* (reprint, New York: McGraw-Hill Book Co., 1949), 1–24. See also Janet James's "Isabel Hampton and the Professionalization of Nursing," in *The Therapeutic Revolution*, 201–44.

37. Barbara Melosh's *"The Physician's Hand": Work, Culture and Conflict in American Nursing* (Philadelphia: Temple University Press, 1982), and Susan Armeny's "Resolute Enthusiasts: The Effort to Professionalize American Nursing, 1880–1915" (PhD Dissertation, University of Missouri-Columbia, 1983).

BOOK REVIEWS

Bargaining for Life: A Social History of Tuberculosis, 1876–1938

By Barbara Bates
(Philadelphia: University of Pennsylvania Press, 1992)

When I first read Barbara Bates's social history of tuberculosis, it was in draft form and bore the title "Searching After Blackberries"—a reference to a line in the poem "John Brown's Body" by Stephen Vincent Benét and, more broadly, to the search of tuberculosis sufferers for a cure. I knew then that the book would find a large audience but that the title would not survive; it would be judged by the marketing department as "too obscure." As much as I miss the subtleties enveloped in the working title, I think *Bargaining for Life* is better and more appropriate, summing up in a brief phrase both the essence of the book and, on a more profound level, the experience of disease.

In *Bargaining for Life* Bates presents two narratives. One is of the life of Dr. Lawrence Flick—himself a sufferer of tuberculosis—who specialized in the treatment of the disease and, more importantly, crusaded on behalf of its sufferers. Flick helped inaugurate Pennsylvania's first sanatorium, pushed for the creation of Rush Hospital for Consumption and Allied Diseases, organized the Phipps Institute for the Study, Prevention and Treatment of Tuberculosis, and played an instrumental role in founding the Pennsylvania Society for the Prevention of Tuberculosis, the first voluntary organization dedicated to the eradication of a disease. Bringing together the disciplines of medicine, public health, and nursing, Flick attacked tuberculosis at every level—fighting for expanded state appropriations to public sanatoriums, promoting various cures and treatments, and overseeing the treatment of patients of all social classes.

While the account of Flick's myriad activities provides a cohesive structure for the book, Flick himself is not the focus of the work. Rather, it is the disease and its sufferers that form the core of *Bargaining for Life*. Using the letters sent to Flick by his patients, Bates documents the experiences of individual tuberculosis sufferers as they searched for health. In an exquisitely detailed chapter entitled "The Final Years of George E. Macklin," Bates recounts the slow death of a Pittsburgh businessman whose decline was recorded in a series of letters written at the turn of the century. Macklin traveled from sanatorium to sanatorium, accompanied by family and caretakers, seeking a cure that proved elusive. At one point Macklin wrote to Flick, "I think I understand my condition. I will never be a strong man again." Throughout his illness, Macklin tried to make bargains. Writing from one sanatorium, for example, he reported that if he had to "stay here for two or three months," he wanted some good poker players around. Later, he attempted to make another deal, stating that he had "made up [his] mind to give up business." Eventually, the letters from Macklin stopped and the reports to Flick were written by his physicians and family. George Macklin's life, like that of so many tuberculosis victims, ebbed away, punctuated by periods of relative comfort but proceeding largely on a downward course in which the symptoms grew increasingly severe and the treatments remained both painful and useless.

Not all of Flick's patients were as unfortunate as George Macklin. Elwell Stockdale recovered sufficiently to become superintendent of the White Haven Sanatorium and eventually opened Pennsylvania's first private sanatorium nearby. Following Stockdale into the sanatorium business were a number of women, some of whom had once been patients and who, later, after they recovered sufficiently, became tuberculosis nurses. Under Flick's leadership, both the Phipps Institute and the White Haven Sanatorium opened training schools for nurses. Many of the candidates did not graduate because their health problems recurred, but those who did found work that others often shunned—caring for tubercular patients.

Most of those afflicted with tuberculosis could not afford to travel from one sanatorium to another, as George Macklin did, nor did they enjoy, if that is the proper word, the constant ministrations of physicians. Tuberculosis was a disease of the poor, many of whom lived at home, working as long as they could, and in the process infecting the members of their families. The poor feared entering consumption wards in hospitals, in part because they knew that after their deaths their bodies would be autopsied. Their reluctance also stemmed from a desire to maintain their families economically. Although the architects of American social welfare policy were obsessively concerned that aid to the poor would pauperize them—leading them and their families to lifetimes on the public dole—in fact, the poor proved extraordinarily reluctant to avail themselves of medical aid, precisely because they feared impoverishing their families. For many poor consumptives, the visiting nurse was the only practitioner they saw. In Bates's words, these women marched "Into the Homes, Minds, and Lives of the Poor," providing them with supportive services and, when necessary, encouraging them to seek help in institutions.

Bates illuminates the present by reflecting on the past and also gives meaning to the past on its own terms. She makes clear the particular configurations of social welfare, medical science, and human need in the late nineteenth and early twentieth centuries that shaped the responses to tuberculosis. At the same time, without drawing explicit comparisons, she tempts readers to consider the parallels between tuberculosis and AIDS. There are many; fear and stigmatization of the sick, then and now, is the most obvious parallel. Another is the ways in which individuals are persuaded to risk their lives to treat the afflicted. For some the lure is a life on the cutting edge of scientific research; for others it is the simple opportunity to do good; and, for a few, both are true. In sum, disease is about bargains. And while the particulars of any illness must be understood in historical context, its transcendent features must also be explored. Bates has offered us the opportunity to do so, and her book, I am certain, will find a broad and appreciative audience.

Janet Golden, PhD
Visiting Scholar
History and Sociology of Science
University of Pennsylvania
Philadelphia, Pa.

The Diary of Emily Jane Green Hollister: Her Nursing Experiences, 1888–1911

Ed. by Deborah D. Smith
(Ann Arbor: University of Michigan Historical Center for the Sciences, 1991)

Emily Jane Hollister (1839–1918) was an untrained nurse in Michigan from 1888 to 1911. In November 1887, "after being visited by sickness, death and misfortune, she was compelled to leave her dear family and go out into the world to seek employment." She sporadically recorded her experiences in notes that were copied in 1913 and given to her son in 1918. In 1955, the son, Richard D. T. Hollister, edited the diary and donated it to the Michigan Historical Society. Deborah D. Smith found the original manuscript and the edited copy in the Bentley Historical Library.

The book actually consists of three parts: a 31-page introduction by

Smith, a 3-page introduction by Richard Hollister, and 139 diary accounts of Hollister's nursing experiences. In her introduction, Smith describes Ann Arbor and the state of nursing during the time Hollister was making her notes. She also gives background information on the Hollister family. Richard Hollister describes the family and what he knew of his mother's need to go to work outside the home. An index and 81 references or explanatory footnotes accompany the introduction and diary entries.

In her recorded notes, Emily Hollister describes her cases with regard to illness, treatment, and outcome. She expresses approval of physician orders and makes comments about the families, their homes, and the care provided. Many of her cases were infant deliveries involving family care for two weeks after the birth. The rest of the cases concerned diseases common to the era. What is amazing is that very few of Hollister's patients died despite the acute nature of the problems she describes.

Smith has been careful to leave the diary accounts in the words of Emily Hollister. She uses the original manuscript rather than the son's edited version in order to provide a more realistic picture of the writing and words used by Hollister in her nursing. As a result, this book gives a firsthand account of private duty nursing at the turn of the century. While it contains biographical information on the Hollister family, in general Hollister's account fits within the realm of literature that describes illness and nursing care at the turn of the century. The incomplete nature of the diary entries makes the book less useful for case study research.

This book will be of interest to all nurses who enjoy reading about nursing care at the turn of the century and to those who like to compare past and present activities. In addition, the personal nature of the entries will make this diary engaging to those who like biography.

Laurie K. Glass, PhD, RN, FAAN
Associate Professor and Director, Historical Gallery
School of Nursing
University of Wisconsin-Milwaukee
Milwaukee, Wi.

Pictures of Health: A Photographic History of Health Care in Philadelphia, 1860–1945

By Janet Golden and Charles E. Rosenberg
(Philadelphia: University of Pennsylvania Press, 1991)

The history of photography, paralleling the development of modern medicine, reflects man's quest for knowledge through applied science and technology. Photography—the word comes from the Greek and means "writing with light"—first appeared in 1839 in the writings of the German astronomer, Von Madler. The quest to capture permanent images on a surface by means other than those of manual drawing required a technical wedding of the camera obscura ("dark chamber") and its glass lens, with an understanding of the principles of light and chemistry. By experimenting with multiple chemical reactions and a variety of surfaces, including metal, canvas, glass, and paper, early photographers learned to make their images permanent and reproducible.

As the success of these first photographers became better known in the 1850s, artists, particularly European painters, began to experiment with photography. The power of the camera to reduce the world to human scale through a single immobilized eye both fascinated artists and provided them with a new art medium. Soon portrait artists opened studios offering famous as well as ordinary citizens an opportunity to possess a permanent image of themselves that just a generation ago only the wealthy could afford. The camera's ability to mirror reality and capture, in a portrait, the minute details of a subject was extolled. It was claimed that the clarity of the image, unencumbered by a painter's vision and skill, added to the truth and reality of photo portraiture.

The growing popularity of photographs encouraged a small group of photographers, still using bulky equipment, to move outdoors and experiment with the recording of political events, wars, and nature. However, it was an American, George Eastman, who in 1888 launched the industrialization of photography and put the camera into the hands of the general public. Eastman, a print manufacturer in Rochester, New York, invented the Kodak hand camera and sold it to the public with the slogan "You press the button, we do the rest." This invention made it possible for ordinary men to photograph the people and the world that surrounded them. The Kodak camera, notes historian Jean-Luc Daval (1982), not only became a commercial success but it profoundly modified and added a new dimension to the use and power of photography. Placed in the hands of ordinary people, cameras would document, record, and preserve the world; in this way, photographs became an extension of man's memory—a historical memory bank.

Pictures of Health: A Photographic History of Health Care in Philadelphia, 1860–1945, by Janet Golden and Charles Rosenberg, is a marvelous example of the richness of this memory bank. Golden and Rosenberg, prominent medical historians, have assembled 170 photographs to create a photo essay on the development of almost a century of health care in Philadelphia.

Rosenberg opens the book with a succinct discussion of the profound changes experienced by urban society and medicine in the era, and of how the camera was used to represent officially the world of Philadelphia medicine. It is a view, or collective image, that depicts medicine's technological and social success over disease and illness.

The scope of this documentary, although neglecting the private office practice of medicine, does encompass hospital-based services and care provided in dispensaries, by visiting nurse associations, in pharmacies, and through municipal health programs. To trace the development of health care over time, the book is divided into three chapters: (1) "Training for the New Professions," (2) "Hospitals: The Delivery of Medical Care," and (3) "Health in the Community."

The first chapter focuses primarily on both the academic education of physicians and the on-the-job training of nurses. The photographs document the physical settings in which education took place, showing medical students in lecture halls and laboratories as well as in operating rooms, hospital wards, and clinics. Student nurses are seen at the patient bedside, on the peripheral edges of surgical teams, in supply rooms, and in the classroom. To acknowledge the important role medications will play in the treatment of illness, there is also a photograph of young men studying to become the pharmacists who will dispense the drugs in the hospitals and community.

The photographs transmit the students' interest—and sometimes, as depicted by women medical students observing surgery (p. 21), their almost palpable intensity and eagerness—in learning their craft. A few glimpses of the students' social lives serve, thankfully, to remind historians that these were youths possessing exuberance and humor. Inclusion of photos of students attending parties or at play lessens the tendency to view them as single-dimensional people and encourages historians to remember that students of the past possess the same human passions of contemporary students.

Golden's introduction to the second chapter describes the proliferation of hospitals in the late nineteenth and early twentieth century that accompanied Philadelphia's growth in wealth and population. The chapter's 75 photos trace the creation of the modern hospital and the medical system that served the diverse needs of patients. The photos reveal how, slowly, the large patient wards were replaced by smaller units and private rooms. Technology, in its stainless steel casings, is portrayed as, for example, scanning the patients, bathing them in light therapy, and helping them to breathe. Finally, the authors document through photos the auxiliary support services necessary to sustain a medical center, including pathology and microbiology labs, patient record rooms, the pharmacy, large kitchens, and laundry rooms.

The final chapter—"Health in the Community"—reviews a wide range of public and voluntary activities that helped protect the health of Philadelphians. Among these activities were the building of sewers, a campaign to destroy rodents, and the provision of maternal and child care in clinics, homes, and schools. Although the public health activities comprise the largest portion of this chapter, industrial health efforts during World War II are also illustrated.

This is a book that can be read and enjoyed on several levels. For those who enjoy viewing photographs of a past era, this is an attractive book. The enlarged photographs provide a richness of detail and clarity not available in similar books, such as Rima Apple's *Illustrated Catalogue of the Slide Archive of Historical Medical Photographs at Stony Brook* (1984).

Pictures of Health will also appeal to historians of nursing and medicine because it combines historical scholarship with a diverse collection of photographs that capture important dimensions of the past. Indeed, this book may encourage historians to reexamine their strong reliance on the written word to interpret the past. As Rosenberg notes, current historians have failed to use visual artifacts, so abundant during the last one hundred years, to study "the cultural assumptions and conscious institutional needs" crucial to the history of the development of the health care system (p. XXV).

The book's collection of photographs will also appeal to the growing numbers of historians who incorporate slides or photographs in their presentations and publications. Stimulation of the visual sense in an audience that has grown accustomed to television and movies to portray reality, they believe, enhances the power of the spoken or written word.

The book successfully illustrates the camera's power to capture on film a slice of reality at a particular point of time. But the images encapsulated in the photographs are more than impartial mirrors of reality. Photographs, as photographers and historians know, are not accidental images but represent a series of choices that shape their captured reality, including the selection of subjects, composition, and means of expression. Photographs, as noted by Oliver Wendell Holmes, are "mirrors with memories" that must be carefully examined to reveal the many dimensions of truth (Davidson and Lytle, 1982). Golden and Rosenberg's insightful historical analysis offers the reader the opportunity to enjoy visually the photographs and to learn how their historical memory bank can be decoded to enhance our understanding of the past.

BARBARA BRODIE, PhD, RN
Professor
School of Nursing
University of Virginia
Charlottesville, Va.

References

Apple, R. *Illustrated Catalogue of the Slide Archive of Historical Medical Photographs at Stony Brook* (Westport, Conn.: Greenwood Press, 1984).
Duval, J. L. *Photography: History of an Art* (New York: Rizzoli International Publication, Inc., 1982), 103.
Davidson, J. and M. Lytle. *After the Fact: The Art of Historical Detection* (New York: Alfred A. Knopp, 1982), 205–29.

As Miss Nightingale Said . . .

Ed. by Monica Baly
(London: Scutari Press, 1991)

Monica Baly's 1986 study, *Florence Nightingale and the Nursing Legacy*, helped to revise radically our picture of Florence Nightingale and of the so-called Nightingale movement in nursing. In *As Miss Nightingale Said . . .*, Baly continues to use primary source material—chiefly personal correspondence—to bring to light Nightingale's life and its historical context and significance.

Prior to Baly's efforts at the British Library and the Greater London Record Office and her examination of the collections of papers at Wilton House, Claydon House, and the Wellcome Institute, most of what was written about Florence Nightingale and nursing relied on the work of Nightingale's official biographer, Sir Edward Cook. Cook's account was essentially a eulogy, written soon after Nightingale's death, in which her failures were swept under the rug and the rough places made smooth.

Personal and legal considerations existed at the time for not exposing conflicts in Nightingale's life; some of the people involved directly or as heirs were still alive and reputations needed to be preserved. Any discussion, for example, that dealt with real differences between Nightingale and the way the St. Thomas Hospital Nursing School operated would have opened up old wounds that Cook wanted to heal. Moreover, the nursing profession, facing competition, needed and wanted a legendary founding figure. Because Cook did his work well and his biography seemed so monumental, few challenged its overall account although many did not agree with his portrayal of Nightingale. Historian Cecil Woodham-Smith modified Cook's portrait of Nightingale considerably nearly forty years later, but she more or less accepted what Cook had to say about St. Thomas Hospital School of Nursing, thereby perpetrating the Nightingale myth and its relation to modern nursing.

The picture that emerged from these early works was that the Nightingale School at St. Thomas Hospital was an independent entity, that Wardroper was an ideal director personally chosen by Nightingale, and that the probationers were carefully chosen, neat, ladylike, above moral suspicion, and trained to train other nurses; none of these conclusions, however, was true. Perhaps if this myth had been challenged early, the course of nursing in America would have been different. Although Nightingale conceived of nurses as more or less independent practitioners, not under the sway of a physician, her ideal was probably approached best in the public health nurse and in the nurse midwife, images far removed from the actual type of nurse trained at St. Thomas. Baly and others have argued that developments in medicine, such as anesthesia and aseptic techniques, as well as the growth of medical specialization, changed the nature of the hospital after the Nightingale School was founded and led to quite a different kind of nursing than Nightingale had envisioned. Even in England, nursing schools served primarily as a way to get inexpensive help for the growing hospitals. Nightingale recognized this but was in no position to change it, although she certainly spoke out against it in her letters.

In discussing Nightingale, Baly wisely places her in the context of her time, looking at changes and developments both in society and in Nightingale's personal life. Baly emphasizes that Nightingale, for example, like most women of her generation, spoke with a great deal of hyperbole, using such terms as "Goddess Baby" or "adored chief," and was careful not to denigrate individuals publicly. In private, however, particularly in personal letters, Nightingale and most of her contemporaries were much more critical and outspoken. Since her letters and other correspondences are voluminous, it is possible to get a Nightingale opinion on almost anything, although her opinions often changed over time.

Nightingale's letters portray Wardroper as a woman in a job she could not fulfill, who was often drunk and who insisted on unnecessary discipline for the probationers. However, because Nightingale saw no alternative, she tolerated Wardroper's behavior and even publicly supported her efforts. Further, Nightingale complained that probationers received negligent and often grossly careless training under unsanitary conditions, but she found it difficult to change these circumstances. Similarly, although Nightingale felt that physicians knew too little about patient care to have control of nursing, she came to realize that the changing hospital situation made physician domination of the nursing profession something she had to accept.

Though in her early years Nightingale was a radical supporter of women's property rights, she later became much more conservative, upset at women who would not follow her example and give up all for the sake of work. She felt that women's efforts to move into male occupations such as medicine only made for "third-rate men" and that women could do more by developing their own nursing role. She believed nurses could achieve this role more effectively as midwives or in public health than in the hospitals. She complained that the more militant suffragettes were vociferous women talking about things of which ordinary women knew nothing at all.

Nonetheless, in spite of her aristocratic manner, Nightingale remained committed to the ordinary people, demanding better care for them in ways that Americans until recently would have labeled socialist. She felt there was nothing wrong with the poor that a good job and a little money would not cure. She was opposed to religious nursing since she felt the job of the nurse was not to care for the souls of the people but their physical ailments. For example, she never wanted Agnes Jones to work at St. Thomas because she feared that Jones's religious zeal would upset the hospital. She later complained about "Agnes and her miracles" and claimed they were the result of visions caused by a lack of sleep and Jones's physical deterioration. However, when Jones died, Nightingale was perfectly willing to accept her as a martyr to nursing and to use her reputation to recruit others.

Nightingale was a woman of many moods, and sometimes they seemed to fluctuate radically. In spite of the many complaints about her family that appear in her letters, for example, she was strongly family oriented, doting on her mother, father, and sister, and on the children of her relatives.

Baly effectively examines these contradictions between the public and private Nightingale in this brief book, focusing on such topics as a Victorian family, the call (to nursing), wars and armies, social policy, hospitals and hospital administration, women, the nature of nursing, nursing education, and nursing management. The book is intended for a general audience, although sources are provided for further research. I would highly recommend it as a brief introduction to the complexities of Nightingale's life and of early nursing. I would hope the book might even find its way into undergraduate issues courses or, where they exist, into nursing history courses, introducing students to a more realistic view of our roots.

VERN L. BULLOUGH, PhD, RN
SUNY Distinguished Professor
of History and Social Studies
SUNY College of Buffalo
Buffalo, N.Y.

References

Baly, Monica. *Florence Nightingale and the Nursing Legacy* (London: Croom Helm/ Routledge, 1986).
Cook, Sir Edward. *The Life of Florence Nightingale*, 2 vols. (London: Macmillan, 1913).
Woodham-Smith, Cecil. *Florence Nightingale* (London: Constable, 1950).

Women at War: The Story of Fifty Military Nurses Who Served in Vietnam

By Elizabeth Norman
(Philadelphia: University of Pennsylvania Press, 1991)

The care of patients within the context of war fascinates nurses. As Elizabeth Norman observes, there is a timelessness to nurses' recollections of wars (p. 27). Whether grappling with the grisly wounds of the American Civil War soldiers, the trenches of World War I, the chaos of the Bataan death march, or the moral dilemmas of Vietnam, combat nursing embodies, in the words of Charles Dickens, "the best of times and the worst of times." War magnifies what military nurses do for a living, and their daily exposure to both the purposeful killing and the desperate saving of human life effectively illuminates the potential of the human spirit and the grim reality of the human condition.

In other wars, combat nurses have been portrayed as romantic martyrs or ministering white angels; however, Norman's graceful analysis of fifty military (Army, Navy, and Air Force) nurses carefully examines the paradoxes of the context and the culture of Vietnam War nursing. With clarity, Norman contrasts the power that nurses held over patients' lives with their helplessness to stop the dying; their humor with the horror of the war; and the nurses' fear of chaos versus their relief in learning that the nursing ideals of perfection have no place in war (p. 159).

The women of this study, part of Norman's dissertation, served in Vietnam from 1965 to 1973, working in over thirty hospitals, ships, and airfields in South Vietnam. This is a narrative about very young nurses, with a mean age of twenty-two; only nine nurses had more than five years of clinical nursing experience. Norman tersely reminds the reader that the study's sample was difficult to locate, for at the onset of the study in 1982, estimates of the number of military nurses who served in Vietnam ranged from 4,000 to 15,000, but "no one knew for sure" (p. 4). As a researcher at the Walter Reed Army Hospital stated, "we never thought that a record of nurses' statistics would be important to keep" (p. 3). This chilling comment reflects Norman's sensitivity to the invisibility of women in wars. While American society has traditionally identified war as a crucible and a right of passage reserved for men, Norman observes that "so too is it for women" (p. 155).

As the title of the book suggests, this is a well-crafted story of war nurses, but it is also a well-researched collective case study that is organized topically to describe the nurses' assignment and arrival in Vietnam, their experiences as women and professionals, their painful homecoming, and their process of coming to terms with the overwhelming sorrow that aged their spirits and impacted on their careers. Just as the public responded with empathy to earlier published autobiographical accounts of Vietnam nurses, the readers of this book may experience a moment of satisfaction and pride in the young nurses' struggles to comfort both patients and fellow nurses in the midst of carnage. For these Vietnam nurses, compassion was not simply a professional cliché, but, as historian Susan Reverby (1989) has suggested, "an obligation to care."

Nonetheless, this book is not a romantic portrayal of nurses that creates its own mythology of altruism. This book is neither sentimental nor sanitized. Norman dares to humanize the nurse, arguing that war is a masculine experience in which men protect women and in which women, in turn, comfort men (p. 67). These traditional roles in Vietnam led to both sexual harassment and sexual liaisons. In war, according to Norman, human bonding is born of isolation and fear, effectively linking passion, youth, trust, and love (p. 71). The Vietnam nurses neither apologized for, nor labeled their personal liaisons with men in Vietnam as promiscuity. In attempting to understand these nurses rather than judge them, Norman eloquently captures the transient and artificial context of war, which redefines the boundaries of acceptable behavior and shapes women's experiences.

The last five chapters of this book, which deal with the events surrounding the nurses' departure from Vietnam and their individual experiences with the aftermath of war, are a major contribution to understanding the social history of Vietnam nurses. Norman goes beyond storytelling to become a hermeneuticist, imposing structure and meaning on a conglomeration of images described by the nurses. To learn something of how nurses create order from chaos gives us information regarding nursing ideology, nurses' ways of establishing autonomy and control, and nurses' construction of reality. Norman identifies some differences between nurses who have served in war and those who have not. She characterizes the combat nurse as possessing a sense of self-reliance that is skeptical of traditional authority, a lack of fear of the future, and a quirky sense of humor. These observations raise questions about emergency-room nurses who also deal with and even thrive on trauma. Is their culture and perspective, like those of war nurses, distinctively different from others?

My only serious reservation about this book concerns Norman's argument that the cultural norms of nursing, which she labels "professional ethos" (p. 165), originate in nursing students' reading of L. Dock and I. Stewart's *A Short History of Nursing* (1932). While students most assuredly experience a rigorous socialization process in nursing schools, the incorporation of values, beliefs, and behaviors is complex and cannot be reduced to a student's exposure to nursing history.

This book is well worth the attention of a wide audience. Its understated drama, insights, and straightforwardness will enlighten nurse clinicians, teachers, and researchers, as well as historians of nursing, of the military, of women's concerns, and of society in general. In addition, this book will be appreciated by the Vietnam nurses who have yet to explore the meaning of their experience, as well as by the colleagues of the eight women whose names are engraved on the Vietnam War Memorial. Norman's thoughtful narrative will no doubt leave an imprint on readers, and the deeply significant subject matter will leave none of our lives untouched.

DIANE HAMILTON, PhD, RN
Associate Professor of Nursing
School of Nursing
University of Rochester
Rochester, N.Y.

References

Dock, L. and I. Stewart. *A Short History of Nursing: From the Earliest Times to the Present Day* (New York: Putnam, 1932).

Reverby, Susan. *Ordered to Care: The Dilemma of American Nursing* (New York: Cambridge University Press, 1987).

The Origins and Rise of Associate Degree Nursing Education

By Patricia T. Haase
(Durham: Duke University Press in Cooperation with the National League for Nursing, 1990)

Associate Degree Nursing Education: An Historical Annotated Bibliography, 1942–1983

By Patricia T. Haase
(Durham: Duke University Press in Cooperation with the National League for Nursing, 1990)

Patricia T. Haase's *The Origins and Rise of Associate Degree Nursing Education* and its companion volume, *Associate Degree Nursing Education: An Historical Annotated Bibliography, 1942–1983*, fill a void in nursing historiography. Both volumes reached print through a cooperative effort of the National League for Nursing and the W. K. Kellogg Foundation, the latter funding a Dissemination Project aimed in part at recounting the foundation's considerable support of Associate Degree (AD) nursing education since World War II.

Sponsored as a way to temper "widespread ignorance" about AD nursing's beginnings and goals, Haase's project responds to the confusion created by the chimera of two-, three-, and four-year education programs, all fixed on Registered Nurse (RN) licensure, and to the failure of RN employers to differentiate graduates of these three kinds of schooling. The study also grew out of the foundation's distress that one issue—entry into practice—has long divided nurses.

Origins and Rise canvasses a generation of American nursing education history. Haase locates the roots of AD nursing in the Nursing Council on National Defense, the Cadet Nurse Corps, and the advent of nurse aides. Post–World War II changes, including advances in medicine, the Hill-Burton Act, a persistent shortage of nurses, the dramatic growth of community colleges, and eventual federal investment in nursing education helped facilitate the emergence of AD nursing education.

As early as 1945, the American Association of Junior Colleges (AAJC), already exploring ways to bring nursing education into community colleges, met with the U.S. Office of Education to discuss postwar community college configuration. The National League of Nursing Education (NLNE), not invited to that meeting, created its own committee in 1946 to consider the implications of community college-based nursing education; two years later Esther Lucile Brown's pivotal report, *Nursing for the Future* (1948), contributed to the unfolding plan.

In the late 1940s and early 1950s, other issues and conditions contributed to the origins of AD nursing: educational initiatives at Teachers College, Columbia University; predictions that the nursing shortage would become severe unless two kinds of nurse workers, professional and technical, were developed; formation of a joint NLNE-AAJC committee; Kellogg Foundation interest in nursing; and Mildred Montag's doctoral dissertation proposing that two-year programs in junior colleges could produce "nursing technicians." Concern about these and other issues led to the formation of the Cooperative Research Project in Junior and Community College Education for Nursing (CRP), directed by Mildred Montag.

Haase details CRP purposes (to define a new type of "technical" nurse and to design an educational program for that nurse) and CRP assumptions, the most important being that nursing work could be gauged along a continuum of simple to complicated functions. Other assumptions were that the nursing shortage could be solved by preparing a new kind of nurse to function around the continuum's midpoint; that community colleges were the most likely places to educate such intermediate or technical workers; and that workers performing nursing tasks at the continuum's simple level were best prepared on-the-job.

Haase describes the seven pilot project community colleges chosen between 1952 and 1955 to demonstrate CRP goals. Early AD nursing programs, seen by Haase as "broad-based . . . radical departures from the traditional nursing curriculum," turned to such innovations as giving pre- and postclinical conferences; assigning more than one student to the same patient; providing programmed instruction; installing campus learning laboratories; and critically evaluating students. Based on Montag's report of CRP success, the Kellogg Foundation agreed to support state-level AD nursing education projects in California, Texas, New York, and Florida. Efforts to improve faculty preparation dominated Kellogg Foundation interest in these years. By the 1960s, the AD nursing education model was successfully established and myriad new programs mushroomed like fast-food franchises.

Nursing leaders assumed that AD nursing programs were terminal and that their graduates were to be viewed as "technical" or "semiprofessional" nurses. Haase devotes a finely developed chapter to examining the proposition that AD graduates were "technical" nurses. She also examines how the American Nurses' Association's (ANA) paper "First Position on Education for Nursing" (1965) and the NLN's more conservative Resolution #5 (1965) influenced the profession's view of AD graduates. Haase's etymology of "technical" deserves wider circulation than it will, regrettably, receive in a history book; misunderstandings over what nursing leaders have meant by "technical" have contributed considerably to a generation's anguish over the entry into practice dispute.

Haase concludes that the ADN movement was highly successful in moving nursing education into America's higher education system and that AD nursing education's crucial contribution to American health care was reducing the nursing shortage since the program's inception in the middle 1950s.

Beyond the research derived from Kellogg Foundation archives, historians of nursing will find little new in *Origins and Rise*. Early chapters benefit from Philip and Beatrice Kalisch's *The Federal Influence and Impact on Nursing* (1980) and Shirley Fondiller's *The Entry Dilemma* (1983). Haase, however, tells the AD education story without the burden of a dense analytical framework that might limit its accessibility only to historians.

Historians of nursing not genuinely excited by *Origins and Rise* will be delighted that Haase, through the Kellogg Foundation Dissemination Project, generated the companion volume, *Associate Degree Nursing Educa-*

tion: An Historical Annotated Bibliography, 1942–1988. Its scope is wide, extending to ANA, NLN, and Kellogg Foundation proceedings, to government documents (including U.S. House and Senate reports), anthologies, and dissertations, and to Educational Resources Information Center (ERIC) and National Technical Information Services (NTIS) references. The index (by title, author, and subject) is thorough and easy to use.

As with any bibliography, individual users might wish more comprehensiveness. For example, Teachers College, Columbia University, and R. Louise McManus figure prominently in Haase's history, but a 1988 dissertation about the McManus years at Teachers College is neither in the history nor in the bibliography. A 1980 dissertation on the history of AD nursing education in Iowa is not listed. Jerome Lysaught's *An Abstract for Action* (1973) is included; missing is the Christy, Poulin, and Hover critique of the Lysaught Report in the *American Journal of Nursing* (1973). The Beletz and Acord article, "Who Should Be the Future SNA Member?" (*Nursing Outlook*, 1987), is omitted. Perhaps a more serious omission is ANA's *Scope of Practice* (1987) distinguishing ADN and BSN competencies. Two authors indexed, "Fagen, C." and "Fagin, C. M.," are one and the same person. There are no references to historians Paul Starr, Rosemary Stevens, Susan Reverby, Darlene Clark Hine, or Barbara Melosh, who are generally viewed as offering useful analyses of nursing's historical context.

Although the two books are described as companion volumes, each agreeably stands alone. Nursing historians will be especially interested in the *Annotated Bibliography* as a tool to extend analytical studies of AD nursing education history but should also find *Origins and Rise* a worthwhile survey of that history. Associate degree nursing educators and their students will surely benefit from reading *Origins and Rise*. This book might also illuminate misconceptions of AD nursing held by baccalaureate faculty and nursing service administrators. Every college of nursing should catalog both books.

With these two volumes, Patricia Haase and the Kellogg Foundation help us understand a decisive period in American nursing education. The educational and organizational structures that emerged in the early 1950s have not substantially changed. Nor, unfortunately, has the consequent discord.

Wendell Oderkirk, PhD, RN
Professor
Bishop Clarkson College
Omaha, Nebr.

References

ANA. "First Position on Education for Nursing." *American Journal of Nursing* 65 (December 1965): 106–11.

Brown, Esther Lucile. *Nursing for the Future* (New York: Russell Sage Foundation, 1948).

Kalisch, Philip, and Beatrice Kalisch. *The Federal Influence and Impact on Nursing* (Hyattsville, Md.: U.S. Department of Health and Human Services, 1980).

A COMMENT

By Mildred L. Montag

Associate Degree Nursing (ADN) has received more attention in articles, speeches, and debates than any other nursing program in history. While the tenor of the current discussions may differ in content and even in intensity from earlier deliberation, the controversy continues. Patricia Haase's book *The Origins and Rise of Associate Degree Nursing Education* does what none has done before: it gives a clear, cogent history of the beginning and the rise of ADN programs. Good reading for those who have recently entered nursing or nursing education, the book is free of the jargon of both nursing and education and offers a positive, forward-looking treatment of associate degree nursing.

Some of what we now take for granted in nursing education did not exist in the 1950s. To make the changes that today seem so commonplace took vision, courage, and stamina on the part of the faculties of the early ADN programs.

The Cooperative Research Project's request to several state boards of nursing in 1952 for permission to design a new education system for a new kind of nurse attests to the vision and courage of early ADN advocates. After much soul-searching, the nursing boards granted their request; this decision not only allowed ADN faculties to design and implement the curriculum they deemed essential, but it had a lasting influence on all curricula as well. For example, it is now expected that boards of nursing will set only general education regulations for programs and will accept college transcripts from graduates as evidence of their ability to take the state licensing examinations. This freeing of regulations, perhaps more than any other feature, was the outcome of ADN faculties' efforts and benefited all nursing programs. It is a development now taken for granted, but to accomplish it involved the enactment of new legislation in some states and changes in regulations in others.

What were called innovations in the early associate degree programs are now standard practice. The faculties were ingenious in developing new instructional technologies and new ways of assigning patients for clinical instruction. For example, the idea of a pre- and postconference with each clinical assignment originated in the first ADN program. These and other innovations are clearly and accurately described in Haase's book; many of the developments described are now part of everyday practice in nursing programs. When students are simply students and not part of the nursing service, many improvements in teaching are possible. Students can then do what Mary Sue Infante (1975) stated so well: they learn to do, instead of doing in order to learn.

Some changes have come quickly, even more quickly than many nursing leaders expected. Debate continues over titles and licensing and over how to distinguish the graduates of the three current programs in order to use them more efficiently and economically.

Even today, not all nurses, nurse educators, or nursing service administrators accept the ADN program. Many still harbor the belief that all registered nurses should have a baccalaureate degree. Associate degree programs were born at a time when nurses were scarce, but they have endured because they fulfill a vital need. Has anyone considered what the nursing situation would be today were it not for the ADN programs and their graduates? Associate degree graduates now exceed those from baccalaureate and diploma programs combined and represent an increasing percentage of the nurses employed in hospitals.

Ginzberg, an economist, cautioned nearly forty years ago that nursing could not advance to professional status if it attempted to have all nurses working at the same level. He believed that patient care needs could be differentiated into two classes; those requiring professional judgments and those of a more elementary nature. He advocated the creation of a large corps of nurses with technical preparation to meet the elementary needs of patients. If this was needed then, how much more needed is it now.

Those who have deplored the growth of ADN programs and who have suggested limiting the number of their graduates probably still do not understand the role of the associate degree nurses in the health care system. Interestingly, the numbers currently projected as desirable from both baccalaureate and associate degree programs are still not based on any research. In addition, only now is there recognition in the profession that "differentiation of functions" is worthy of study. Perhaps the continuing notion that "a nurse is a nurse is a nurse" has contributed to our delay in recognizing the need for a clearer distinction between the baccalaureate and associate degree programs. Haase's clear explanation of what associate degree programs can produce should help the profession in this regard.

A note must be made about the role of the community college in developing and implementing the ADN program. From the beginning, community college administrators and the American Association of Junior Colleges (now the American Association of Community Junior Colleges) were interested and supportive. While it is true that junior colleges existed since the early 1900s, the community college, as we know it now, had its beginning in the early 1950s. It was fortunate that the ADN program fit so well and in such a timely way into the purposes of the community college.

Haase has stated that "the future of the AD program is bright." Current National League for Nursing (NLN) data support this statement. The programs now number 829 and more are contemplated. The growth of ADN programs from 2 in 1952 to over 800 in 1990 is impressive. The movement from hospital-based diploma programs to instruction in educational institutions has also been more rapid than many anticipated.

Haase concludes that "the future role of the ADN graduate is quite clear." While not everyone would agree with this statement, the ADN Council is clear in its articulation of objectives and outcomes as outlined in its statement on graduates' competencies. Might it not resolve some of the current confusion if the other nursing programs had such succinctly stated outcomes? One thing does seem certain: graduates of ADN programs are and will remain the most numerous. The profession's challenge, then, is to use these graduates effectively so that the nursing needs of patients can be met.

MILDRED L. MONTAG, EdD, RN, FAAN
46 Kilburn Rd.
Garden City, N.Y.

Reference

Infante, Mary Sue. *The Clinical Laboratory in Nursing Education* (New York: John Wiley, 1975).

Black Women in White: Racial Conflict and Cooperation in the Nursing Profession, 1890–1950

By Darlene Clark Hine
(Bloomington: Indiana University Press, 1989)

How have race and racism affected the nursing profession? What has it been like for famous and not-so-famous black women nurses struggling to find their place in the world of health care? Darlene Clark Hine's *Black Women in White* examines these and other issues in a compelling exploration of the experiences and history of African-American nurses.

Hine, who is the John A. Hannah Professor of History at Michigan State University, envisions this book as the first of several volumes exploring black health care professionals. She tells her story as any rigorous historian would, but with a sense of pride in being an African-American and a great joy in being able to give us this piece of our history. This groundbreaking study does a great service to historians of nursing and pays high tribute to black nurses.

The book does not follow a strictly chronological order. After a short introduction, major phases in the struggles of black nurses from the early 1800s into the 1950s are presented, with some time overlap among the chapters. The book surveys major historical events of our nation's history as they relate to nursing: slavery, the Civil War, the World Wars, legal registration of nurses, the upgrading of nurse education, and the creation of professional nursing organizations. The history Hine relates runs parallel to the one with which we are most familiar, but one which has largely been told from the perspective of white nursing.

Hine focuses on the efforts of African-American health care professionals, particularly black women nurses, to combat racism inside the medical establishment. She begins her account early in the history of the United States, with the arrival of black slaves in the New World. Hine relates how many black women slaves cared not only for the sick in their own slave communities but also for the white families who enslaved them.

Hine places this history, and other health care and professional issues particular to the black community and its would-be nurses, into the context of the Nightingale tradition and the development of white nursing. For example, because blacks were forbidden care in white hospitals and because blacks could not be educated in white schools, African-Americans were forced to develop their own hospitals and schools of nursing. Black self-help initiatives and white philanthropic largesse led to the establishment of about a dozen major black hospitals and nursing schools by the turn of the century.

We learn of the people involved in and the circumstances surrounding the rise, and in some cases the fall, of these hospitals. Hine describes the nursing personalities and the nature and quality of nursing education at southern schools such as Lincoln Hospital, Durham, N.C. (1901); Freedman's in Washington, D.C. (1894); Tuskegee Institute in Alabama (1892); Dixie Hospital and Training School at Hampton, Va. (1891); and the Phyllis Wheatley Sanitarium and Training School for Nurses in New Orleans (1896).

The phenomenon of separate races in nursing was not restricted to the South. Hine tells the stories of Provident Hospital School of Nursing in Chicago (1891); Frederick Douglas Memorial Hospital Training School (1895) and Mercy Hospital School of Nurses (1907), both in Philadelphia; and the nursing schools at Lincoln Hospital (1896) and Harlem Hospital (1923) in New York City. In addition, Hine briefly mentions hospitals that treated patients and educated nurses of both races separately at the same institution. Hine also takes time to examine the role that white philanthropic foundations played in developing and upgrading black hospitals and schools of nursing, in particular the activities of the General Education Board, the Rockefeller Foundation, and the Julius Rosenwald Fund.

Hine examines the quality of nursing education as well as the life of the black student nurse in the early twentieth century. Because black women at the time were thought by many to be immoral, student nurses were often subjected to strict disciplinary rules in order to protect the reputation of both themselves and the hospitals with which they were associated.

With black as with white, nursing education moved from diploma schools to collegiate institutions. Hine offers an example of this transition in her in-depth review of the creation of collegiate nursing education at Dillard University in New Orleans in 1935.

Professional affiliation was as important for black nurses as for white. We learn of the admittance of black nurses to the National Organization for Public Health Nursing in 1912 and of their rejection by the American Nurses' Association (ANA) in 1916. Black nurses responded to the closed door of the ANA by establishing the National Association of Colored Graduate Nurses (NACGN). When black nurses were admitted to the ANA in 1951, the NACGN dissolved. The two women so important to the life of the NACGN, Mable Keaton Staupers and Estelle Massey Riddle Osborne, are discussed in depth regarding their struggle for the integration of black nurses into the mainstream of American professional nursing.

Before the conclusion, we are treated to the experience of black nurses in the Cadet Nurses Corps and to the lives and careers of four black nurses who "exemplify the striving and measured achievement of black nursing."

The history of racism in the nursing profession is a long and complex one. Dr. Darlene Clark Hine's book, which won the American Association for the History of Nursing's 1990 Lavinia Dock Award, is a valuable addition to existing nursing history literature. This book should be found on the syllabi of all undergraduate and graduate courses in nursing history. *Black Women in White* is also an invitation to other historians of nursing to continue to explore the role of race and racism in the nursing profession.

Carla M. Schissel, PhD, RN
Nurse Practitioner
Northwest Grady Clinic
Atlanta, Ga.

Caring and Responsibility: The Crossroads Between Holistic Practice and Traditional Medicine

By June S. Lowenberg
(Philadelphia: University of Pennsylvania Press, 1989)

This award-winning book (*Choice* magazine, 1989–1990 Outstanding Books) reports the findings of an extensive ethnographic field study of the holistic health movement and its relationship to traditional allopathic medical practice. The book will hold the interest of scholars and students of nursing, medicine, medical sociology, public health, and anthropology, and that of other health care professionals regardless of their orientation to practice.

Although *Caring and Responsibility* presents little of the substantive history surrounding its themes, it is an important resource for historians of nursing and health care. Lowenberg's study touches on timeless and intriguing historical questions. Much has been written by historians, for example, of nursing's traditional, womanly, and caring commitment to minister to sick patients. Lowenberg does not challenge this caring stance. Rather, her work has the potential to expand this analysis as it subtly suggests that the professionalization of nursing in the early twentieth century may both have shaped and have been shaped by the shifting meanings of volition and personal responsibility for illness and its prevention.

Chapter 1 is an introduction to the study; it includes the assumptions on which the inquiry was based, its methodology and rationale for the field study approach, and a comprehensive description of the field setting. The methodology is continued in two appendixes that contain the interview guide for patients and providers, and respondent profiles. The book goes on to present a detailed discussion of the differences in the underlying beliefs and approaches of holistic and allopathic medicine (Chapter 2), as well as a credible recent history of the holistic health movement (Chapter 3). Lowenberg's presentation of the ideology, meanings, and values underlying holistic health contributes substantially to the reader's understanding of the views and practices of those who participate in this model of care. Moreover, Lowenberg sensitizes the reader to the power and the politics of the health care system, pointing out that a shift away from allopathic medicine and toward a holistic health model could result in more power for nursing.

Chapters 4, 5, and 6 focus on the role of the sick within the holistic health movement and on the shifts that have occurred in the practitioner-client relationship and in responsibility for illness as a result of the inroads holistic health ideology is making into allopathic medicine. Lowenberg's findings indicate that physicians continue to control patient-practitioner interactions and absolve patients of guilt for illness regardless of orientation. But, despite physician input, the findings indicate that patients do experience blame and guilt because of the diffusion of holistic notions into society as a whole.

In Chapter 7, Lowenberg presents her most penetrating analysis of the data and goes beyond the myths and jargon of both holistic health and allopathic medicine to reveal a potential for denial of available resources to ill people. More specifically, Lowenberg points out that the holistic health movement has led to a subtle moral life-style crusade and a punitive societal trend, not unlike that of the mid-nineteenth century, that have resulted in condemnation and withdrawal of resources in the face of illness or life-style "lapses."

The findings reported in this book provide answers to fundamental questions about the relationship between the consumer and the health care professional, including changes and problems with the application of the holistic health model, transformations in the sick role associated with holistic practice, and the attribution of blame for illness. These questions are posed and answered as contemporary concerns, but historians will easily recognize their timeless significance.

At the same time, *Caring and Responsibility* raises as many questions as it answers. The reader is left with an understanding of the pervasiveness of the holistic health movement in his or her thinking about responsibility for illness and for the care of ill persons. But the reader is also left with a concern for ill people who may be trapped in a web of tension generated by attempts to integrate holistic concepts with traditional medical practice.

JACQUELINE FAWCETT, PhD, RN, FAAN
Professor
School of Nursing
University of Pennsylvania
Philadelphia, Pa.

PATRICIA O'BRIEN D'ANTONIO, PhD, RN
231 Avon Road
Merion, Pa. 19072

Intimate Adversaries: Cultural Conflict Between Doctors and Women Patients

By Alexandra Dundas Todd
(Philadelphia: University of Pennsylvania Press, 1989)

The purpose of this sociological study is to explore the role of language in face-to-face interactions between male gynecologists and their female patients. A second purpose is to link such communications to their social and historical context in order to discover the way power relationships in the health care system are expressed and to explore their social consequences. Todd limits her study of medical conversations to those involving contraceptive care because she presumes these women patients are essentially healthy and because she believes contraception use reflects a general worldview rather than purely a medical concern.

The introduction and first two chapters provide the background for the study, with observations about the current system of health care based on the prevailing "medical model for illness." Todd traces the emergence of a medical profession imbued with the values of a capitalistic economic system and insulated by a culture infused with elitism, racism, sexism, and hierarchy. Recognizing that prior studies point out the role that women play through their collective socialization to be "good girls," Todd ends this part of the discussion by raising research questions about the way the "diseasing of reproduction" actually occurs when the patient is a woman.

Chapters 3 and 4, which present the study, make up the heart of the book. Covering a two-and-one-half year period of observation, interviews, and taping of actual discourse from doctor-patient medical encounters, this study takes place in two large urban settings: a women's clinic in a community health center and the office of a private gynecologist. The data base consists of observational and interview notes from this period, together with a detailed sociolinguistic analysis of twenty tapes, ten from each setting. Todd states that the study was designed neither to reveal universal truths about health care delivery nor to identify statistically significant facts. Todd's major premise is that a cultural adversarial relationship exists between doctors and patients that is exacerbated when a female patient is seeking contraceptive advice and care from a male physician. This adversarial relationship, stemming from history, is nurtured by internalized assumptions about gender roles and is supported by social/cultural institutions. The experiences of four patients are used to illustrate major linguistic patterns and perceptual differences between the doctor and patient.

Pointing out that "language is an active force in the understanding of social life" (p. 52), the negotiated process revealed in social interaction can reflect and uncover the gender-informed power relationships existing between the female patient and her male gynecologist. Todd hypothesizes that by adapting speech act theory to fit the specific requirements for tabulating and analyzing speech acts—such as statements, directives, questions, reactions, and answers—communication patterns and content that reflect and perpetuate male dominance and female ambivalent communication in medical care could be found. Through sociolinguistic analysis of such communication patterns, Todd hopes to "raise the issues, to continue the discussion and thereby increase the knowledge and political activism" necessary to transform the current medical illness model into a "social model for health" (p. 152).

The study's findings confirm that women share the prevailing cultural gender-informed understanding of power and authority. Women do not confront, contradict, or fail to follow doctors' orders regarding their own health care. This is true in spite of the fact discovered by Todd in follow-up interviews that the concerns of many female patients were not even recognized, much less addressed by their male doctors. Sociological questions remain as to why these patterns persist so systematically, and as to why the ideological attachment exists to such ideas as the fragmented person separated from social life. Todd reflects on these mysteries in an interesting review of the epistemological underpinnings of the scientific worldview, its pervasiveness in both individual and social assumptions, and their consequences. Todd ties her perceptions of the medical profession to the capitalistic model and the prevailing scientific worldview. These ideas, she argues, make it possible to reduce women and their reproductive concerns to mechanistic biological parts. This entire system of beliefs, shared by men and women in this society, fragments the whole person and promotes the "diseasing of reproduction." Chapter 5, "Good Doctors in a Bad Model," where these matters are discussed, is one of the most rewarding and insightful in the book.

The last chapter, "Across a Crowded Room: Some Problems, Some Solutions," reflects what this reviewer considers to be the major inadequacy of the book. The book's perspective is feminist and scholarly, and while it is very readable and well documented, it fails to acknowledge the contemporary nursing profession, including its historical contributions, its social activist role, and its caring goals for society. The existence of the modern nursing profession remains one of the world's best kept secrets. Todd's bibliography notes only two citations attributed to nursing publications, dated 1966 and 1975, raising the issue of a historical distortion in Todd's understanding of the health care delivery system.

It is also difficult for Todd to bring together the two extremes in her research goals. A microanalysis of discourse between a dyad is linked with society-level political activism. A much more extensive exploration of the social levels between the two poles of health care delivery would seem to be required. Nevertheless, her attempt demonstrates creative research with interesting possibilities if we can discover the ways that language shapes our attitudes, and by extension, our institutions.

While the book is provocative reading for the general and academic audience, the historian (particularly the nurse-historian) might find frustrations. This is not a historical study. In her review of the historical emergence of contemporary health care, the author draws on contemporary literature, chiefly from sociology and feminist sources. Almost all historical references are taken from secondary sources. Only one bibliographic citation is dated earlier than 1900. Despite its weaknesses, however, this study raises significant feminist issues for the historian and deepens the appreciation for linguistic meanings and their historical significance. This alone makes *Intimate Adversaries* very worthwhile reading.

Wanda Heistand, EdD, RN
Professor of Community Health Nursing
Lienhard School of Nursing
Pace University
Pleasantville, N.Y.

Clara Barton: Professional Angel

By Elizabeth Brown Pryor
(Philadelphia: University of Pennsylvania Press, 1987)

Clara Barton, founder of the American Red Cross, has been perceived as a Victorian heroine by many nineteenth- and twentieth-century writers. Elizabeth Brown Pryor's full-length, feminist biography does nothing to contradict that image. It does, however, present the reader with minute details of one woman's apparently lifelong struggle for independence and meaningful work. The audience for the book will probably be women interested in this burgeoning genre of writing that communicates the often painful, but always instructive, details of a life. Many nurses will be interested because of Barton's Civil War and Red Cross nursing experiences—although Barton herself denied that she had ever been a nurse.

From her birth in 1821 until her death at age ninety in 1912, Barton's life spanned a remarkable period in American and global history. Unfortunately, because the untitled chapters offer a chronological account of Barton's personal life, important historical events, characters, and themes are often difficult to trace. Without a clearly delineated historical context for its biographical details, the book's 370 pages sometimes make tedious reading. When the author says that she has devoted her "entire adult life" to writing the book (p. xv), the reader occasionally feels the weight of this burden!

Pryor is a master at teasing out the tensions and contradictions both in Barton's psychological makeup and in her "sad" childhood. Indeed, the book places all of Barton's accomplishments in the context of her personality—"a complex combination of insecurity and forthrightness, rigidity and flexibility . . . frequently at odds with itself" (p. 213). The overall impression given in this book, sustained to the last, is that of Barton as a heroic, tragic figure whose "whole life had been spent in a search for the public acclaim that served as a salve for the indifference of her family" (p. x).

In many ways, however, Barton's life and upbringing resembled that of her middle-class contemporaries (Florence Nightingale, for example). In the genre of the best new feminist biography, Pryor describes a life that began with a liberal, eccentric, often chaotic family in a small, Puritan, Massachusetts town. The Bartons inculcated philanthropy and a "taste for masculine accomplishments and pursuits" (p. 13) in their youngest daughter. In her early adult years, Barton identified strongly with her father and with men, as well as with work, "almost as if it were a religion" (p. 16).

Already intense and sensitive at age eleven, she started nursing her ill brother and "refused to leave his side for nearly two years" (p. 17). Although her formal education was scant, Barton was extremely bright and began teaching school, one of the few respectable occupations for single women, at age eighteen. She taught successfully until about age thirty, when she was passed over by a man for the headship of a school she had founded. Disillusioned, chronically depressed, and bitter, she moved to Washington, D.C., in 1854 and became an office worker. She was one of the few women in the Patent Office to earn the same salary as the male clerks and quickly established herself both professionally and socially as a force with which to be reckoned.

Always flaunting social mores and acceptable behavior for women, she became embroiled in what would today be labeled "office politics" (this proclivity, as well as her poor judgment of people, would plague her for the rest of her life). The Civil War, as well as her family's illnesses and tragedies, rescued Barton from office work, and she discovered the adventure of following the Union Army and providing relief and nursing care. She also met Elizabeth Cady Stanton and Susan B. Anthony, embracing feminism along with an appreciation of female friendship.

After the Civil War, Barton was again searching anxiously for meaningful work, fighting depression and physical breakdown. Traveling in Europe in the 1860s, she first learned about the International Red Cross, and became involved in organizing relief work in the Franco-Prussian War. Again, she discovered her love of and need to rescue others. As Pryor points out: "This was Clara Barton as she liked best to picture herself: the Lady Bountiful, sowing dignity and hope to the afflicted, reaping loyalty and love in return" (p. 171). Her efforts gained her powerful friends and royal honors, and by the late 1870s she had become a heroine to ordinary Americans who read of her in the popular press.

The story of Barton's attempt to establish and legitimize the American Red Cross fills half of the book. One loses sight of much of the history, however, in the myriad names and places that entered Barton's life and work; readers seeking a clear picture of the Red Cross and its ideological origins should look elsewhere (for example, to John Hutchinson's "Rethinking the Origins of the Red Cross," 1989). The conclusion of the book is sad indeed as Barton struggles to maintain control of the philanthropic organization she had brought to life amid personal scandals and takeovers. Acknowledging that she had become "a target on the skirmish lines" (p. 343), she finally resigned from the permanent presidency of the Red

Cross in 1904. It is clear where Pryor's sympathies lie as she depicts Barton dying in 1912, bereft of friends and estranged from her family.

This book makes a solid contribution to the historiography of Victorian women's lives, to the field of women's work, and to the history of philanthropy. There are fascinating details of Barton's attempt to "aid but not pauperize" (p. 249) and of how Barton flaunted the concept of the "worthy poor" in her relief aid to Sea Island blacks. The author has delved into the treasure trove of Barton's diaries (found sealed behind a wall of the Clara Barton National Historic Site) to marvelous advantage, and the book is well worth reading.

Meryn E. Stuart, PhD, RN
Assistant Professor, School of Nursing
Adjunct Hannah Professor, Faculty of Medicine
University of Ottawa
Ottawa, Ontario
Canada

References

Hutchinson, John. "Rethinking the Origins of the Red Cross." *Bulletin of the History of Medicine* (1989) 69:557–78.

SUBJECT INDEX

GUIDELINES FOR CONTRIBUTORS

To facilitate publication of your contribution, we ask that you follow these guidelines in preparing your manuscript. For solicited articles, length guidelines and submission deadlines will be specified in the solicitation letter. Unsolicited submissions are welcome at any time and will be acknowledged promptly; manuscript length should be appropriate to the topic of the submission.

The entire manuscript (including notes, quoted or set-off text, and references) must be typed fully double spaced. Single-spaced typescripts will be returned to the author for retyping. All typescripts must be prepared with a typewriter or letter-quality computer printer. Draft-quality dot-matrix printouts will not be accepted for publication. Margins of at least one inch on all sides must be maintained. Please submit the original (ribbon) copy of the typescript and three photocopies. All pages, including reference pages, should be numbered consecutively. Please omit any author identification lines on manuscript pages to facilitate blind review.

The cover page for your article must include the following: article title (no more than two parts: title and subtitle); full names of author(s) as meant to appear in print; the address, telephone number, and fax number for the corresponding author; brief acknowledgments of support or assistance; and at least six key words or phrases to be used in subject indexing.

Up to three levels of text headings may be used in your typescript; these must be differentiated clearly in your manuscript by distinct and consistent indentations and capitalization. For questions of note style, please follow the guidelines for numbered endnotes in *The Chicago Manual of Style* (13th edition). All notes must be double-spaced and typed separately from the text (i.e., placed at the end of the article rather than as footnotes). Reference lists should be used solely to provide bibliographic data for sources cited in the text.

Tables must be typed double-spaced, each on a separate sheet, and must be accompanied by a title and/or legend. Figures (line drawings, photographs, etc.) must be submitted as black-and-white camera-ready glossy prints. All drawings, graphs, and charts must be professional-quality. Illustrations prepared with computerized graphic programs will not be accepted unless they are indistinguishable from professional-quality artwork drawn by a graphic artist. Glossy prints must be labeled on the back with the name of the article, author(s), and figure number. Photographs must be accompanied by an appropriate credit line (name of photographer, archive, or collection). Captions or legends for all figures must be typed double-spaced and provided on a sheet separate from the figures themselves. Be sure to make explicit reference to each figure and table within the text, but attach all tables and figures to the end of the typescript.

If more than 500 words of text are quoted from a scholarly book or 250 words from a scholarly article, or if a table or figure has been previously published, the article manuscript must be accompanied by written permission from the copyright owner (who is not necessarily the author of the quote, table, or figure). It is the responsibility of the author to determine who owns the copyright and to submit the appropriate permission letters. Final acceptance of the manuscript will be withheld until all necessary permission letters are received.

All correspondence concerning your submission should be sent to: Joan E. Lynaugh, Editor, *Nursing History Review,* University of Pennsylvania, 420 Guardian Drive, Room 307, Philadelphia, Pa. 19104-6096. Phone: (215) 898-4502; Fax: (215) 573-2168

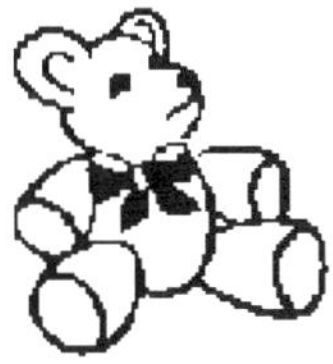

American Association

You are invited to join the American Association for the History of Nursing, whose mission is to preserve, promote, and disseminate information about the history and heritage of the nursing profession.

What are the purposes of the AAHN?

- Stimulate national and international interest in the history of nursing, promote collaboration among its supporters, and encourage research in the history of nursing.
- Promote the development of centers for the preservation and use of materials of historical importance to nursing.
- Serve as a resource for information related to nursing history.
- Produce and distribute materials related to the history and heritage of the nursing profession.

What are the benefits of AAHN membership?

- Receive the official AAHN journal *Nursing History Review*, published annually in January and devoted to the history of nursing and health care: *Long neglected, the history of nursing has recently become the focus of a considerable amount of attention. Over the past decade, developments in the history of medicine, the history of women—particularly of women's work—and nursing itself have resulted in a new recognition of the importance of the subject.*

As the official journal of the American Association for the History of Nursing, Nursing History Review *enables those interested in nursing and health care history to trace new and developing work in the field. The* Review *publishes significant scholarly work in all aspects of nursing history as well as reviews of recent books and updates on national and international activities in health care history.*

- Establish linkages with others who are ardent about the history of the nursing profession.
- Receive the AAHN quarterly *Bulletin*, which keeps you informed about calls for abstracts, fellowship and grant opportunities, conferences, book releases, and other news related to the history of nursing and the AAHN.
- Attend annual AAHN conferences where refereed papers and posters on a wide range of history of nursing subjects are presented, a book mart of historical reference material is conducted, and an auction consisting mainly of nursing memorabilia is held.
- Extend your professional insight through dialogues with colleagues.
- Learn how to compete for the annual prestigious Lavinia L. Dock and Teresa E. Christy awards, which recognize exemplary historical research and writing related to nursing history.